# Levison's
# Textbook for Dental Nu

# Levison's Textbook for Dental Nurses

## TENTH EDITION

Carole Hollins BDS

General Dental Practitioner
Member of the Panel of Examiners, National Examining Board for Dental Nurses

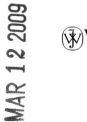
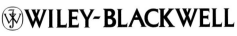WILEY-BLACKWELL

A John Wiley & Sons, Ltd., Publication

This edition first published 2008
© 2004, 2008 Blackwell Munksgaard
© 1960, 1963, 1969, 1971, 1978, 1985, 1991, 1997 Blackwell Science Ltd

Blackwell Munksgaard, formerly an imprint of Blackwell Publishing, was acquired by John Wiley & Sons in February 2007. Blackwell's publishing programme has been merged with Wiley's global Scientific, Technical, and Medical business to form Wiley-Blackwell.

*Registered office*
John Wiley & Sons Ltd, The Atrium, Southern Gate, Chichester, West Sussex, PO19 8SQ, United Kingdom

*Editorial offices*
9600 Garsington Road, Oxford, OX4 2DQ, United Kingdom
2121 State Avenue, Ames, Iowa 50014-8300, USA

| | |
|---|---|
| First edition published 1960 | Sixth edition published 1985 |
| Second edition published 1963 | Seventh edition published 1991 |
| Third edition published 1969 | Eighth edition published 1997 |
| Fourth edition published 1971 | Ninth edition published 2004 |
| Fifth edition published 1978 | Tenth edition published 2008 |

For details of our global editorial offices, for customer services and for information about how to apply for permission to reuse the copyright material in this book please see our website at www.wiley.com/wiley-blackwell.

The right of the author to be identified as the author of this work has been asserted in accordance with the Copyright, Designs and Patents Act 1988.

Library of Congress Cataloging-in-Publication Data
Hollins, Carole.
   Levison's textbook for dental nurses / Carole Hollins. – 10th ed.
          p. ; cm.
   Includes index.
   Rev. ed. of: Textbook for dental nurses / H. Levison. 9th ed. 2004.
   ISBN 978-1-4051-7557-9 (pbk. : alk. paper)   1. Dental assistants.   2. Dentistry.   I. Levison, H. (Henry)
II. Levison, H. (Henry). Textbook for dental nurses.   III. Title.   IV. Title: Textbook for dental nurses.
   [DNLM:   1. Dental Assistants.   2. Dental Care.   WU 90 H741L 2008]
   RK60.5L43 2008
   617.6′0233—dc22
                                                                                    2008018008

A catalogue record for this book is available from the British Library

Set in 9.5/12pt Palatino by Graphicraft Limited, Hong Kong
Printed in Spain by GraphyCems

1   2008

# Contents

# Introduction to the Tenth Edition

This edition has been updated and produced just as dental nursing enters the most exciting of times – full recognition as a profession in its own right, and with compulsory registration of its members with the General Dental Council from August 2008. Registerable qualifications via the National Certificate or the Level 3 National Vocational Qualification (NVQ) ensure that dental nurses have access to the necessary quality of training to begin their career pathways as vital members of the dental team. This edition provides the updated underpinning knowledge for both qualifications, with information on where to find further knowledge and areas of study as necessary, for the NVQ and for the post-registration qualifications provided by the National Examining Board for Dental Nurses (NEBDN).

Further revision and updating of the text has embraced the concepts of continuing professional development and lifelong learning for dental nurses, with the aim of assisting them in constantly seeking to improve their skills as healthcare professionals. New legislation and syllabus updates to the National Certificate qualification have also been included, with information on accessing their definitive charting and instrument identification guidelines, as well as full details of the National Certificate examination and the newly introduced Record of Experience. For the first time, the full syllabus for this qualification has been included in the text, with the very kind permission of NEBDN.

It is hoped that all dental nurses in training will find this edition informative, easy to use, and beneficial to their studies.

*Carole Hollins*

# Introduction to the First Edition

This book is designed to cover the syllabus for the British Dental Nurses and Assistants Examination. Although written primarily for nurses preparing for this examination, it also provides an outline of dental surgery for those embarking on a career of dental nursing; thus helping them gain a greater understanding of the nature and aims of their duties. For examination purposes, the subject matter is deliberately presented in a dogmatic fashion and, to aid final revision, there is a summary after each chapter.

The text was prepared during a winter spent in the North Isles of Shetland with the School Health Service mobile dental unit; and for helpful advice and encouragement throughout, I am indebted to my former dental nurse, Miss M.E. Isbister. I wish to thank my wife for typing the manuscript; my sister, Miss B. Levison, for the drawings; the Amalgamated Dental Trade Distributors Ltd for providing some new blocks; and Mr P. Saugman of Blackwell Science for his guidance.

*H. Levison*

# Acknowledgements

Sincere gratitude and thanks must go to H. Levison for the inception and superb continuation of this marvellous book, which has become known as 'the bible' for dental nurses. It has helped generations of them to follow their chosen career in dental nursing, and is set to continue to do so for many years to come.

In updating this edition, I am indebted to my sister (again!) for her computer expertise, and to the Kidsgrove dental practice staff and patients for their eagerness in posing for various photographs.

I also thank the National Examining Board for Dental Nurses and the General Dental Council for their very kind permission to reproduce various items within the text, and I must express great appreciation for the continued support of previous illustrators too.

Finally, I sincerely wish to thank the staff of Wiley-Blackwell for their unstinting help and support during the updating process, and especially to Amy Brown – whose endless enthusiasm makes her a pleasure to work with.

# Abbreviations

| | |
|---|---|
| AIDS | acquired immune deficiency syndrome |
| ALARA | as low as reasonably achievable |
| ALS | advanced life support |
| ANUG | acute necrotising ulcerative gingivitis |
| BADN | British Association of Dental Nurses |
| BDA | British Dental Association |
| BDJ | British Dental Journal |
| BDS | Bachelor of Dental Surgery |
| BLS | basic life support |
| *BNF* | *British National Formulary* |
| BPE | basic periodontal examination |
| COSHH | control of substances hazardous to health |
| CPD | continuing professional development |
| CPITN | community periodontal index of treatment needs |
| CPR | cardiopulmonary resuscitation |
| DCP | dental care professional |
| DDPH | Diploma in Dental Public Health |
| DDR | Diploma in Dental Radiology |
| DGDP | Diploma in General Dental Practice |
| DMF | decayed, missing, filled |
| DNSTAB | Dental Nurses Standards and Training Advisory Board |
| do | distal occlusal |
| DPB | Dental Practice Board (name change to Business Services Agency, changing again imminently) |
| *DPF* | *Dental Practitioners' Formulary* |
| DPT | dental panoramic tomograph |
| DRABC | dangers, response, airway, breathing, circulation |
| DRO | Dental Reference Officer |
| EAV | expired air ventilation |
| ECC | external cardiac compression |
| ECG | electrocardiogram |
| EDH | Enrolled Dental Hygienist |
| EDT | Enrolled Dental Therapist |
| EOT | extra-oral traction |

| | |
|---|---|
| F/ | full upper denture |
| F/F | full upper and lower dentures |
| /F | lower full denture |
| FDI | International Dental Federation |
| FDS | Fellow in Dental Surgery |
| FGC | full gold crown |
| GA | general anaesthesia |
| GDC | General Dental Council |
| GI | gold inlay |
| GIC | glass ionomer cement |
| GP | gutta percha |
| HBV | hepatitis B virus |
| HCV | hepatitis C virus |
| HIV | human immunodeficiency virus |
| IOTN | Index of Orthodontic Treatment Need |
| IV | intravenous |
| LA | local anaesthesia (analgesia) |
| LDS | Licentiate in Dental Surgery |
| MCCD | Membership in Clinical Community Dentistry |
| M Clin Dent | Master of Clinical Dentistry |
| MDS | Master of Dental Surgery |
| MFDS | Member of the Faculty of Dental Surgery |
| MGDP | Membership in General Dental Practice |
| MGDS | Membership in General Dental Surgery |
| MIMS | Monthly Index of Medical Specialties |
| MJDF | Membership of the Joint Dental Faculties |
| mo | mesial occlusal |
| mod | mesial occlusal distal |
| MOrth | Membership in Orthodontics |
| M Paed Dent | Membership in Paediatric Dentistry |
| MRD | Membership in Restorative Dentistry |
| MSc | Master of Science |
| NEBDN | National Examining Board for Dental Nurses |
| NHS | National Health Service |
| NME | non-milk extrinsic (sugar) |
| NRPB | National Radiological Protection Board |
| NSAID | non-steroidal anti-inflammatory drug |
| NVQ | National Vocational Qualification |
| OPG | dental panoramic tomograph (orthopantomograph) |
| P/ | partial upper denture |
| P/P | partial upper and lower dentures |
| /P | partial lower denture |
| PBC | porcelain bonded crown |
| PCT | primary care trust |
| PE | partially erupted |

| | |
|---|---|
| PJC | porcelain jacket crown |
| PoM | prescription-only medicine |
| ppm | parts per million |
| PV | porcelain veneer |
| RA | relative analgesia (now known as inhalation sedation) |
| RDN | Registered Dental Nurse |
| RDT | Registered Dental Technician |
| RIDDOR | Reporting of Injuries, Diseases and Dangerous Occurrences Regulations |
| rINN | recommended international non-proprietary name |
| RPA | radiation protection advisor |
| RPS | radiation protection supervisor |
| TMJ | temporo-mandibular joint |
| UE | unerupted |
| ZOE | zinc oxide and eugenol cement |

# 1  Structure of the Dental Profession

## The dentist

Dentists undergo five years of undergraduate training at a university dental school. On passing their final examinations, students are awarded the degree of Bachelor of Dental Surgery (BDS). But they cannot use the title of dentist or practise the profession until their names have been entered in **The Dentists Register**.

The register is kept by the **General Dental Council** (GDC) and contains the name, address and qualification(s) of every person legally entitled to practise dentistry in the United Kingdom. Such persons may describe themselves as dentist, dental surgeon or dental practitioner. There is no difference between these titles. Dentists may also use the courtesy title of Doctor but must not imply that they are anything other than dentists. Following qualification all dentists are legally required to continue their professional education until their retirement from practice, in order to maintain and update their skills.

Registered dentists have a wide choice of opportunities within the profession: general practice, community dental service, hospital service, university teaching and research, industrial dental service and the armed forces. They may also take additional higher qualifications and become specialists in a particular branch of dentistry. Some examples of such qualifications are:

- Fellowship in Dental Surgery (FDS)
- Master of Science (MSc) in a specialty
- Master of Dental Surgery (MDS)
- Master of Clinical Dentistry (M Clin Dent)
- Membership in General Dental Practice (MGDP)
- Membership in the Joint Dental Faculties (MJDF)
- Membership in Orthodontics (MOrth)
- Membership in Clinical Community Dentistry (MCCD)
- Membership in Restorative Dentistry (MRD)
- Membership in Paediatric Dentistry (M Paed Dent)
- Membership of the Faculty of Dental Surgery (MFDS)
- Diploma in Dental Public Health (DDPH)
- Diploma in Dental Radiology (DDR)

- Diploma in General Dental Practice (DGDP)
- Diploma in Orthodontics (DOrth)

These qualifications are provided by the faculties of dental surgery, and the faculty of general dental practitioners, of the royal colleges of surgery.

Having obtained the relevant higher qualifications, dentists may join the Specialist Lists for their particular specialty. The following lists are included in the Dentists Register:

- Oral and maxillofacial surgery
- Surgical dentistry
- Dental and maxillofacial radiology
- Dental public health
- Oral medicine
- Oral microbiology
- Oral pathology
- Orthodontics
- Periodontics
- Prosthodontics
- Restorative dentistry

## General Dental Council

The GDC is the governing body of the dental profession and its duties are set out in legislation. These duties are to promote high standards of professional education and professional conduct among dentists, and dental care professionals (DCPs), throughout their entire practising career. It thereby ensures that the status of the profession in the community is upheld and that a proper code of conduct is maintained for the protection of the public. In essence, its remit is to protect patients and to regulate the dental team.

In performance of these duties the GDC must be satisfied that courses of study at dental schools and the qualifying examinations are adequate, and the same applies to postgraduate education.

It is the policy of the GDC for all dentists, after qualification, to serve one year of vocational training before starting independent practice. Such training schemes are already in force in National Health Service (NHS) general practice, the community and hospital services, and also on a voluntary basis in non-NHS practice. As soon as adequate resources and facilities are available, it will be mandatory for all dentists to undergo vocational training after qualification.

The GDC is empowered to remove or suspend from the register any dentist or DCP who has been convicted of a criminal offence or is guilty of serious professional misconduct. It may also suspend any dentist whose fitness to practise is seriously impaired because of physical or mental conditions.

Apart from registered dentists, the only other persons permitted to undertake dental treatment are **dental hygienists** and **dental therapists**. The GDC is responsible for these DCPs in much the same way as for dentists. After qualification they must be enrolled by the GDC in the DCP register. The limited range of dental treatment which they are permitted to undertake is laid down in the Dental Auxiliaries Regulations.

## The dental team

Dentists' training enables them to undertake, without assistance, all treatment necessary for patients, including construction of their dentures, crowns and bridges, etc. Except for the actual treatment performed within the mouth, much of the work which a dentist is qualified to do can be performed by others. For example, a chairside **dental nurse** provides an extra pair of hands for preparing and mixing filling and impression materials, and for helping with suction, retraction and illumination to keep the operative field clear and dry for the dentist and comfortable for the patient. A **dental technician** can make dentures, crowns and bridges ready for the dentist to fit, while dental hygienists and therapists are permitted to undertake limited forms of dental treatment.

By utilising all this assistance, a dentist becomes the leader of a team which can practise in the most efficient way. Dentists carry out all the treatment which they alone can perform, while the other members of the team – hygienist, therapist, dental nurses and technician – perform all the work which a dentist can delegate. Compared with a single-handed dentist, the dental team can provide far more treatment each day with less effort and fatigue for all concerned, and thereby give a better total service to the patient and the community.

This description of a clinical dental team, consisting of a dentist, dental nurse and dental auxiliaries (hygienist and therapist), is no longer valid for the new millennium. An enlarged team of dentist and DCPs is superseding it. This new group of team members will eventually comprise:

- Dental nurses
- Dental hygienists
- Dental therapists
- Orthodontic therapists
- Dental technicians
- Clinical dental technicians
- Maxillofacial prosthetists and technologists

All the above will be registered by the GDC and have specific training programmes, extended duties and professional responsibilities for continuing professional development and professional conduct similar to those of dentists. Further information is available from: General Dental Council, 37 Wimpole Street, London

W1G 8DQ; tel: 020 7887 3800; fax: 020 7224 3294; e-mail: information@gdc-uk.org; website: www.gdc-uk.org.

## Dental care professionals

This section introduces the new dental team of dentist and GDC registered DCPs for the new millennium.

### Dental hygienist

After two years' training at a dental hospital, or in the armed forces, hygienists are awarded a Diploma in Dental Hygiene. They can then become registered by the GDC and use the title of Enrolled Dental Hygienist (EDH). They are permitted to undertake a number of dental procedures prescribed by a dentist, and for which they have been trained. These duties include:

- Scaling and polishing teeth
- Use of local anaesthesia
- Application of fluorides and fissure sealants
- Treating patients under conscious sedation, provided that a dentist is present in the room
- Emergency replacement of dislodged crowns, using temporary cement
- Removal of excess cement
- Application of a temporary filling if one becomes dislodged while under treatment
- Taking impressions

Apart from their treatment role, hygienists are also trained to be proficient dental health educators.

### Dental therapist

Dental therapists undertake a two-year course at a dental hospital. They are awarded a Diploma in Dental Therapy and having obtained GDC registration, they may use the title of Enrolled Dental Therapist (EDT). They are permitted to carry out the same treatment as hygienists and can also undertake a wider range of procedures such as:

- Simple fillings
- Pulp treatment of deciduous teeth
- Extraction of deciduous teeth
- Fitting preformed crowns on deciduous teeth

Hygienists and therapists are required to have prior experience as a dental nurse and a National Certificate or NVQ for admission to dental hospital training courses. Some of these courses provide for dual qualification as hygienist and therapist, and many include training in dental radiography. As with hygienists, an important part of the dental therapist's role is dental health education.

## Dental technician

Dental technicians are highly skilled craftsmen who construct dentures, crowns, bridges, inlays, orthodontic appliances, splints and replacements for fractured or diseased parts of the face and jaws. They work to the dentist's prescription in a dental laboratory. Training consists of a full-time course in a dental hospital or technical college, or an apprenticeship with part-time attendance at a technical college. From July 2008, only registered clinical dental technicians will be able to carry out laboratory work as they become recognised as another category of DCP by the GDC.

## Dental nurse

The role of dental nurses, their duties and training facilities are covered in Chapter 2.

# The National Health Service

Dental treatment in the United Kingdom is provided either privately or through the NHS. Private patients obtain treatment from a practitioner of their choice and pay a fee to the practitioner for professional services given.

NHS dental treatment differs from private practice in the range of treatment provided and the method of payment for such treatment. Certain types of treatment available in private practice are restricted in the NHS. Payments to the dentist are controlled by the NHS, with patients' contributions ranging from nil to a set maximum.

Currently, NHS treatment available to the public is split into three bands, as follows:

- Band 1 – simple treatments such as examinations, radiographs, scalings
- Band 2 – routine treatments such as fillings, extractions, root treatments
- Band 3 – complex treatments involving laboratory work such as crowns, bridges, dentures

A set fee is charged to the patient for each of the bands, regardless of the amount of treatment carried out, so for instance the same fee is paid for one filling or 10 fillings, if provided during the same course of treatment.

The cost of the NHS is borne by the state, and the government department responsible for it is the Department of Health. The Department of Health delegates operational management of the service to the NHS Executive. For administrative purposes the country is divided into a number of large **strategic health authorities** for overall planning. These are subdivided at a local level into a large number of smaller authorities called **NHS trusts** for hospital services and **primary care trusts** (PCTs) for community clinics and general practitioner services. PCTs have the responsibility of deciding the level of need for NHS dentistry in their area, as well as providing emergency out-of-hours dental care to the public.

## Community dental service

The community dental service was formerly called the school dental service, providing examination and treatment for children and expectant and nursing mothers. It still meets the same needs but has acquired additional responsibilities. These vary according to local demand but can include: treatment for special needs patients of all ages; treatment of older people; provision for general anaesthesia; conscious sedation and orthodontic treatment for patients of general practitioners; and dental health programmes for the community at large.

The community dental service is administered by an NHS trust or PCT and co-operates with hospital staff and general practitioners in planning and co-ordinating all dental services in the district. Salaried community dental officers provide treatment in clinics with equipment and materials supplied by the trust or PCT.

## Hospital dental service

Hospitals are administered by an NHS trust. Dental services are provided by the consultant oral surgeon and consultant orthodontist. They provide specialist advice and treatment to patients referred by practitioners outside the hospital and to patients referred from other departments of the hospital. They are also in overall charge of dental care for long-stay inpatients. In addition, most consultants provide postgraduate courses and part-time training posts for general practitioners.

## General dental service

This is the general practitioner service which provides a significant share of all dental treatment in the United Kingdom. It is administered by the local PCT which holds dentists' contracts and is responsible for NHS disciplinary procedures.

The Dental Practice Division of the Business Services Authority (previously the Dental Practice Board) authorises payment of treatment fees to practitioners. It can also arrange for patients to be examined by its dental reference officers (DROs).

General practitioners set up and equip their practices at their own expense and can treat private patients as well as NHS patients.

New legislation (Health and Social Care Act) will, over the next few years, introduce major changes to improve NHS dental services, for patients and the practices providing it.

## Clinical governance

Clinical governance requires every NHS practice principal to have a quality assurance system for the practice, in order to ensure a consistent quality of care. It must cover:

- Infection control (see Chapter 7)
- All legal obligations of health and safety law in the practice (see Chapter 23)
- All legal obligations for radiation protection (see Chapter 14)
- Compliance with GDC requirements for continuing professional development (see Chapter 2)

The practice must:

- Appoint a member of the staff to be responsible for operating the system
- Display a written practice quality policy for patients
- Provide the PCT with an annual report on the quality assurance system

## Clinical audit and peer review

Clinical audit is an essential feature of clinical governance that came into force for NHS dentists in 2001. Its purpose is to ensure that individual dentists assess different aspects of their practice, make changes where needed, and thereby improve service and care for their patients.

Peer review is an optional alternative to clinical audit for dentists who prefer to undertake their practice assessments within a group of other dentists, and thereby share the benefit of the group's combined experience.

Whichever option is chosen for implementing these requirements, it is subject to approval by a local assessment panel, and submission of a report on completion.

# British Dental Association

The British Dental Association (BDA) is the professional body representing the majority of dentists in the United Kingdom. It publishes the *British Dental Journal* (*BDJ*) and negotiates for the profession with the government and other bodies where dental interests are concerned. Membership of the BDA is voluntary and open to all dentists.

# 2  The Dental Nurse

Employers requiring a dental nurse look for the following attributes:

- Ability to communicate
- Intelligence
- Ability to show initiative
- Friendliness
- Sense of loyalty and responsibility
- Awareness that the first priority in a practice is the patient

Of the above attributes, the ability to communicate and show initiative is more likely to be regarded as important than academic knowledge, since all dental nurses have to be qualified or in training to be able to work in practice, so an accepted level of intelligence is mandatory anyway. However, a command of written and spoken English is essential as poor grammar, spelling and speech reflect badly on a practice, as well as creating communication difficulties.

Although the duties of a dental nurse vary from practice to practice, according to its size and number of staff employed, they may be classified under the headings of surgery and office duties. To perform these efficiently, dental nurses must possess certain personal qualities and a knowledge of the law and dental ethics.

## Personal qualities

The dental nurse is usually the first person to receive a patient. This is an important occasion as a patient's confidence in the practice may well be influenced by the appearance and manner of the dental nurse.

### Appearance

A dental nurse should be smartly dressed without going to extremes of fashion. Attention to personal hygiene is essential, not only as it affects appearance, but also to ensure good results and prevent cross-infection in the surgery. Hair should be short, or secured away from the face, to prevent contact with working areas or equipment during close chairside assistance. Similarly, jewellery and wrist watches should not be worn as they can be unhygienic or liable to damage surgical gloves.

## Personality

A calm, courteous and sympathetic manner, combined with a cheerful and friendly disposition, is an obvious necessity when dealing with anxious patients. It will gain their confidence, and allow the dental nurse to keep cool under all conditions and cope with any emergency which may arise. Handling patients in a busy practice can be trying and requires much patience and tact.

## Speech

The voice must be calm to inspire confidence, and clear enough to be understood on the telephone. Instructions to patients should be given in simple language to avoid misunderstanding.

## Concentration

Concentration requires an alert mind and attention to detail. Mistakes must not be made in patients' records, appointments, telephone messages, assisting with treatment or dealing with emergencies.

## Punctuality

The smooth running of a busy practice depends on the staff and patients keeping appointments on time. Dental nurses must set an example by observing strict punctuality on duty.

# The law

All nurses are affected directly or indirectly by two enactments: the Dentists Act (see below), and the Health and Safety at Work Act, which is covered in Chapter 23.

## Dentists Act

Under the Act, the General Dental Council is given the important function of maintaining high standards of professional conduct among dentists and DCPs, with responsibility to their patients as the first priority. Anyone found guilty of a criminal offence or serious professional misconduct is liable to be removed or suspended from the register kept by the GDC, and is thereby legally forbidden to practise. This now applies to dental nurses and other DCPs, and requires them to be registered with the GDC and their adherence to standards of professionalism similar to those already applying to dentists, hygienists and dental therapists. These standards are set out in the GDC's 'Standards Guidance' booklets, which are available to all dental professionals. The key points are covered in Chapter 15.

## Ethical practice

All members of the dental team are required to:

- Put patients' interests first
- Respect patients' dignity and choices
- Protect patients' confidential information
- Co-operate with other members of the dental team and other healthcare colleagues in the interests of patients
- Maintain their professional knowledge and competence
- Be trustworthy

## Applying ethical principles

The practical application of these ethical principles requires you to:

- Apply them in your work as a dental professional, whether or not you routinely treat patients
- Understand that you are professionally responsible for your actions and must be able to account for them
- Put patients' interests before your own or those of your colleagues
- Apply these principles when handling queries and complaints from patients and in all other aspects of non-clinical professional service
- Maintain your GDC registration and work only within the limits of your knowledge, professional competence and physical capability
- Take effective action to protect patients if you believe they are being put at risk by: your health, behaviour or professional performance; or those of a colleague; or by any aspect of the practice clinical environment
- If in doubt, obtain advice from senior staff, appropriate professional body or the GDC
- Treat patients with respect, courtesy and awareness of their dignity and rights
- Understand and promote patients' responsibility for making decisions about their bodies, their priorities and their care, and obtain their consent before any treatment is undertaken
- Provide all the information, including the risks, benefits, costs and alternative options, upon which they can make their decision
- Ensure that there is no discrimination against patients regarding their race, ethnic origin, age, sex, disability, special needs, sexuality, lifestyle, beliefs and economic status
- Treat all information about patients as confidential, and for use only for the purposes for which it was provided

■  Ensure that such material is kept securely to prevent any accidental or un-authorised access to it

GDC registration completes the first stage of your professional career. Thereafter:

■  Compliance with your legal obligations, knowledge, skills and professional competence must be maintained and updated by verifiable continuous professional development
■  Justify your professional status, and the trust of your patients and colleagues, by honesty and fairness in all your professional and personal activities
■  Apply all these ethical principles to clinical and professional relationships, and to any commercial or business dealings in which you may be involved
■  Maintain proper standards of personal behaviour in all aspects of your life, and thereby promote patients' confidence in you and public confidence in the dental profession

It is illegal at present for dental nurses and technicians to carry out any work in a patient's mouth. Dental nurses are not allowed to take X-rays unless they have been specially trained for this purpose. Further details are given in this chapter and in Chapter 14.

A dentist may delegate to a dental nurse the responsibility for giving patients instruction in oral hygiene, provided that:

1  The dentist is satisfied that the dental nurse is fully competent to do so.
2  Suitable and documented training has been given in this area, showing that the dental nurse has been deemed competent by more senior colleagues.
3  It is understood that the dentist is personally responsible for whatever instruction is given.

## Continuing professional development

Continuing professional development (CPD) and lifelong learning are now statutory requirements for the continuing registration of DCPs, and will become compulsory for dental nurses from July 2008. It aims to guide an individual in updating their skills and education throughout their working life, to ensure that they stay abreast of all the changes and updates in their chosen career. This should then ensure that they provide the best care and service as is possible to patients.

CPD is either verifiable or non-verifiable. Verifiable CPD is that offered formally, with specific learning outcomes stated. Certificates of attendance and participation in verifiable CPD activities are issued and must be kept as evidence of complying with the GDC's requirements, they may even have to be produced as evidence of verifiable CPD activity. Examples of verifiable CPD are:

■  Attendance on postgraduate courses
■  Attendance at local meetings organised by postgraduate tutors

- Distance-learning programmes, with stated learning outcomes
- Computer-aided learning programmes (CAL)
- Attendance at conferences with stated learning outcomes
- Studying and taking formal examinations in dental-related subjects
- Completing tests set on articles published in dental journals

From July 2008, mandatory CPD will begin for dental nurses on a five-year cycle, similar to that for dentists. Dental nurses will be required to undertake and record a minimum of 50 hours of verifiable CPD over this period, which must include:

- Medical emergencies – 10 hours
- Disinfection and decontamination – 5 hours
- Radiography and radiological protection – 5 hours
- Legal and ethical issues – if dealing with patients on a regular basis
- Complaints handling – if dealing with patients on a regular basis

Non-verifiable CPD is that done on an informal basis, often purely for reasons of personal interest. Although new information may well be learned during these activities, it cannot be tested nor proved that specific learning outcomes have been achieved. Examples include:

- Reading dental journals, with no testing of the contents of any articles
- Reading post-graduate textbooks
- Accessing dentistry-related websites and downloading information
- Attendance at staff meetings
- Completion of 'in-house' training
- Completion of staff appraisals

When carried out correctly, organised CPD events covering the mandatory areas of dental practice, as well as a wider range of subjects relevant to the role of the dental nurse, which are of great benefit to the individual. It should enable recognition of areas that are of interest as well as areas where more knowledge is required, as dentistry is an ever-changing discipline where new materials and techniques are constantly being developed. Completion of CPD should produce some of the following for all dental nurses:

- Increased job satisfaction
- Identification of problem areas
- Improved communication with colleagues
- Improved efficiency
- Improved career prospects
- Greater commitment to the workplace

The planning and undertaking of CPD should be given careful thought by the dental nurse to ensure that not only the mandatory requirements of the GDC are met, but also that any other CPD undertaken is of use to themselves. While the temptation exists to only attend courses of personal interest, a broader coverage of subjects is more desirable and useful to the development of the dental nurse. The following points should also be taken into consideration when planning CPD activities:

- It can be time-consuming, and may involve personal expense
- It requires self-discipline to carry out and complete
- It must be structured and organised to be of any real value
- There must be a real educational benefit to undertaking it
- Appropriate courses may not be available locally
- Courses may run during work time, so employers must be amenable to participation
- Courses may also run outside work time, so leisure time will be affected

A staff training and development system must be in place in all dental workplaces, whereby the skills held by all staff are reviewed on a one-to-one basis so that individual training needs can be identified. This is usually carried out as an annual staff appraisal process.

Records should be kept of the points discussed during the appraisal, as well as any needs that have been identified and any methods discussed for meeting those needs. These points can be developed into a Personal Development Plan (PDP), where the necessary CPD requirements can be looked into and successfully accessed, and the individual PDP can be updated accordingly. This is then available to the GDC, or prospective new employers, as evidence that the dental nurse not only has ambitions and identified training needs, but that they have successfully carried them out.

## Ethics

As already described, all registered dental nurses will soon become legally recognised DCPs with the same responsibilities as other registered members of the dental team. Meanwhile they are expected to obey their own code of ethics which was introduced before the middle of the past century.

1   They must be honest and loyal, and serve their employers and patients to the best of their ability.
2   They must hold in strict confidence all details of professional services rendered by their employers. This is not only an ethical obligation but a legal one too. Confidentiality of patients' records is compulsory. This is covered in more detail in Chapter 15. Dental nurses must realise that breach of confidentiality constitutes grounds for dismissal.
3   They should strive to improve their own professional ability and that of their team colleagues, and inform their employer of any duties they feel unable to undertake satisfactorily.

4   They should disclose to an appropriate person any circumstances adversely affecting proper patient care or staff health and safety.

## Duties of a dental nurse

It is of the utmost importance for dental nurses to realise the extent of patients' perception of the efficiency of a practice. The livelihood of a dental nurse, as well as that of a dentist, depends on meticulous attention by the entire practice staff to the following requirements:

- Maintenance of a high standard of cleanliness throughout
- Adequate heating and ventilation
- Careful planning of appointments and an efficient recall system. Patients' time is just as important as that of dentists, and appointment times should accurately cater for varying lengths of visit. Some visits are unavoidably longer than planned and any patients kept waiting should be informed of delays and offered help if inconvenienced
- Strict confidentiality at all times. This includes preventing medical histories, conversations, financial transactions and reactions to treatment being overheard
- No delays in communicating information to patients or dentist. This entails: rapid retrieval of filed records, radiographs, models and correspondence; legible handwriting, proper typing format, good English and correct spelling; keeping written records of telephone messages; and adequate back-up copies of computerised records
- Ready availability of addresses and telephone numbers of emergency, building and equipment maintenance services, taxis, public transport and welfare facilities
- Updated stock and maintenance records, to ensure that materials are never out of stock, equipment is always working properly, and a full range of spares is immediately available
- Orders for materials are precise, unambiguous and give correct catalogue descriptions
- Efficient liaison with the dental laboratory to prevent delays in despatch and receipt of work, and to ensure that work prescriptions for the technician include all required details
- Staff know how to maintain and service their equipment
- All practice staff are trained and regularly practised in the safety policies concerning infection control, X-rays, mercury hygiene, resuscitation, emergency procedures and fire drill (Chapter 23)

### Office duties

The reception, clerical and administrative duties of a dental nurse may be summarised as follows:

- Responsibility for, and supervision of general cleanliness
- Reception of patients and dental company representatives
- Arrangement of current and recall appointments
- Completion and filing of patients' records
- Recording of all attendances and treatment
- Ordering and storage of supplies
- Management of financial records
- Correspondence
- Knowledge of NHS regulations and organisation

Much of the secretarial work can be handled far more quickly and efficiently with a computer. This has not only taken over the role of typewriter, but also that of accounts ledger and filing cabinet; it has also revolutionised the keeping, filing, storage, retrieval, display, printing and security of all types of practice records.

## Surgery duties

Specific surgery duties are covered in the appropriate chapters but general preparation of the surgery is common to all procedures. Thorough preparation of the surgery is essential before the day starts, between patients, and at the end of a treatment session.

## Beginning of the day

- Dental nurses should be well groomed with clean nails, clean uniform and with minimum jewellery.
- Switch on power, water and air supply to all equipment. Check temperature, ventilation and lighting throughout premises.
- Check that domestic staff have cleaned the premises thoroughly.
- Run, and record result of, autoclave test.
- Disinfect all working surfaces.
- Discharge water for two minutes through three-in-one syringe and handpieces with water spray. Refill ultrasonic cleaner with fresh fluid.
- Set out clean uniforms and linen as appropriate.
- Check that all other equipment is working satisfactorily.
- Ensure that appointment book, day book, patients' notes, radiographs, laboratory work, emergency kit and all materials for the day are ready.
- Prepare surgery for first patient: fit new disposable covers where necessary; provide protective spectacles and supply of disposable masks and gloves; lay out mirror, probe and tweezers.

## Reception and treatment of patient

Before a patient enters the surgery, adjust the dental chair and move any mobile equipment so that the patient will have no difficulty with access. Ensure that you and the dentist know the patient's name, title, purpose of visit and length of appointment.

- Check that the dentist has the patient's notes and relevant records such as medical history, radiographs and models.
- Remind the dentist of any particular aspects of the patient, such as anxiety about treatment, nausea during impressions, fainting tendency, special medical history, time of patient's transport home, etc.
- All unnecessary instruments should be out of view with no sign of a previous patient's visit. The surgery should always appear to patients as if their appointment is the first of the day.
- Always greet patients by name, and with a smile, and introduce them to the dentist by name. Relieve the patient of any excessive clothing or bags, and hang them in the office section of the surgery.
- Seat the patient comfortably, fit a new disposable bib, supply a new disposable beaker of warm mouthwash, a receptacle for the patient's denture, and a new disposable napkin for removal of lipstick or drying the lips after rinsing. Protective spectacles are provided for patients treated in the supine position.
- Always remember that what is all in a day's work for a dental nurse may well be a very worrying experience for a patient. The surgery atmosphere must be one of friendly communication, appreciation of the patient's feelings, and relaxed efficiency.
- If the appointment is for examination only, the dental nurse records and charts the examination findings.
- For treatment, the dental nurse provides the dentist with a clear, dry operative field by attending to illumination, suction and retraction of cheeks, lips and tongue.
- Instruments and materials are passed to the dentist, materials mixed and assistance given in all procedures throughout the visit.
- In addition, the dental nurse closely observes the patient so as to anticipate and forewarn the dentist of any impending complications such as fainting or sickness.
- At the end of the visit the dental nurse ensures that no sign of the treatment is left on the patient's face or clothing. The next appointment is arranged and given in writing to the patient. Any post-operative instructions given by the dentist are repeated by the dental nurse, and given in writing, when necessary, before the patient leaves.
- Any work for the dental laboratory is disinfected, carefully packed and documented ready for despatch.
- Treatment is entered in the daybook, and used notes and records set aside ready for filing.
- The surgery is then prepared for the next patient so that no traces of the previous visit remain.
- Used instruments are cleaned and sterilised, or set aside, away from treatment zones, ready for bulk cleaning and sterilisation. Waste is placed in the

appropriate containers, as covered in the next section. Spittoon and work surfaces are cleaned and disinfected. Water is discharged for 30 seconds from the three-in-one syringe and a new disposable tip fitted.

■ New disposables are provided, and sterile handpieces flushed with water.

■ Instruments and records are then set out ready for the next patient.

## End of the day

■ Instruments used on the last patient are cleaned and sterilised. Handpieces are cleaned and lubricated in accordance with manufacturer's instructions and then sterilised. The aspirator bottle is emptied and the whole drainage system flushed with disinfectant. The spittoon, unit and work surfaces are also cleaned and disinfected. All non-disposable instruments and materials are then returned to their proper place.

■ Laboratory work is disinfected (see Chapter 19), checked for proper documentation and carefully prepared for despatch to the technician.

■ Exposed X-ray films are checked for proper documentation and processed (Chapter 14).

■ Treatment of the last patient is entered in the daybook, all patient notes and records are filed, and back-up copies of computer records are made.

■ Waste disposal is then undertaken. Ordinary domestic and office waste is stored in bin bags ready for the local waste collection service.

■ Non-sharp hazardous waste is ordinary surgery waste that may or may not be contaminated with saliva, and/or blood. It includes *empty* plastic local anaesthetic cartridges. It is stored and sealed in special hazard labelled containers.

■ Sharp waste contains empty glass local anaesthetic cartridges, syringe and suture needles, scalpel blades, burs, metal matrix bands, root canal instruments and anything else that could perforate, scratch or cut exposed skin or gloves. It may only be collected in rigid puncture-proof containers.

■ A new class of hazardous waste called **special waste** must be stored in separate rigid approved containers. Special waste includes: prescribed medicines; harmful, irritant, toxic and corrosive substances; X-ray processing solutions; and local anaesthetic cartridges that still contain some of the anaesthetic.

■ Special arrangements must be made for disposal of mercury and amalgam waste. This includes extracted teeth with amalgam fillings. It cannot be incinerated like hazardous waste, as it would liberate poisonous mercury vapour. Chapter 16 covers this aspect of waste disposal.

■ Full records must be kept of all types of hazardous waste collection by authorised contractors, as covered again in Chapter 23.

■ The appointment book is used for making out the next day's page in the daybook and getting notes and records ready.

■ A check is made of security arrangements, such as: locking drug and filing cabinets, store cupboards, drawers, doors and windows.

■ Finally, all electric, gas, water and air services to surgery equipment are switched off.

All these daily surgery duties may be summarised as follows:

- Care and maintenance of equipment and instruments
- Care of drugs
- Preparation of surgery and setting out instruments
- Sterilisation and prevention of cross-infection
- Recording and charting
- Chairside assistance during all operative procedures
- Pre- and post-operative care of patients
- Processing and mounting radiographs
- Oral hygiene instruction

## Legal aspects

In addition to the chairside duties mentioned, a dental nurse also performs the indispensable roles of chaperone and witness. Dentists are sometimes accused of improper or negligent conduct and, for this reason, a dental nurse must always be present in the surgery when the dentist is attending a patient. The presence of a third party has great legal value and protects both dentist and patient. If temporary absence is unavoidable, the door should be left open until the dental nurse returns or another member of staff stands in.

### Consent to treatment

Any form of dental examination or treatment without appropriate consent is an assault which could lead to legal proceedings. Consent to treatment from any person of 16 years of age and over (unless mentally incapacitated) is legally valid, but only if the necessity, nature, complications, alternative options and treatment costs have been personally explained by the dentist, and are understood by the patient. This is called **informed consent**.

Consent may be verbal or written, but whenever possible it should be written. This is essential for general anaesthesia, sedation, and other procedures with significant risks or side-effects, or involving high fees. Written consent must be signed and dated by the patient and dentist. For patients under 16 (or mentally incapacitated), parental consent is required.

## British Association of Dental Nurses

The British Association of Dental Nurses (BADN) aims to: assist, protect and represent its members; improve education, training and career opportunities; promote and defend their professional status; and liaise with all appropriate bodies in pursuit of these aims.

It is in the best interests of all nurses to join the BADN and take an active part therein. Full details of membership and the facilities it can provide are obtainable from: BADN, Hillhouse International Business Centre, PO Box 4, Room 200, Thornton-Cleveleys, Lancashire FY5 4QD; tel: 01253 338360; e-mail: admin@badn.org.uk; website: www.badn.org.uk.

## National Examining Board for Dental Nurses

Since 1943 the National Examining Board for Dental Nurses (NEBDN) has been the body solely responsible for the examination for the National Certificate for Dental Nurses. It consists of examiners from all branches of practice, and nurses representing the BADN. All the examiners are either dentists or registered nurses and they are elected to the Panel of Examiners by the NEBDN, again ensuring that all branches of dentistry are represented. All examiners must have been qualified for at least seven years.

This long and successful history of pioneering the first professional qualification for UK dental nurses has now been changed by the arrival of new legislation to enhance their status and career prospects, by requiring all dental nurses to be registered as DCPs and subject to the same professional obligations as other DCPs. Trainee dental nurses will not be allowed to use the title of registered dental nurse (RDN) until they have passed their qualifying examination and joined the DCP register.

The original National Certificate examination will continue, but a new National Vocational Qualifications (NVQ) examination for dental nurses offers them an alternative training scheme. It transfers the emphasis of training from the academic environment to the workplace (the dental practice). Dental nurses can now choose whether their path to registration as DCPs is via the NEBDN or the NVQ route. As there is some difference between the syllabuses for each qualification, dental nurses considering the NVQ route to qualification are advised to also read the textbook *NVQs for Dental Nurses* by Carole Hollins (published by Blackwell Munksgaard). The second edition covering recent syllabus changes will be available soon.

Meanwhile, dental nurses who already hold the National Certificate but have not enrolled on the voluntary register should do so as soon as possible. Dental nurses who do not hold the National Certificate may opt for this or the NVQ route to qualify as a DCP. However, for an interim period of two years until July 2008, unqualified but experienced dental nurses have been able to register on the grounds of their existing experience. For more information on the National Voluntary Register, call 01253 773270.

The National Certificate examination will continue in its present form alongside, but separate from, the NVQ process. Dental nurses requiring clarification should contact the BADN (page 19) or the NEBDN (page 21). More information on NVQs is obtainable from: City and Guilds, 1 Giltspur Street, London EC1A 9DD; tel: 020 7294 2468; fax: 020 7294 2400; website: www.city-and-guilds.co.uk.

### The National Certificate Examination

The examination for the National Certificate is held twice a year, in May and November, at many centres throughout the country. It may be taken at any age, with any amount of experience and without any educational qualifications. However, the certificate cannot currently be awarded until a nurse has two years' full-time (or equivalent part-time) chairside experience. Although the NEBDN may, at any time, alter the syllabus or vary the form of the examination, it consists at present of written, spotter, practical and oral sections, as well as the imminent introduction of a work-based Record of Experience.

The current syllabus, which has recently been updated in line with GDC requirements, is given in the Appendix. All areas are covered in this textbook, but the reader is advised to develop a broad base of underpinning knowledge of dental nursing by accessing theoretical information from any other sources available too, if necessary.

Candidates for the examination may obtain copies of the syllabus and regulations, an entry form, past examination papers and any further details from: NEBDN, 110 London Street, Fleetwood, Lancashire FY7 6EU; tel: 01253 778417; fax: 01253 777268; e-mail: admin@nebdn.org; website: www.nebdn.org.

The purpose of the examination day is to be successfully tested by various examiners, to prove that the dental nurse has a full knowledge of their role in the workplace and that they are safe to work as a dental nurse. Before the examination day, the Record of Experience must also have been fully completed by each candidate to show written evidence of practical experience in the required areas of dental nursing, as set out by NEBDN.

## Written examination

This is currently two hours long and consists of two parts, Part A and Part B, both of which must be completed within the time limit.

### Part A

This has four sections.

#### Section 1
Fifteen multiple choice questions (MCQs), where the one most suitable answer from four choices is marked with a cross. For example:

A barbed broach is used in endodontics to:

1  Smooth the canal walls
2  Determine the canal length
3  Remove the canal contents ×
4  Locate the canal entrance

#### Section 2
A diagram is provided which requires labelling, and with several related short answer questions for completion. So for example, a diagram of the mandible will be shown with various anatomical points to be labelled, and then some

short answer questions about related nerve supplies to various teeth to be answered.

Section 3
Up to 10 more unrelated short answer questions where you are required to complete the statements given, for example: RIDDOR stands for ......……..

Section 4
A blank dental chart is given, with instructions to record various items of treatment that are present and various items to be carried out. Each must be correctly recorded on the chart, in the definitive manner set out in the Dental Charting Booklet available from NEBDN.

The whole of Part A should take no longer than 30 minutes to complete.

*Part B*

Part B consists of five questions, of which only four have to be answered. Answers may be written in essay or note form. They must be clear and well ordered, and take no longer than about 20 minutes each to write.
   Examples of various styles of long answer questions are:

■ Name five types of commonly used dental radiograph and say how each is used
■ What precautions should be taken to protect the patient and staff from overexposure?

Write short notes on each of the following:

1   Cleaning the dental clinical environment
2   Cleaning handpieces and instruments
3   The use of PPE

   Use of abbreviations can save time in written answers. Show the examiner that you know their meaning by using the full name first, followed by the abbreviation in brackets. Thereafter just use the abbreviation. A list of abbreviations is given at the beginning of this book.
   There is a comprehensive revision guide covering the whole syllabus in the form of all the types of question used in the written examination. Model answers to these questions are provided at the end of each section. The title of this recommended guide is *Questions and Answers for Dental Nurses*, 2nd edition, by Carole Hollins (published by Blackwell Munksgaard).

*Practical examination*

Each candidate will have been given an attendance time for the afternoon practical session at their chosen examination centre, and this must be adhered to.

There are four elements to the practical session, and each one has to be attended by every candidate.

This is a timed exercise over five minutes where each candidate passes along a 'spotter track', which has been laid out with any 20 items from the definitive spotter list produced by NEBDN. The items are arranged in five groups of four, and each has to be correctly identified in writing by the candidate, allowing 15 seconds for each one. An excellently illustrated book, specially produced to help nurses prepare for the spotter, is the *Dental Instrument Guide*, by dental nurse tutor Dawn Matthews, and is obtainable from: Orpington College, The Walnuts, Orpington, Kent BR6 0TE; tel: 01689 899700; fax: 01689 877949; e-mail: enquiries@orpington.ac.uk; website: www.orpington.ac.uk.

These are split into test A and test B, where test A is always a material mixing test (such as an impression material or a luting cement), and test B is to identify and describe the function of various items used in a stated dental procedure (such as a surgical extraction or a scale and polish). Each test should take about 2.5 minutes to complete, and candidates have to choose their A and B tests from two options written on the underside of the test cards.

Manufacturers' instructions will be available to read if any of the materials are unfamiliar to candidates, but any material covered by the syllabus may be used for examination purposes and unfamiliarity by the candidate is not accepted as a reason not to perform the mixing test. It is accepted, however, that candidates will be nervous during the examination and may produce a poor mix, but as long as this is pointed out to the examiners and the candidate can demonstrate knowledge of what should have been produced, the test will be marked favourably.

Examples are:

Test A choice 1: Mix sufficient of the material provided to take an upper impression for an orthodontic study model. Load into the correct tray and present it to the examiner.

Test A choice 2: Mix sufficient of the material provided to take an impression for a lower full denture. Load into the correct tray and present it to the examiner.

Test B choice 1: The dentist is to provide oral hygiene instruction to the patient. Choose five items that may be required and explain their function to the examiner.

Test B choice 2: The dentist is about to apply rubber dam. Choose five items that may be required and explain their function to the examiner.

*Oral (viva)*

The remaining eight minutes of the practical session is a viva, where one examiner asks the candidate questions on any part of the syllabus and the candidate gives verbal answers. A table with items is available for the examiners to use as prompts if they require, and usually has a skull, selections of moisture control items, X-ray film packets, local anaesthetic cartridges, forceps, extracted teeth, and oral health items. The questions will not be limited to these areas, however, as the viva is designed to cover any points from the syllabus that are not covered elsewhere.

The examination as a whole then is designed to test both the theoretical knowledge and practical skills of each candidate in as many areas of dental nursing as is possible.

*Record of Experience*

This is a new development in the National Certificate examination, which will become compulsory for all candidates to complete from September 2008. Entry to the actual examination days in 2009 onward will depend on the existence of a fully completed Record of Experience (R of E) by every candidate.

The R of E is designed to show evidence of the dental nurse's practical skills in all chairside procedures and in some reception duties. They are recorded as Practical Experience Record Sheets (PERS) in varying numbers for each set task, and split into five units covering the required areas of the syllabus. Each unit also has various Supplementary Outcomes attached, which are designed to be completed after the dental nurse has researched and found the necessary information to be recorded within their own work environment. The five units are as follows:

*Unit 1*

- Preparation of the clinical environment
- Management and maintenance of the clinical environment
- Sterilization process
- Disinfecting impressions
- Supplementary outcomes

*Unit 2*

- Assisting in preventive techniques
- Booking dental appointments
- Supplementary outcomes

*Unit 3*

- Assisting in clinical assessments
- Assisting in the taking of radiographs
- Processing and mounting radiographs
- Supplementary outcomes

- Assisting in cavity restoration procedures
- Assisting in endodontic procedures
- Assisting in the preparation and fitting of fixed prostheses
- Assisting in the preparation and fitting of removable prostheses
- Supplementary outcomes

*Unit 5*

- Assisting in the extraction of a tooth/root
- Setting up a local anaesthetic syringe
- Supplementary outcomes

In addition, and to complete the R of E, a case study also has to be written by every candidate, which is based around a treatment session from one of the following:

- Surgical procedure
- Restorative procedure
- Provision of a fixed prosthesis
- Provision of a removable prosthesis

The case study should be limited to 1000 to 1500 words and be presented in a computer-printed format. This not only makes the study more legible to read, but also makes use of the IT skills of the dental nurse. Candidates are encouraged to include relevant documents, such as post-operative instruction sheets, in the case study presentation so that a full account of the treatment session is produced. The case study is designed to encourage modern candidates to approach dental nursing as an holistic profession, rather than as a series of inflexible set duties at the chairside that rarely overlap.

All the PERS have to be signed off in the workplace by a GDC registrant (dentist, hygienist, dental nurse) to validate them as being successfully carried out by the candidate, and the whole R of E must be available for checking and moderation at the candidate's training centre, by trained NEBDN members.

Training centres will apply to NEBDN for an R of E for each of their candidates, in the early stages of their training course. The supplementary outcomes will be updated and changed periodically to prevent any attempts by new candidates to merely copy other candidates' work.

The process of moderating the R of E will begin in September 2008, but only at accredited training centres. Candidates from non-accredited training centres will therefore be unable to sit the National Certificate examination.

## Training centres

Full-time and part-time day or evening courses are held at some dental hospitals and technical colleges, or run privately at various locations, such as health centres.

Conditions of entry and duration of these courses vary from place to place but full details may be obtained on application. NEBDN holds a list of all accredited training centres throughout the country that offer training courses for the National Certificate.

Although previously dental nurses could enter and pass the examination without attending a course, this is no longer possible since registration of dental nurses became compulsory in July 2008. To ensure that training courses offering the National Certificate provide an agreed standard of training to dental nurses, a process of accreditation has been introduced whereby every approved course has to follow guidelines and standards set down to ensure that a consistently high quality of training is provided. Only these training centres and courses are then recommended by NEBDN as suitable for candidates wishing to study and train as dental nurses.

## National Vocational Qualifications

The NVQ dental nursing qualification is an optional alternative to the NEBDN National Certificate for registration as a DCP. The NVQ equivalent of the National Certificate is called NVQ Level 3 Oral Health Care: Dental Nursing.

The NVQ requires a similar amount of knowledge as its forerunner but is entirely different in the way the knowledge is tested. Whereas the National Certificate examination takes place in a dental hospital or college of further education, lasts one day, and the examiners are mainly unknown to the candidates, most of an NVQ testing takes place in the familiar and less stressful surroundings of a candidate's own workplace: their employer's surgery.

The required knowledge is split into a series of units that are completed and tested in the workplace by local assessors and witnesses who may be dentists or registered DCPs, but will not be your particular employer. Candidates complete their tasks at their own rate but must keep comprehensive records of their progress for the assessments. Various colleges and companies hold courses to cover NVQ requirements and assessments, but they are not an essential requirement. The final test for the dental nurse is a shorter version of the written part of the National Certificate examination. It is set and marked by NEBDN examiners, and held at an NEBDN examination centre. It currently consists of:

- Multi-choice short answer questions
- Medical history questions
- Dental charting

An advantageous feature of the NVQ structure is that it simplifies acquisition of other healthcare qualifications, as many of these share units already included in the dental nursing requirements. The NVQ units have recently been updated and renamed and the excellent book by Carole Hollins, *NVQs for Dental Nurses* (published by Blackwell Munksgaard) is also being updated to cover the new format.

## Extra qualifications

After obtaining their National Certificate, dental nurses can take further courses of study to qualify them for work in specialised fields such as conscious sedation, radiography, orthodontics, special care and oral health education. These courses lead to a special certificate and are arranged by the NEBDN in conjunction with the Dental Nurses Standards and Training Advisory Board (DNSTAB) and other interested bodies. Full details are obtainable from the NEBDN or BADN.

Although it is not necessary to attend a course for entry to these post-qualification examinations, all candidates must be on The Dental Nurses Register described on page 10.

Dental nurses with the National Certificate are also eligible to train as hospital dental nurse tutors, hygienists and therapists. Those wishing to become tutors may need a Further Education Teachers' Certificate. Courses for this are held at local colleges of further education.

Details of hygienist and therapist training are mentioned in Chapter 1 and further information is obtainable from: General Dental Council, 37 Wimpole Street, London W1G 8DQ; tel: 020 7887 3800; fax: 020 7224 3294; e-mail: information@gdc-uk.org; website: www.gdc-uk.org.

## Certificate in Oral Health Education

As mentioned on page 12, dental nurses are permitted to give patients instruction in oral hygiene, provided a dentist is satisfied that they are competent to do so.

Although it is not necessary for dental nurses to have passed any examination for a dentist to be satisfied of their competence, they can prove it by obtaining the NEBDN Certificate in Oral Health Education. It covers the knowledge and experience necessary to comply with GDC requirements for dentists wishing to delegate this important function to their dental nurses.

## Certificate in Dental Sedation Nursing

The examination covers the basic principles of conscious sedation and patient care, and the knowledge and skills necessary to comply with GDC requirements for dentists to have fully trained and experienced dental nurses for these procedures.

## Certificate in Special Care Dental Nursing

This qualification is intended for dental nurses whose work involves assisting in dental treatment of patients whose health and social care needs require special provision.

## Certificate in Orthodontic Nursing

This qualification covers the special knowledge and skills necessary for a dental nurse to assist an orthodontist, and to undertake associated tasks that can be delegated by the orthodontist. It will also serve as an introduction to a future class of DCP called an **orthodontic therapist**.

## Dental Radiography Certificate

The College of Radiographers and DNSTAB have arranged courses and an examination for dental nurses which satisfy the legal requirements for dentists who train their nurses to take and process radiographs. Details of courses are obtainable from: Society and College of Radiographers, 207 Providence Square, Mill Street, London SE21 2EQ; tel: 020 7740 7200; website: www.sor.org.

# Registration

For admission to the Register, a dental nurse must have passed one of the following:

- The NEBDN National Certificate examination
- An examination recognised by the dental hospitals
- The NVQ Level 3 Oral Health Care: Dental Nursing qualification
- Any other dental nursing examination approved by the GDC

For more information on registration, call 01253 773270.

# 3 Outline of Physiology

This chapter deals with the biology and relevant physiology (that is, the functioning) of the human organism, to provide the necessary underpinning knowledge and understanding of the body as a whole in relation to dentistry and dental nursing.

The basic unit of living organisms is the cell, and all (except red blood cells) contain a nucleus that has the individual DNA that makes each of us unique. The DNA is held as chromosomes which separate and duplicate during cell division and growth.

Many cells specialise to perform certain roles, and when similar cells group together they are referred to as tissues. Groups of tissues that perform different functions are called organs – such as the heart, or the liver – while those that have related functions are called systems – such as the digestive system or the respiratory system.

There are four basic types of cell in the human body:

- **Muscle cells** – these generate forces and produce motion; they may be attached to bones to allow limb movement, or enclose hollow cavities so that their forces cause expulsion of the cavity contents (such as the movement of food through the digestive tract)
- **Nerve cells** – these can initiate and carry electrical impulses to distant areas of the body along their length to produce many actions, such as to cause muscle cells to contract, or to cause glands to release chemicals or fluids in the body (such as the salivary glands)
- **Epithelial cells** – these cover the body surface as skin, or surround organs or line hollow structures within the body; they act to separate areas of the body from each other and from the external environment, to prevent the uncontrolled movement of harmful micro-organisms
- **Connective tissue cells** – these connect various parts of the body together by anchorage and support, such as in the whole bony skeleton and tendons and ligaments

All of these cells require a source of fuel to produce the energy they need to be able to work and carry out their individual functions, and the fuel is provided by the food that we eat. The energy in the food is released for use by the cells by the action of food digestion in the digestive system, and is used for any of the following:

- Maintenance of body temperature above or below that of the surroundings – this is called **homeostasis**
- Production of movement to allow food gathering, and therefore the production of more energy
- Reproduction for the survival of the species

In addition, the body cells require a source of oxygen to be able to burn the food eaten to produce the energy they require to function. Oxygen is brought into the body through the respiratory system, and transported by the circulatory system around the body to every cell that needs it. These three major organ systems (digestive, respiratory and circulatory) will be discussed in Chapter 4.

The human body has 10 organ systems, each with various components and specific functions to allow the continuation of life. The organ systems are listed below.

- **Circulatory system** – composed of heart, blood vessels, blood; functions to allow the rapid bulk flow of blood around the body tissues.
- **Respiratory system** – composed of nose, throat, larynx, trachea, lungs; functions to allow the exchange of oxygen and carbon dioxide between the body and the external environment.
- **Digestive system** – composed of mouth, pharynx, oesophagus, stomach, intestines, pancreas, salivary glands, liver, gall bladder; functions to digest, process and absorb nutrients, and to excrete waste products.
- **Urinary system** – composed of kidneys, ureter, bladder, urethra; functions to regulate blood plasma and excrete waste products.
- **Musculo-skeletal system** – composed of cartilage, bone, ligaments, tendons, joints, skeletal muscle; functions to support and protect the internal organs, and allow movement.
- **Immune system** – composed of white blood cells, lymph, spleen, bone marrow, thymus gland; functions to defend against infection, and produce red and white blood cells.
- **Nervous system** – composed of brain, spinal cord, nerves, sensory organs (eye, ear, etc.); functions to give consciousness, and regulate and coordinate body activities.
- **Endocrine system** – composed of all the glands that secrete hormones; functions to regulate and coordinate the workings of the whole body.
- **Reproductive system** – composed of the male or female sex organs; functions to allow reproduction and the continuation of the human species.
- **Integumentary system** – composed of the skin; functions to protect against injury and dehydration, and maintain the body temperature.

# 4 Circulation, Respiration and Digestion

## Circulation

The main component of the circulatory system is the heart, a muscular pumping organ situated in the thorax (chest cavity). It is connected by blood vessels to every tissue in the body, and carries out the following functions:

- Pumping oxygenated blood from the lungs to the body tissues so that they can work
- Collecting deoxygenated blood from the body and transporting it to the lungs where the waste products are excreted, by being breathed out

The heart has four chambers within, the upper two called the atria and the lower two the ventricles. The atria and ventricles are separated by one-way valves that allow blood flow in the direction of atria to ventricles only, and the left and right side of the heart have no communication between them. The right side of the heart transports only deoxygenated blood, from the body to the lungs, while the left side of the heart transports only oxygenated blood, from the lungs to the rest of the body again (Figure 4.1).

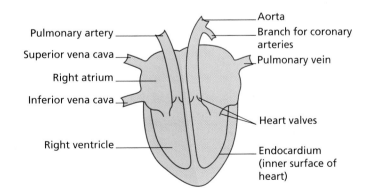

Figure 4.1 The heart.

## Action of the heart

Deoxygenated blood is collected from the whole body through the veins and transported to the right atrium via the **inferior and superior venae cavae**. As the heart beats, it pumps this blood through the one-way valve between the two right heart chambers (tricuspid valve) and into the right ventricle. The next beat pumps it out of the right ventricle and into the **pulmonary artery** where it passes to the lungs for reoxygenation.

Once oxygenated, the blood returns to the left atrium through the **pulmonary vein**, then it is pumped through the one-way valve (mitral valve) into the left ventricle. The next heart beat pushes this blood out of the heart into the **aorta**, and then back around the whole body to reoxygenate all the cells and tissues and allow them to continue their normal functions.

The heart beat itself begins on the top surface of the right atrium in a group of specialised muscle cells called the **pace-maker**. These cells receive electrical stimulation from two sets of nerves from the brain; one set speeds up the rate of the heart beat and the other set slows it down. In this way the heart rate is regulated to allow both exercise and rest as necessary. After each heart beat, the blood is prevented from flowing backwards again by the one-way valves within the heart itself, which snap shut as the blood pressure increases within the heart chambers.

## Circulatory system

The circulatory system is an enclosed loop of blood vessels, with the heart at its centre. The blood vessels taking oxygenated blood around the body are the **arteries**, the largest of which is the aorta, and these gradually decrease in size away from the heart to arterioles and then **capillaries**. The capillaries are just one cell thick, and this allows the oxygen that they carry to be released into the surrounding tissues so that it can be used to burn food nutrients and create energy.

As oxygen passes out of the capillaries, the waste product of the energy production – carbon dioxide – passes from the surrounding tissues into the capillaries. This gas exchange process is called **internal respiration** (Figure 4.2). The deoxygenated

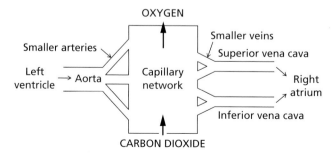

Figure 4.2 Internal respiration.

blood then travels from the capillaries into small veins called venules, then into larger **veins** until it reaches the heart in one of the largest veins, the vena cava. Deoxygenated blood from the upper body is transported to the superior vena cava, and from the lower body to the inferior vena cava. This is the **systemic circulation**.

At the same time, and with each heart beat, the deoxygenated blood in the right side of the heart is pumped to the lungs through the **pulmonary artery** (the only artery to carry deoxygenated blood). Here, the carbon dioxide is released into the lungs to be breathed out while oxygen that has been breathed in travels from the lungs into the blood capillaries, so that the blood is reoxygenated again. This gas exchange is called **external respiration** (Figure 4.3). The oxygenated blood is then transported to the left side of the heart in the **pulmonary vein** (the only vein to carry oxygenated blood) so that it can then be pumped back around the body. This is the **pulmonary circulation** (Figure 4.4).

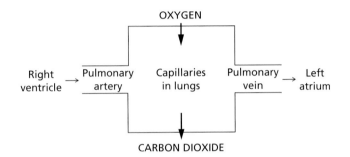

Figure 4.3 External respiration.

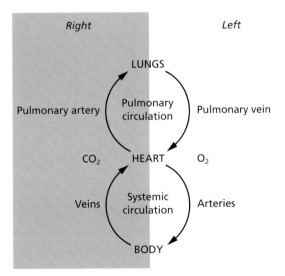

Figure 4.4 Circulation (deoxygenated blood shaded blue).
Source: *Emergency Procedures and First Aid for Nurses*, M. Skeet, Blackwell Science Ltd, Oxford.

## Blood vessels

When the blood leaves the heart in the arteries it is under greatest pressure as a result of the heart beat, so the walls of the arteries are elastic to allow them to expand as the powerful surge of blood passes along them. Once the initial wave of the pumped blood has passed, the artery walls relax back to their normal size again until the next heart beat. This difference in pressure within the arteries can be measured using a **sphygmomanometer** to record a person's **blood pressure**. The highest reading occurs when the heart contracts, and the lowest reading occurs when the heart relaxes; so in a healthy adult at rest the blood pressure is measured at around 120/80.

Also, when the artery passes over bone, the blood surge can be felt as the pulse at various sites around the body:

- **Carotid pulse** – at either side of the neck where the carotid arteries lie across the neck vertebrae
- **Brachial pulse** – at the inner surface of the elbow where the brachial arteries lie over the elbow joints
- **Radial pulse** – at the inner surface of the wrists as the radial arteries lie over the radius bone of the lower arms
- **Femoral pulse** – at the top of the inner thighs as the femoral arteries lie over the femoral bone of the upper legs

In comparison the veins are not elastic, as the pressure of the blood surge is greatly reduced here, being so far away from the source of the heart beat. Indeed, they contain one-way valves along their length to prevent the blood from flowing backwards between heart beats, in a similar way to the valves within the heart itself.

## Blood

The circulatory system is filled with about 5 L of blood in an adult, and it is regulated and kept around a temperature of 37°C by the process of homeostasis. It consists of several cell types floating in a straw-coloured fluid called **plasma**:

- **Erythrocytes** – red blood cells
- **Leucocytes** – white blood cells
- **Platelets** – thrombocytes, which are fragments of larger blood cells called megakaryocytes

**Erythrocytes** are disc-shaped cells with no nucleus, so they cannot divide and replace themselves, but have to be constantly produced in the body by the red marrow of certain bones. Their lack of nucleus and their shape provides the maximum space available for them to carry out their main task – to transport oxygen around the body. They achieve this by attaching oxygen to the red pigment they contain – **haemoglobin**. As discussed previously, oxygen is vital to all cells to be able to produce energy and carry out their various functions. It is picked up by the erythrocytes in the capillaries of the lungs during external respiration, transported around the body by the circulatory system to wherever it is needed, and then released into the tissues during internal respiration.

**Leucocyte** is the collective name for a group of several cells that are mainly concerned with defending the body against micro-organisms and disease. They are made in several areas of the immune system, such as the lymph nodes and bone marrow, and circulate throughout the body at all times. However, when the body comes under attack from micro-organisms, massive numbers of leucocytes pass along the circulatory system to the area of disease, and then squeeze through the capillary walls to the tissues under attack. Here, they surround and destroy the micro-organisms so that the disease is prevented from spreading. In very severe infections, the leucocytes are helped to destroy the invaders by antibodies released from the body's immune system.

**Platelets** (or thrombocytes) also contain no nucleus, as they are just separate fragments of a larger blood cell found in the red bone marrow. Platelets are concerned with the coagulation of blood at the site of injury to prevent excessive blood loss. They achieve this by physically helping to plug damaged blood vessels by acting as a meshwork for the successful formation of a blood clot, as well as by releasing powerful chemicals that assist further in clot formation.

**Plasma** is the fluid part of the blood that carries the blood cells within it. It consists of about 90% water, with powerful chemicals called plasma proteins floating within, as well as the three types of blood cells. Plasma acts as the transport system of the body, by carrying numerous cells and chemicals from one area to another as they are needed. A summary of its functions is as follows:

- Transport of erythrocytes to allow oxygenation of the body tissues
- Transport of waste carbon dioxide, dissolved in the plasma, from the body tissues to the lungs for exhalation and removal from the body via the respiratory system
- Transport of digested food nutrients from the digestive system to the body tissues, for use as fuel to create energy
- Transport of waste products from these cells to the kidneys, where they are filtered out as urine which is then excreted from the body through the urinary system
- Transport of leucocytes to the site of any micro-organism attack, to allow the body to defend itself from disease
- Formation of antibodies and antitoxins from special plasma proteins called **globulins**, which help the body resist more severe infections
- Transport of powerful chemicals called **hormones**, from the glands where they are made to the area of the body where they are required
- Transport of the plasma protein **fibrinogen** to the site of any injury, to assist in blood clotting

## Relevant disorders of the circulatory system

Several disorders are relevant to the dental nurse, as they may have consequences to the dental treatment offered, the suitability of local anaesthetics or conscious sedation techniques used, and the possibility of patients presenting as a medical emergency during treatment. The more common disorders are outlined below.

### Coronary artery disease

The coronary arteries supply oxygenated blood to the heart itself, branching off the aorta as soon as it leaves the left side of the heart. Any internal damage to these vessels, such as by the presence of fatty cholesterol deposits, prevent platelets from behaving normally and only clotting at the site of injury. Instead, they form clots within the coronary arteries that result in the following:

- Partial obstruction of oxygenated blood flow, causing **angina**
- Full obstruction of oxygenated blood flow, causing **myocardial infarction** (heart attack)

If the clot (or **thrombus** as it is correctly termed) forms in another blood vessel, it will have similar effects on the organ it supplies (if an artery) or it may become dislodged within a vein and ultimately travel to the pulmonary artery and block the blood flow to the lungs. This is called a **pulmonary embolism** and can be fatal.

### Cardiac arrest

The sudden failure of the heart to beat at all (**asystole**), or to beat ineffectively without pumping the blood (**fibrillation**). This may occur due to the presence of a thrombus, or for other reasons including severe anxiety – a state that can be seen in some dental patients who have a profound fear of dental treatment.

### Rheumatic fever

An illness suffered by the patient previously that causes damage to the heart valves. Any future episodes of bacteraemia (bacteria in the blood) such as those caused by invasive dental treatment, including scaling, can cause inflammation of the inside of the heart (**bacterial endocarditis**) with possibly fatal consequences.

### Anaemias

One of several disorders affecting the oxygen-carrying capacity of erythrocytes. This may occur due to heavy blood loss, to lack of sufficient erythrocyte production by the red bone marrow (including due to **iron deficiency**), to excessive destruction of erythrocytes by the body, or to the production of abnormal haemoglobin as occurs in **sickle cell anaemia**. The ultimate result is that the patient has poor tissue oxygenation, which may result in a simple faint, or may be life-threatening if they undergo dental treatment using sedation or general anaesthetic techniques.

### Bleeding

This may occur excessively in patients with clotting disorders (such as **haemophiliacs**), or in patients prone to thrombus formation who have been prescribed anti-clotting drugs such as **warfarin**. Routine invasive dental treatment in these patients (especially extractions) could result in uncontrolled and life-threatening blood loss.

## Respiration

The main components of the respiratory system are the two lungs, which are immense air-filled sacs situated in the thorax. The heart lies partially over the upper surface of the left lung (Figure 4.5). The lungs are connected to the external environment by a system of air sacs and tubes deep within their structure called **alveoli** and **bronchioles** respectively, which join to larger tubes that ultimately become the two main **bronchi**, and these in turn connect to the **trachea**, or windpipe (Figure 4.6). This travels up the neck and joins the respiratory system to the atmosphere through the **larynx** in the throat, which connects to the **naso-pharynx** at the back of the mouth and nose (Figure 4.7).

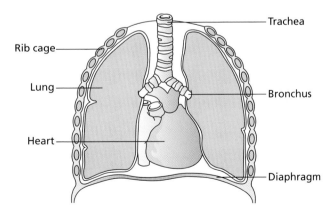

**Figure 4.5** The chest. Adapted from source: *Lecture Notes: Human Physiology*, 5th edn, 2006, O.H. Petersen (ed.), Blackwell Publishing, Oxford.

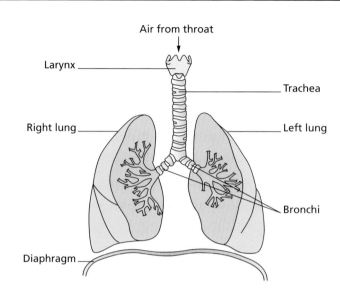

Figure 4.6 Respiratory system.

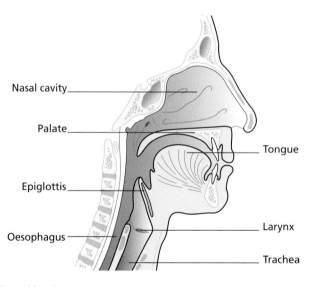

Figure 4.7 Air and food passages.

The functions of the respiratory system are as follows:

- Inhalation of air to provide oxygen for absorption into the circulatory system
- Expiration of the respiratory waste product, carbon dioxide, from the body
- Warming and filtering of the inspired air, to remove foreign body particles and prevent irritation of the lung tissues

The exchange of oxygen and carbon dioxide (**external respiration**) occurs within the alveoli, which are microscopic air-filled sacs just one cell thick and surrounded by capillaries from the pulmonary artery. The pulmonary artery transports deoxygenated blood from the whole body to the alveoli, via the right side of the heart. Air breathed in (**inspired**) from the atmosphere contains 20% oxygen and tiny amounts of carbon dioxide, while that breathed out (**expired**) contains just 16% oxygen, as the body tissues use the 4% difference to help produce energy to function. Expired air contains 4% carbon dioxide too.

At the same time, the deoxygenated blood contains carbon dioxide dissolved in the plasma as a waste product formed when the energy was produced by the body tissues. This gas has no function in the body, indeed its presence can cause considerable damage to the cells and organs if not removed, so it passes out of the capillaries into the alveoli and is exhaled with each breath.

## Breathing

The action of inspiring and expiring – breathing – can occur because the thorax is a sealed chamber whose volume can be increased and decreased by the action of the muscles involved with the chest cavity. The thorax is made up of the ribcage with the **sternum** (breast bone) between, and connected at the back to the spine. The bottom of the ribcage is sealed from the abdominal cavity by a sheet of muscle called the **diaphragm**.

The contraction of the muscles between the ribs causes them to expand outwards, pulling the lungs out with them as they are attached to the chest wall. At the same time, the diaphragm contracts and pulls the lungs downwards so that the overall result is an increase in the volume of the chest cavity, and also the lungs that are attached to it. Consequently, air rushes into the expanded lungs and the process of external respiration occurs. Relaxation of the muscles causes a reduction in the volume of the lungs, and expired air is pushed out of them as the person breathes out.

This process of **ventilation** occurs approximately 16 times a minute in an adult at rest, with an exchange of about a half litre of air at each breath. The rate and depth of breathing increases dramatically during exercise, and also when the person is exposed to fearful or anxious situations.

## Protective mechanisms

The respiratory system is the only means of supplying the body tissues with oxygen, and as life cannot exist without oxygen, several protective mechanisms have evolved to ensure that the system remains open and functions correctly.

The nose, larynx, trachea and bronchi are all lined with **cartilage**, a stiff gristly material that ensures these areas of the respiratory system remain open at all times. The nostrils are also lined by **hairs** to trap foreign particles that have been breathed in, and the rich blood supply to the nose helps to warm the air as it passes through. Warm air is less irritating to the respiratory tissues than cold air. Larger foreign particles are removed from the nose by **sneezing**, and from the lower respiratory tract by **coughing**.

Above the larynx, the respiratory and digestive systems split off into their own routes, with air passing down the trachea and food and drink travelling into the **oesophagus** and so to the stomach. A special flap of cartilage called the **epiglottis** falls across the top of the larynx during the action of swallowing, so closing the trachea momentarily and preventing food or drink from passing into the lungs (Figure 4.8).

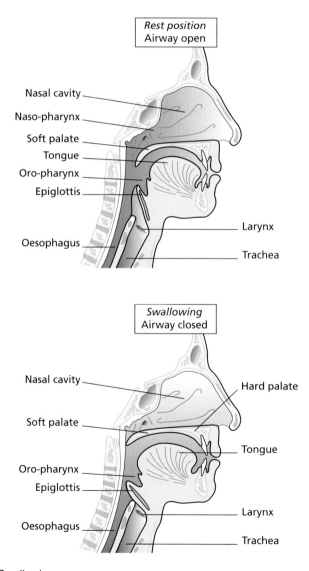

Figure 4.8 Swallowing.

In addition, the whole respiratory tract is lined by cells that produce a sticky coating called **mucus**, and have microscopic hair-like projections called **cilia** that together trap any finer particles of dust and dirt, and then waft them back up the respiratory system away from the lungs. The foreign particles are expelled from the body by coughing or by blowing the nose.

## Relevant disorders of the respiratory system

Again, several disorders are of relevance to the dental nurse as they may affect the choices available for dental treatment as well as the manner in which the treatment can be provided.

## Bronchial asthma

A hypersensitivity response to inhaled particles that compromises the patient's breathing by constricting their airways. Asthma attacks can be brought on by anxiety (including the prospect of dental treatment) and can be life-threatening if the airways are not quickly reopened.

## Anaphylaxis

Although not strictly a respiratory disorder, the severe allergic reaction of anaphylaxis has a catastrophic effect in shutting down the airways and preventing adequate breathing and tissue oxygenation. Death can occur quickly from suffocation.

## Bronchitis

Inflammation of the bronchi, following a respiratory infection (acute bronchitis) or as a slow-onset disease especially in smokers (chronic bronchitis). The airways are narrowed and copious amounts of sputum are coughed up on practically a daily basis. These patients are unsuitable for treatment under conscious sedation in practice, and under general anaesthetic only as a last resort.

## Emphysema

Widening of the alveoli, preventing the adequate occurrence of external respiration without the additional help of oxygen supplies. Bronchitis and emphysema occurring together is called **chronic obstructive airways disease**.

## Inhaled foreign body

This can occur at any time, but the dental patient is especially vulnerable during treatment, as fine instruments are used and the patient is often lying supine. If a foreign body is inhaled, it tends to fall into the right bronchus as this lies in a near vertical line with the trachea. The removal of the foreign body may well involve chest surgery.

## Digestion

The main components of the digestive system are the stomach, intestines, liver and pancreas. They all lie in the abdominal cavity and are connected to either end of the body by the mouth and oesophagus, and the rectum (Figure 4.9). Their aims are to:

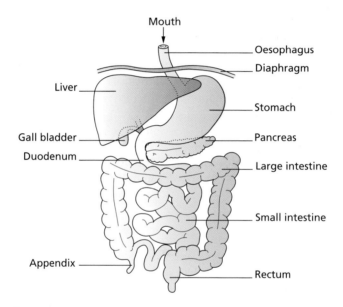

**Figure 4.9** Digestive system.

- Break down and absorb the nutrients within food
- Transfer these nutrients to the circulatory system for transport to all areas of the body
- Detoxify any substances not required by the body
- Remove any solid waste products from the body

All living organisms need food for the following purposes:

- Growth
- Replacement of worn and damaged cells

■ As a source of energy to enable normal bodily functions to occur, for the organism to live

The food we eat cannot be used directly by the tissues to produce energy, but has to be **digested** and broken down into nutrients by the action of powerful chemicals called **enzymes**. The enzymes involved are very specific for the classes of food eaten, and these classes can be grouped as shown below.

■ **Proteins** – these are found in meat, fish, eggs, milk, cheese, beans, and some cereals; they are necessary for cell growth and repair.
■ **Carbohydrates** – these are found in sugars from fruit, vegetables, and processed foods, or in starch from bread, cereals and potatoes; they are necessary for cell energy production.
■ **Fats** – these are found in meat, milk, cheese and butter from animals, or seed and fruit oils from plants; they are necessary for energy production and, when stored beneath the skin, as insulation against a cold environment so helping to maintain the body temperature.
■ **Vitamins** – several different vitamins are required for health but only in small quantities; specifically vitamins A, B group, C and D.
■ **Minerals** – in very small quantities again; specifically calcium, phosphates, fluoride, sodium, and iron.
■ **Water** – more than 80% of the body is made up of water, and it is required by all cells and tissues for normal bodily functions.

## Digestive system

All food and drink enters the body through the mouth, where it is **masticated** (chewed) by the teeth and mixed with saliva to begin carbohydrate digestion, before being swallowed. The teeth and saliva are covered in detail elsewhere. As stated earlier, swallowed particles are directed towards the **oesophagus** and prevented from entering the trachea by the action of the epiglottis in the larynx. In a similar way, the particles are prevented from entering the nose by the sealing action of the soft palate across the **naso-pharynx**.

The muscular action of the oesophagus (**peristalsis**) pushes the swallowed foods down the throat, through the thorax (behind the heart and lungs) and into the abdominal cavity to the **stomach**. The acid and enzymes in the stomach begin digesting any proteins and fats, and removing any iron available for haemoglobin production, before the food passes out into the **small intestine**, where digestion is completed. The acidic stomach contents are neutralised by **bile** from the **liver**, via the **gall bladder**, and the **pancreas** also assists digestion by passing some enzymes into the small intestine too.

The indigestible mass that remains is moved by peristalsis into the **large intestine**, where water and minerals are absorbed before the mass is excreted through the **rectum**.

*Liver*

As the foods are broken down and digested, they are absorbed through the stomach and intestines into the underlying blood capillaries. The capillaries join to become the **portal vein** which carries the nutrient-rich blood to the liver for storage. The nutrients are then released by the liver as required by the body cells. The liver acts as the chemical factory of the body, and its functions are as follows:

- Storage and distribution of carbohydrates
- Storage of vitamins
- Manufacture of bile for fat digestion and neutralisation of stomach acid
- Manufacture of plasma proteins for the blood
- Detoxification of drugs and alcohol
- Disposal of waste products
- Storage and distribution of iron

*Relevant disorders of the digestive system*

Any disorder or condition causing **regurgitation** of the stomach contents, or vomiting, will have a direct effect on the teeth as the enamel surface becomes eroded. Other actual disorders may have direct effects, or indirect through the medication being taken.

*Regurgitation*

This is due to conditions such as gastric reflux and hiatus hernia.

*Bulimia*

This is self-induced vomiting after eating, due to a profound fear of being fat.

*Diabetes*

Insufficient production of the hormone **insulin** by the pancreas, causing an increased amount of circulating glucose rather than it being stored in the liver and in fat cells. The more severe form, **type I diabetes**, occurs in younger patients who are dependent on insulin injections for control of the disorder. The milder form, **type II diabetes**, can be controlled with tablets or by eating a carefully controlled diet. It occurs in older patients and is also linked with obesity.

*Liver disease*

No matter what the cause, liver disease is likely to affect the ability of the patient to store and use food nutrients efficiently, and the liver may be unable to detoxify some drugs, including sedatives and anaesthetics.

### Crohn's disease

This is chronic inflammation of any part of the digestive tract, preventing adequate absorption of food nutrients, with possible intestinal blockages in severe cases. Patients may be taking long-term steroid treatment.

### Ulcerative colitis

This is chronic inflammation and ulceration of the large intestine and rectal linings. Again, patients may be taking long-term steroid treatment.

# 5  Medical Emergencies

Medical emergencies can occur anywhere, at any time, but some may be more likely to occur in the dental surgery setting due to the nature of dental treatment and the anxiety it evokes in some patients. The anxiety that some patients experience may have the following effects:

- Lowering the pain threshold so that 'discomfort' is experienced as 'pain', producing an agitated or even unco-operative patient
- Perception of being about to feel pain, so that stress levels and the anxiety state are raised – this can then put a huge strain on the patient's body, especially the heart and circulatory system
- Fear and anxiety at the prospect of dental treatment may worry the patient enough to prevent them eating beforehand, for fear of vomiting – the patient will then have a low blood sugar and be more prone to fainting, and in diabetic patients the low blood sugar is likely to precipitate a hypoglycaemic attack

In addition, the following points also have to be considered:

- Many dental treatments involve the injection of a local anaesthetic, and these may interact with some common patient medications
- Any of the materials, antibiotics or local anaesthetics used in dentistry have the potential to cause an allergic reaction in the patient, the worst case scenario being a full **anaphylactic reaction**
- Many dental treatments are carried out with the patient lying **supine** (flat) in the dental chair, and this leaves their airway potentially vulnerable to foreign object inhalation, choking and a full respiratory obstruction emergency

The dental team can do much to reduce the anxiety levels of their patients merely by creating a friendly, welcoming and pleasant atmosphere at the practice. Showing sympathy to an anxious patient helps to reduce their stress levels, and alleviates their concerns over appearing 'foolish' to the staff and to other patients. For those patients whose anxiety is so great that it borders on **phobia** (an exaggerated and illogical fear), all methods of pain and anxiety control techniques should be considered by the dental team, and offered where appropriate.

This ensures that these patients will still attend and undergo dental treatment routinely.

However, patients who pose the greatest concern with regard to medical emergencies are those with diagnosed risk factors, such as:

- Heart conditions and **hypertension** (high blood pressure)
- Liver or kidney disorders
- Diabetes
- Allergies
- Certain medications known to react with local anaesthetics, etc.
- Previous history of complications during dental treatment
- Long-term steroid treatment

These patients will be identified by the accurate completion and recording of a medical history before dental treatment begins. This medical history can then be stored with the patient records (either computerised or paper, or both) and updated at the beginning of every course of treatment.

Nevertheless, medical emergencies can, and do, occur in the dental surgery environment and the dental team must be able to recognise them and support life where necessary until specialist help arrives (that is, paramedics). All members of the dental team are expected to hold a **Basic Life Support** (**BLS**) certificate if working with patients, and to undertake the necessary continuing professional development (CPD) requirements to update their medical emergencies knowledge as laid down in the Standards Guidance documentation of the General Dental Council (GDC).

The correct recognition of the cause of any emergency is vital if the casualty is to be correctly treated and their life supported until the emergency services can attend. This is done by being able to recognise the **signs** and **symptoms** of an emergency.

Signs are what the rescuer can see with regard to the casualty, such as:

- Skin colour
- Breathlessness
- Suddenness of any collapse
- Actions before collapse, such as clutching the chest
- Condition of the pulse

At the same time, the casualty will feel symptoms, which may be asked about if they are not unconscious, such as:

- Any pain and its location
- Nausea
- Drowsiness
- Difficulty breathing
- Dizziness

By assessing the casualty, and noting the signs and symptoms exhibited, the rescuer can determine their next course of action, and often this will be to reassure the conscious casualty and to summon more experienced help. However, there are two signs that should prompt any rescuer to begin BLS immediately:

- **Unconsciousness**
- **Abnormal breathing**

These two signs indicate that the casualty's life is at risk: sudden unconsciousness may indicate that the heart has stopped beating (**asystole**) or is beating ineffectively (**fibrillating**), and abnormal breathing indicates a compromised airway and possible lack of oxygen to the brain (**hypoxia**). The presence of any of these signs may result in the death of the casualty if not dealt with quickly by the rescuer. The aim of BLS is to achieve both of the following:

- Carry out **rescue breathing** to supply oxygen to the lungs
- Circulate the oxygen to the body tissues by **external chest compressions**

In the panic of an emergency situation, it helps to follow a well-rehearsed and methodical plan of action, so that all actions necessary are taken and in the correct sequence. This not only gives the casualty the best chance of survival, but also protects the rescuer from harm themselves, as well as justifying their actions to others. Currently, the BLS sequence to be followed can be remembered as: D R S A B C.

> **Dangers** – assess any likely source of danger to the rescuer, such as fire, chemical spillage, dangerous electrical supplies.
> **Responsiveness** – call to the casualty and shake them to assess their level of consciousness.
> **Shout for help** – help will be required to carry out BLS if the casualty is unresponsive/unconscious, as it is physically exhausting for the rescuer to perform BLS alone.
> **Airway** – open the casualty's airway by tilting the head back and lifting the chin, or by thrusting the lower jaw forwards, and remove any visible debris by drainage or the surgery suction unit.
> **Breathing** – take 10 seconds to look, listen and feel for signs of spontaneous breathing, if breathing is abnormal or absent the emergency services must be called.
> **Circulation** – any residual oxygenated blood must be quickly pumped around the body and brain by performing 30 chest compressions at a rate of 100 per minute. After these first 30 compressions, two rescue breaths are given, and then the 30:2 algorithm is continued by the rescuers until specialist help arrives.

External chest compressions are carried out as described below (Figure 5.1).

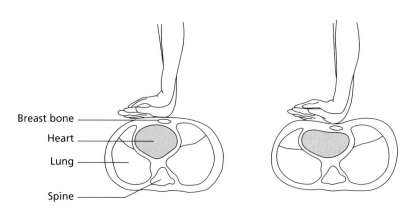

Breast bone

Heart

Lung

Spine

**Figure 5.1** External cardiac compression.
Source: *Emergency Procedures and First Aid for Nurses*, 2nd edn, M. Skeet, Blackwell Science Ltd, Oxford.

1   Heart must be compressed between the sternum and the spine, to mimic a heart beat and produce a circulatory flow, at the rate of 100 per minute.
2   The base of the sternum can be felt in the midline of the chest by following the bottom edge of the ribcage to the centre.
3   The heel of one hand is placed two finger widths above this point, towards the head.
4   The hands are locked together over this point and pressed down with a sharp rocking motion.
5   The rocking motion is performed 30 times.

If breathing is abnormal (intermittent, gasping, wheezy) or absent, two rescue breaths are now given as described below (Figure 5.2).

1   Airway is opened by tilting the head back and lifting the chin, or by thrusting the mandible forwards on both sides.

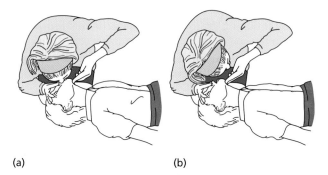

(a)                              (b)

**Figure 5.2** Expired air ventilation. (a) Inflation. (b) Expiration.
Source: *Lecture Notes on Anaesthetics*, J.N. Lunn, Blackwell Science Ltd, Oxford.

2   Nostrils are pinched closed and rescuer's mouth is sealed over the casualty's mouth, or a resuscitation mask is sealed over the casualty's mouth and nose together.
3   Open airway is maintained while two steady exhalations containing 16% oxygen are given, and the chest is observed for upwards movement.
    Casualty is checked for signs of spontaneous breathing.

The various causes of the collapse of a casualty must be known and understood by the dental nurse, so that they can assist usefully in the emergency treatment of these individuals should the need arise. While knowing and understanding the functions of the emergency equipment that all dental surgeries must hold, the dental nurse would not be expected to administer any of the drugs available.

In this chapter, the following medical emergencies will be covered:

- Faint (vaso-vagal syncope)
- Asthma attack
- Anaphylaxis
- Epileptic seizure
- Diabetic hypoglycaemia or coma
- Angina attack that may lead to myocardial infarction
- Choking

All of the above are potentially life-threatening emergencies, except for the simple faint. This is such a common occurrence in dental surgeries however, that it is important the dental nurse can recognise and treat it successfully. The emergency drugs that all dental practices must hold are shown below, and while the dental nurse should be aware of them and their emergency usages, their dosage and skill of administration is not expected to be known to them.

| Emergency | Drug and dose | Route given |
| --- | --- | --- |
| Asthma attack | Salbutamol metered dose 0.1 mg | Inhaler |
| | Oxygen | Face mask |
| Anaphylaxis | Adrenaline 1:1000 | Intramuscular (IM) injection |
| | Oxygen | Face mask |
| | Hydrocortisone 100 mg | IM injection |
| | Chlorphenamine 10 mg/ml | IM injection |
| Epileptic fit | Oxygen if possible | Face mask |
| | Diazepam 10 mg/2 ml if fit is prolonged | IM injection |
| Hypoglycaemia | Conscious – GlucoGel | Oral |
| | Unconscious – glucagon 1 mg | IM injection |
| Angina | Glyceryl trinitrate (GTN) metered dose 0.4 mg | Sublingual |
| | Oxygen | Face mask |
| Myocardial infarction | Aspirin 300 mg | Oral |
| | Oxygen | Face mask |

## Faint

This is a brief loss of consciousness due to a temporary reduction in oxygenated blood to the brain (**hypoxia**), and is the likeliest medical emergency to be encountered in the dental surgery.

**Signs** – pale and clammy skin, weak and thready pulse, loss of consciousness
**Symptoms** – dizziness, tunnel vision, nausea
**Treatment**:

- If unconscious – lay casualty flat with their legs raised above the head to restore blood flow to the brain
- Maintain airway and loosen tight clothing
- Provide fresh air flow or oxygen
- If conscious – sit casualty with head down, loosen tight clothing, provide fresh air
- Give GlucoGel or dextrose tablet when consciousness returns to restore the blood sugar levels

## Asthma attack

Asthma is a diagnosed hypersensitivity condition affecting the respiratory airways. The airways narrow in response to exposure to inhaled particles, so that exhaled air has to be forced out of the respiratory system and the casualty has difficulty breathing. The same response can occur in stressful or fearful situations, or with exercise, especially if the casualty has a respiratory tract infection.

**Signs** – breathless with wheezing on expiration, cyanosis (blueness of lips), restlessness
**Symptoms** – difficulty in breathing, sensation of suffocating or drowning
**Treatment**:

- Administer **salbutamol inhaler** from emergency drug box
- Give oxygen
- Calm and reassure the casualty
- Call 999 if the casualty does not make a rapid recovery

## Anaphylaxis

This is a severe allergic reaction by the casualty's immune system to an allergen, such as with an allergy to penicillin, latex, or food products such as nuts. The immune system over-reacts to the allergen, causing severe swelling of the head and neck in particular, and a sudden fall in blood pressure (**hypotension**) causing collapse.

**Signs** – rapid facial swelling, formation of a rash, gasping, collapse
**Symptoms** – sudden onset breathing difficulties, becoming severe, tingling of extremities
**Treatment**:

– Call 999 urgently
– Trained rescuer to administer **adrenaline** from emergency drug box
– Also administer steroid and anti-histamine if necessary
– Maintain airway and give **oxygen**
– Perform **BLS** if necessary until specialist help arrives

## Epileptic fit

This is a condition in which there is a brief disruption of the normal electrical activity within the brain, causing a fit. The fits can occur mildly (**petit mal**) and the casualty may appear as though they are just daydreaming, or they may occur in a major form (**grand mal**).

**Signs** – sudden loss of consciousness, followed by 'tonic–clonic' seizure, possible incontinence. Tonic phase – casualty becomes rigid, clonic phase – casualty convulses
**Symptoms** – casualty may experience an altered mood (**aura**) just before the fit begins, dazed on recovery, with no memory of the fit
**Treatment**:

– Protect the casualty from injury, but make no attempt to move them
– Remove onlookers from the area and maintain the casualty's dignity
– Allow their recovery, then ensure they are escorted home
– If no recovery within seven minutes, call 999
– Trained rescuer to administer **diazepam** from emergency drug box, with great caution

## Hypoglycaemia and diabetic coma

These two conditions may occur in patients diagnosed as having diabetes, who have either not followed their insulin regimen correctly, or who have not eaten at the correct times. The resulting drop in their blood glucose levels can be catastrophic and cause collapse. The timing of dental treatments involving local anaesthesia is crucial for these patients, as they will be unable to eat without traumatising their oral soft tissues until the anaesthetic has worn off. The dental team must therefore ensure that appointment times fit around the diabetic patient's normal insulin and meal regimes.

**Signs** – trembling, cold and clammy skin, becoming irritable to the point of being aggressive, drowsy, slurred speech, may mistakenly appear to be drunk
**Symptoms** – confusion, disorientated, blurred or double vision
**Treatment**:

- If conscious, give **GlucoGel sachet** from emergency drug box
- If unconscious, trained rescuer to administer **glucagon** from emergency drug box
- Maintain airway and give **oxygen**
- Call 999 if no recovery

## Angina

This usually occurs in patients diagnosed as having coronary artery disease, in whom these blood vessels, which supply the heart, are narrowed due to the presence of cholesterol or a thrombus (blood clot). During times of stress, anxiety, or while exercising, the reduced oxygenated blood supply to the heart is insufficient to allow full functioning, and the casualty will experience chest pains ranging in severity from indigestion to a heart attack.

**Signs** – congested facial appearance, casualty clutching chest or left arm, irregular pulse, shallow breathing
**Symptoms** – crushing chest pain that may travel into left arm or jaw, nausea, breathlessness
**Treatment**:

- Administer **glyceryl trinitrate (GTN) spray** under tongue, from emergency drug box
- Give oxygen
- Keep sitting upright, but maintain airway
- Calm and reassure the casualty
- Call 999 urgently if no recovery or consciousness is lost – suspect cardiac arrest

## Myocardial infarction

This usually occurs in patients with a history of heart disease, especially angina, when either their drug regimen has not been followed correctly, or they have been exposed to anxiety or stress.

During an angina attack, the turbulence caused by the increased coronary artery blood flow may be sufficient to dislodge any blood clots present, and these may lodge and completely obstruct the blood vessel. This will prevent oxygenated blood from supplying that section of the heart muscle, which will then die.

Signs – sudden clutching of chest, grey appearance, possible collapse
Symptoms – sudden crushing chest pain that is not relieved by GTN spray
Treatment:

- Call 999 urgently
- Administer **aspirin** from emergency drug box
- Give **oxygen** and keep casualty sitting upright
- Maintain airway
- Calm and reassure casualty
- Perform **BLS** if necessary until specialist help arrives

## Choking

Like the simple faint, choking is an emergency that may occur in the dental surgery due to the nature of dental treatment. However, unlike the simple faint, choking is a very serious situation that could result in the death of the casualty if not dealt with promptly. It can occur in both the conscious or unconscious casualty, by the partial or full blockage of the respiratory tract causing lack of blood oxygenation. The body tissues will become **hypoxic**, and this can be catastrophic when the brain or heart is affected.

Signs – sudden coughing or wheezing, laboured breathing, inability to speak, blue lips
Symptoms – aware of respiratory obstruction, breathing difficulties, dizziness
Treatment:

- Calm and reassure the casualty
- Support them leaning forward and encourage coughing
- Give five **back slaps** between the shoulder blades to dislodge the obstruction
- Begin **abdominal thrusts (Heimlich's manoeuvre)** to cause artificial coughing if the obstruction is still present
- If the casualty becomes unconscious, clear and open the airway as for **BLS**
- Call 999 if this is unsuccessful

The technique of giving abdominal thrusts is as follows:

1   Stand behind the casualty
2   Rescuer wraps their arms around the casualty, just below their ribcage
3   Fist is formed with one hand and grasped by the other, positioning both in the upper abdomen

4    Both hands are pulled in sharply, to cause an artificial cough
5    Air will whoosh out at each thrust, hopefully dislodging the obstruction

## Preparation of the dental team for medical emergencies

Besides the legal obligation of complying with the GDC's 'Standards Guidance' regulations, ensuring that all team members have current BLS certificates and that they are updated regularly, the dental team can do much to prepare for a medical emergency event.

In particular, the team can have regular 'in-house' emergency training practice sessions that are carried out and recorded accurately.

In addition, a policy must be in place that covers all of the following points:

- Designation of the team leader (usually the senior dentist)
- All staff must stop work and be available to assist with the emergency immediately
- The location of the emergency drugs box and oxygen cylinders must be known by all staff
- Duties will be delegated by the team leader and must be carried out correctly by those involved – in particular, duties to collect the emergency drugs box, the oxygen, to call 999, to clear other patients away, to direct the specialist emergency personnel to the casualty
- Staff should not undertake duties they are not specifically trained for
- All staff must be competent in BLS and able to assist as necessary
- Commands from the team leader must be followed immediately and accurately
- Duty of care to the casualty must be upheld at all times

The dental team members are also well advised to familiarise themselves with the emergency equipment, and to practise the use of it on a regular basis. In particular:

- Use of the resuscitation masks and Ambu bags
- Use of the portable suction unit for clearing the airway
- Use of artificial airways
- Switching on the oxygen supply, and connecting the tubing and masks correctly
- Opening drug vials and correctly drawing up their contents

If a medical emergency does occur, accurate written records must be kept of the whole event for legal reasons. Any failure to do so, or any altering of the record contents, would cause the offender to be liable to GDC proceedings, or even prosecution in serious cases. The dental nurse would be personally responsible for their own actions, and can no longer assume that the senior dentist would be vicariously liable, and held to account for everyone else's performance.

The importance of a full written account thus cannot be over-stressed, not only for the protection of the public, but also for all staff. If it is shown that everything possible was done to avoid an emergency, and that the full and correct actions were taken by all when one occurred, no one can be held to account for what is then an unfortunate and unavoidable accident.

# 6 Microbiology and Pathology

Pathology is the study of disease, and disease is the condition of suffering from an illness. Many diseases are caused by contamination of the body cells by microscopic living organisms, collectively called **micro-organisms**. The three main groups of micro-organisms are as follows:

- **Bacteria** – microscopic single cell organisms that survive as **spores** when conditions are not favourable for them to grow and reproduce.
- **Viruses** – ultra-microscopic organisms that live within the cells of other organisms.
- **Fungi** – a type of microscopic plant organism that grows across cells and tissues as an extensive branching network of fungal tissue.

There is a fourth type of micro-organism, called **protozoan**, but this has no relevance to dentistry.

In addition, recent research has uncovered the existence of **prions**, which are not micro-organisms but rather a type of special protein that is capable of causing disease. Those diseases discovered so far include 'mad cow disease' and the human variation of it which is called '**Creutzfeldt–Jakob Disease**' (CJD). The transmission of CJD is becoming more of a concern in dentistry as prions are not affected by the usual decontamination and sterilisation techniques used in the dental surgery environment. This means that an infected patient could pass on CJD to another patient when supposedly sterile instruments are re-used. As the prions are known to specifically affect nerve tissue, all endodontic instruments (root canal treatment) now have to be considered as single-use disposable items in dentistry, as they come into contact with the nerve tissue found within the pulp of the teeth. The instruments must all be safely discarded in sharps boxes after being used on just one patient, and then new instruments are used on the next patient. This avoids the possibility of passing prions from the first patient to the second.

The oral cavity provides the ideal conditions for micro-organisms to live, especially bacteria, being warm and well oxygenated, and providing many sheltered areas for them to lodge in, without being disturbed and removed. Many are harmless, but many more cause disease within the oral cavity when their numbers increase. Other micro-organisms not normally present in health can be transferred to the oral cavity and cause disease, such as by using contaminated crockery or cutlery, or by sharing a toothbrush between individuals. The micro-organisms relevant to dentistry are described below.

## Bacteria

These single cell micro-organisms have a rigid outer wall which determines their shape and helps to categorise them into named groups (Figure 6.1):

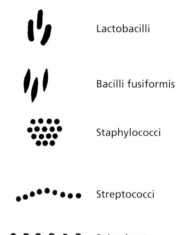

Lactobacilli

Bacilli fusiformis

Staphylococci

Streptococci

Spirochaete

Figure 6.1 Bacteria found in the mouth.

- **Cocci** – are circular; colonies living in clusters are called **staphylococci**, while those living in chains are called **streptococci**
- **Bacilli** – are rod-shaped with pointed ends, round-ended ones are called **lactobacilli**
- **Spirochaetes** – are spiral shaped

When their living conditions are not ideal for the colony to grow and expand, bacteria survive as **spores**, in a similar way that plants produce seeds to survive the winter while the parent plant dies from the cold. The spores have a very hard outer coating that protects the bacteria within from chemicals, drought and wide variations in temperature. Many can therefore survive the action of disinfecting chemicals used in dentistry, and the only sure way of removing the risk of bacterial contamination on dental instruments is to either sterilise them or to only use them once before they are discarded. Dental instruments are expensive to buy, so wherever possible they are manufactured to withstand the sterilisation process and be re-used safely.

Although the body's natural defence mechanisms will help to protect it to some extent from attack by micro-organisms, by the existence of its **natural immunity**, drugs have also been developed to be used to fight against them. For bacteria the important drug groups are:

- **Antibiotics** – these are taken to kill bacteria causing a severe illness, but can also kill some of the helpful bacteria within the body, especially those in the digestive system. Treatment with antibiotics is therefore often associated with stomach pain or diarrhoea.
- **Bacteriocidal agents** – these are chemicals that act to kill bacteria and are used to clean externally (such as surgery work surfaces).
- **Bacteriostatic agents** – these are chemicals that do not kill bacteria but prevent them reproducing and multiplying, and used to clean externally.

Some of the more important bacteria associated with dentistry are shown below.

| Bacteria name | Associated disease |
| --- | --- |
| *Streptococcus mutans* | Dental caries |
| *Lactobacillus* | |
| *Actinomyces* | Periodontal disease |
| *Porphyromonas gingivalis* | |
| *Prevotella intermedia* | |
| *Treponema denticola* | |
| *Staphylococci* | Skin and gingival boils |
| *Bacillus fusiformis* | Acute necrotising ulcerative gingivitis |
| *Borrelia vincenti* | |

## Viruses

Viruses are far smaller than bacteria, being visible only with an electron microscope. They live within the cells of other organisms, such as humans, existing as a protein capsule that contains all of the chemicals they need to reproduce within the cells of their host (Figure 6.2). The protein capsule is unique for every virus, and causes the body cells to react against it while trying to fight off the disease that the virus has produced.

Viral diseases are more difficult to cure than those caused by other micro-organisms because very few drugs have been developed against them, although some anti-viral agents do exist. Fortunately, **vaccinations** have been developed to prevent many viral diseases instead. They consist of a harmless dose of the dead virus or its protein capsules which are injected into the individual, or given orally. The presence of the dead virus or capsules causes the host body's immune system to fight against them by making **antibodies**, although the disease itself cannot develop. If the individual is then exposed to the same viral disease again, these

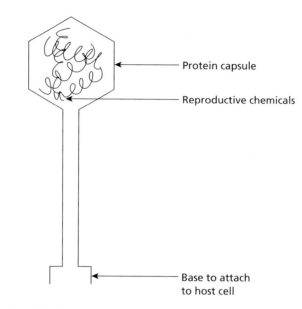

**Figure 6.2** Structure of a virus.

antibodies already present will fight off the viral attack and prevent the individual from becoming ill. This is called **acquired immunity**.

Viruses are also more difficult to kill than bacteria, and either the process of sterilisation or the use of some specialised viricidal chemicals are required to do so.

Some of the more important viral infections are shown below.

| Virus name | Associated disease |
| --- | --- |
| Hepatitis A, B, C, etc. | Various inflammatory liver diseases, some fatal |
| | Hepatitis B vaccinations for all dental personnel |
| Herpes varicella | Chickenpox |
| Human immunodeficiency virus (HIV) | Acquired immune deficiency syndrome (AIDS) |
| Herpes zoster | Shingles |
| Herpes simplex type I | Cold sores |
| Epstein–Barr | Glandular fever |
| Paramyxovirus | Mumps |

## Fungi

Fungi are plant-like organisms similar to microscopic colonies of mushrooms or toadstools. They grow as an extensive network of branches lying across the body tissues (called hyphae) and reproduce by budding out from the ends of the hyphae, or by the production of spores from fruiting bodies (like microscopic mushrooms). They tend to live on the outer surface of the body, such as on the skin, the oral cavity lining, the nails, and the surface of the eye, rather than growing within the body tissues.

The only fungal infection of dental importance is that caused by *Candida albicans*, which is responsible for:

- **Oral thrush** – this appears as a removable white film with underlying sore patches on the soft tissues of the oral cavity, and is associated with general ill health, especially in older people or those with other serious diseases such as AIDS.
- **Denture stomatitis** – this is also known as 'denture sore mouth', and occurs beneath both dentures and orthodontic appliances as a red sore. It is associated with poor appliance hygiene, allowing the fungus to colonise the underlying oral tissues.

Fungal infections are treated with anti-fungal agents, usually taken as a pastille to be sucked in the mouth. Underlying illnesses also need diagnosing and treating, and appliance hygiene needs to be reinforced by the dental team in cases of denture stomatitis.

## General effects of disease on the body

Micro-organisms that have the capability of producing a disease are referred to as **pathogenic organisms** or **pathogens**, as opposed to those that cannot cause illness or disease and which are called **non-pathogens**. When pathogens attack the body they may have several effects on the body cells and tissues, causing any of the reactions listed below.

- **Infection** – the actual invasion of the body cells by the pathogens, resulting in an **inflammatory response** of the cells which produces the five signs of inflammation: **heat, swelling, pain, redness, loss of function**.
- **Ulcer** – a shallow break in the skin or mucous membrane, leaving a raw and painful circular base that may bleed when touched.
- **Cyst** – an abnormal sac of fluid that develops within the body tissues over a period of time.
- **Tumour** – a swelling within any body tissue due to an uncontrolled and abnormal overgrowth of the body cells; when the swelling causes no harm other than to displace any surrounding structures it is called **benign**, but when the swelling invades and damages the surrounding structures it is called **malignant**, and is usually referred to as **cancer**.

## Response of the body to pathogen attack

The body has three natural lines of defence against attack by pathogens, which in fit and healthy individuals are often enough to prevent a serious illness developing:

- Intact skin and mucous membrane which acts as a physical barrier against the pathogens
- Surface secretions that help to dilute and neutralise the pathogens and their poisons (**toxins**), such as saliva in the mouth, gastric juice in the stomach, sweat on the skin, and tears in the eyes
- Inflammatory response if the body tissues are breached

Problems may occur in individuals who are not fit and healthy when their body is attacked by pathogens, as they may be unable to defend themselves so that a disease takes hold and they become ill. Those most likely to suffer are:

- **Older people** – the functioning of the body cells in older patients is not as efficient as when they were younger; cells and tissues wear out with age and cannot be replaced as easily, and other age-related disorders may be present that affect the ability of the body to repair itself.
- **Young children** – including babies, whose natural immune systems will not be functioning fully for some time, so they are more prone to developing diseases after attacks by pathogens, as well as not having received their full vaccination programme until older.
- **Debilitated** – those patients of any age who are said to be **immuno-compromised** because they have an underlying illness that affects the ability of their immune system to fight off pathogens; these include people with diabetes, those suffering from a range of illnesses such as leukaemia, kidney failure, AIDS and various cancers, and those taking drugs that act to suppress their immune system for the purpose of organ transplantation or cancer treatment.

## Inflammatory response

If the body tissues are breached by the pathogen, an inflammatory response occurs. This is the normal reaction of the body to exposure to an irritant such as an infective micro-organism, but it may also occur when exposed to physical and chemical irritants such as cuts, fire burns or chemical burns. Microscopically, the reaction of the body is the same.

- Huge increase in the blood flow to the affected area, so that many leucocytes can be transported there to fight the pathogens.
- The sudden increase in blood volume in the area will cause the tissues to appear **red** and **swollen**, and feel **hot** to touch.

- The swollen tissues will also press against the surrounding nerve cells, causing **pain**, and the affected area will then become too painful to use, resulting in **loss of function**.
- Leucocytes pass out of the capillaries and into the invaded body tissues to fight the pathogens by surrounding and eating them.
- They are helped by the movement of blood plasma into the tissues, containing antibodies and antitoxins which act to neutralise the poisons produced by the pathogens.
- Toxin production by the pathogens may be severe enough to cause a rise in body temperature from the normal 37°C, indicating an intense infection.
- During the battle, both leucocytes and pathogens are killed, and their debris collects to form **pus** in the body tissues.
- If the pus remains contained in the area of invasion it forms an **abscess**, but if it manages to spread into the surrounding tissues it is called **cellulitis**.
- When the inflammatory process occurs as above, it is described as **acute infection**, but when it occurs over a long period of time with few of the symptoms (especially pain) being evident, it is described as **chronic infection**.
- If the infecting micro-organism is powerful and difficult for the inflammatory response to control, it is described as **virulent**.
- Older, young, and debilitated patients may be unable to fight off an infection without the use of drugs such as **antibiotics**, **anti-virals**, or **anti-fungals**, and these may also have to be used in healthy individuals when a virulent organism is involved.

When the inflammatory response occurs in the absence of micro-organisms, no infection will occur, nor pus form, and the body tissues will repair any damage caused by the irritant.

## Tissue repair

Once the inflammatory response has overcome the infecting micro-organisms, or the physical or chemical irritant has been removed, the body will repair itself. New leucocytes will travel to the area and remove any damaged or dead tissue, and they will then lay down a temporary layer of repair cells called **granulation tissue**. This consists of basic tissue cells and capillaries which form a fibrous framework for the more specialised tissue cells to grow and develop onto. So if the damage occurred in skin, skin cells will be formed, if in bone, bone cells will be formed, and so on.

If a chronic infection is persistently present, the body's attempts to repair the damage will only be partially successful, and a state will exist where tissue is being repaired at the same time as chronic infection is still present. This is the usual case with infections such as periodontal disease. The infecting micro-organisms are never completely eradicated, the chronic infection is always present and its severity swings between low grade and held at bay, with intermittent acute episodes that require treatment and drug therapy to overcome.

## Immunity

During the inflammatory response, certain leucocytes are not involved in fighting the micro-organisms, but are stimulated to release **antibodies and antitoxins** into the blood plasma instead. The stimulation occurs because these leucocytes recognise the invaders as being foreign to the normal body tissues; they are identified as **antigens**. Other antigens that will cause a similar response are transplanted organs, foreign bodies, toxins from plant and animal tissues, and incompatible blood transfusions.

The antibodies and anti-toxins are quite specific for an invading micro-organism, and some are present from birth by being inherited randomly (called **natural immunity**) or by the specific inheritance of a mother's own antibodies and anti-toxins (called **passive immunity**). Once a micro-organism has been encountered and the infection fought off, the necessary antibodies and anti-toxins will remain in the individual's blood for life to prevent any recurrence of the same infection. This is called **acquired immunity**. Unfortunately, this does not occur for every micro-organism and in addition, many of them (especially viruses) can go through a process called **mutation**, where they change their chemical make-up slightly to effectively produce a new variation of a disease. The individual will then have to be exposed to this new variant before suitable antibodies and anti-toxins can be made by their leucocytes.

Where acquired immunity is possible for a micro-organism, it can be produced artificially by injecting the individual with a dose of the dead micro-organisms. This will stimulate the leucocytes to develop the necessary antibodies and anti-toxins to fight off the disease, but without actually infecting the individual with that disease. This is called **vaccination**. In this way, individuals can be protected against serious and fatal infections without having to be exposed to, and survive, the actual attack. The close-up and hands-on nature of dental treatment exposes the team to many infections daily and with the risk of catching any of them. Consequently, all team members must be vaccinated against the following:

- Hepatitis B
- MMR – measles, mumps and rubella (German measles)
- Tuberculosis and whooping cough (pertussis)
- Poliomyelitis
- Diphtheria and tetanus
- Chickenpox (if not already naturally immune)
- Meningitis

No vaccinations are available at present for some serious and fatal diseases, and one of the most important ones in relation to the dental team is AIDS, as this is transmitted mainly by blood, and many dental procedures produce bleeding. Avoidance of infection by any micro-organism can only occur if procedures are in place with regard to the following:

- Staff vaccination
- Use of protective wear during treatment and cleaning procedures
- Use of single-use disposables where possible
- Correct cleaning methods

## Allergy

Occasionally the immune response over-reacts to the presence of an antigen, with sudden swelling of the tissues and copious production of fluids occurring. This is called an **allergic reaction**. It can range in severity from a mild rash to a full anaphylactic shock episode, which is potentially fatal. (See Chapter 4.)

Often, individuals prone to an allergic reaction will already suffer from disorders such as asthma, eczema or hay fever, so they should be able to be identified from their medical history. During dental treatment, areas of caution involve the use of latex products (such as gloves and rubber dam sheets), and the prescribing of some drugs, especially the antibiotic penicillin and its derivatives.

## Dentally related pathology

Several pathological lesions can be seen in the oral cavity, some more common than others, and these are summarised below. Oral cancer will be discussed in detail.

- **Dental caries** – bacterial infection of the hard tissues of the tooth.
- **Periodontal disease** – bacterial infection of the gingivae and periodontal supporting tissues.
- **Oral thrush** – fungal infection of the oral soft tissues.
- **Periapical abscess** – bacterial infection of the tooth pulp causing abscess formation at the apex (can be acute or chronic).
- **Periodontal abscess** – bacterial infection within a periodontal pocket causing abscess formation.
- **Aphthous ulcers** – ulceration of the oral soft tissues that is not related to infection.
- **Herpetic ulceration** – viral infection of the oral soft tissues causing ulceration.
- **Acute necrotising ulcerative gingivitis** – acute bacterial infection of the gingivae causing ulceration.
- **Dental cyst** – cyst formation associated with a tooth, either erupted or unerupted.
- **Alveolar bone cyst** – cyst formation within the jaw bone.
- **Pericoronitis** – acute bacterial infection of the soft tissues (operculum) associated with a partially erupted tooth.
- **Localised osteitis** – bacterial infection of the bony walls of an extraction socket (also called **dry socket**).

- **Cellulitis** – spreading bacterial infection from a tooth into the surrounding deep soft tissue structures.
- **Cleft palate** – developmental defect of the palate (roof of the mouth) where the two bony halves fail to join together completely.
- **Oral cancer** – malignant tumour usually affecting the oral soft tissues initially.

## Oral cancer

Oral cancer can affect various areas of the mouth: the soft tissues, the salivary glands, or the jaw bones. Ninety per cent of oral cancers affect the soft tissues initially, as a lesion called **squamous cell carcinoma** (SCC). The suggested causative factors are:

- **Tobacco habits** – all tobacco products contain chemicals capable of causing cancer (**carcinogens**).
- **High alcohol consumption** – alcohol acts as a solvent for the carcinogens, and allows their easier entry into the soft tissues.
- **Both together** – smokers who also drink heavily are at most risk of SCC.
- **Sunlight** – in fair-skinned people, sunlight is associated with SCC affecting the lower lip.
- **Diet** – research is ongoing into links between SCC and diets high in fats and red meat, or low in vitamin A and iron intake.
- **Genetics** – some people are genetically predisposed to developing SCC.

The signs and symptoms of SCC include the following, and should be specifically looked for during routine dental examinations by the dentist:

- Painless ulcer that has no obvious cause, and fails to heal within three weeks
- Ulcer especially occurring beneath or on the side of the tongue, or in the floor of the mouth
- Presence of a white or red patch associated with the ulcer

The risk factors shown previously make the occurrence of the signs and symptoms far more serious in these individuals, and any suspicious lesions must be referred to an oral surgery hospital department for investigation immediately. Even then, the five-year survival rate from SCC is only around 55%, and is dependent on early detection and aggressive treatment.

The dental team has a vital role not only in early detection of SCC but also in patient education of the risk factors, especially in high-risk patients. This is especially important with smoking and tobacco usage, including the habitual chewing of betel nuts and tobacco *paan* in some Asian societies. In addition, the effects of smoking on dental and general health should also be discussed with suitable patients, as follows:

- Oral cancer
- Development of oral pre-cancerous lesions
- Periodontal disease
- Poor wound healing, especially after extraction
- Tendency to develop 'dry socket' after extraction
- Stained teeth
- Heart disease
- Respiratory disease
- Other cancers

## Drugs used in dentistry

The drugs discussed in this section are those used in dentistry to fight disease, specifically those used against micro-organisms. Many other drugs are used for other purposes by the dentist while providing treatment, and they are discussed in relevant chapters.

Drugs are classified into groups with a specific action, although some may have more than one use. Those of relevance here are:

- **Antibiotics**
- **Anti-virals**
- **Anti-fungals**
- **Analgesics**

All drugs available for prescription by the dentist to a patient, or available over the counter, are detailed in a publication called the *Dental Practitioners' Formulary* (*DPF*), which is issued to all practising dentists by the Department of Health. It is an invaluable guide to the drugs available, as well as giving details of their actions, dosages, contra-indications and side effects.

Drugs may be applied externally, such as ointments and creams, or taken internally, such as tablets and capsules. When applied externally their strength tends to be recorded as a percentage, while those used internally are recorded as milligrams for solids or millilitres for liquids. The more frequently used drugs to fight micro-organisms and alleviate the symptoms of infection are discussed below.

### Antibiotics

Antibiotics are drugs used specifically to fight against infection by **bacteria**. Many different bacteria exist that can cause dental problems: dental caries, periodontal disease, dental abscesses, and pericoronitis for instance. Some bacteria thrive in the oxygen-rich environment of the mouth, but others prefer to live in oxygen-poor areas such as deep within the periodontal pockets of a patient with periodontal disease. This second type of bacteria are called **anaerobes**, and they often require the use of different antibiotics for their eradication.

The bacteria involved can become immune to the antibiotics if used over a pro-longed period or inappropriately, so their use must always be justified.

Typical antibiotics used in dentistry are as follows:

- **Penicillin** – this is used against the spread of infection in pericoronitis, cellulitis, and to prevent secondary infection after oral surgery procedures. Typical dose is 250 mg taken four times daily for three to five days. Can cause allergic reaction in some patients (even anaphylaxis), and reacts with the drug methotrexate.
- **Amoxicillin** – this is a type of penicillin with a wider range of action. Typical dose is 250 mg four times daily and may be increased to 500 mg taken three times daily for up to five days in severe infections. Also used as a prophylaxis against infective endocarditis in susceptible patients, as a single 3 g liquid dose taken one hour before dental treatment.
- **Erythromycin** – this is an alternative for penicillin and its derivatives, in patients who are allergic to them.
- **Clindamycin** – this is an alternative for prophylaxis against infective endo-carditis in patients allergic to amoxicillin, given as a single 600 mg dose one hour before dental treatment.
- **Metronidazole** – this is used against anaerobic bacteria often associated with pericoronitis, periodontal disease, and acute ulcerative necrotising gingivitis. Typical dose is 200–400 mg taken three times daily for three days, depending on the severity of the infection. Has a severe reaction with alcohol, so patients must be suitably warned.

## Anti-virals

These are drugs used specifically against infections caused by a virus, but the only infection of dental relevance is the 'cold sore' on the lip that occurs after infection with the herpes simplex type I. An anti-viral cream containing **aciclovir** applied to the lesion several times a day may prevent the full development and blistering of the cold sore infection. The lesions are highly infective while present, and the dental team must protect themselves by wearing full personal protective equip-ment during treatment. Ideally, the patient should not be treated while a cold sore is present, unless for emergency treatment.

## Anti-fungals

These are drugs used specifically against fungal infections, and the relevant dental lesion is in cases of infection causing oral thrush. This may appear as denture stomatitis beneath removable appliances, or as sores at the angle of the mouth called **angular cheilitis**. Both are due to infection with the fungus *Candida albicans*. When present within the mouth, patients are prescribed anti-fungal lozenges or pastilles to suck while their appliance is out, or capsules to be taken internally, and all of the following are available:

- **Fluconazole** – this is used in severe infections as a daily 50 mg capsule dose for between seven and 14 days.
- **Nystatin** – this is used as an oral suspension or as lozenges taken four times daily after food for seven days.
- **Amphotericin** – this is used as 10 mg lozenges to be slowly dissolved in the mouth, four times daily for between 10 and 15 days.
- **Miconazole** – this is used as an oral gel to be swilled around the mouth four times daily.

## Analgesics

Analgesics are drugs used to relieve pain primarily, although some have other effects too. They are invaluable to dental patients experiencing pain (especially toothache) although dental treatment is often required to solve the problem and eliminate the pain completely. All should be avoided during pregnancy. The following are all available as over-the-counter analgesics:

- **Paracetamol** – this is an analgesic and has **anti-pyretic** properties – it reduces body temperature when fever is present. It has no anti-inflammatory effect. It causes serious liver damage if the recommended dose is exceeded, and this may be fatal.
- **Ibuprofen** – this is a non-steroidal anti-inflammatory and analgesic which is safer than paracetamol but can cause stomach ulcers if used to excess. It should not be given to asthmatic people.
- **Aspirin** – this is an analgesic with anti-inflammatory properties. It has several contraindications that limit its use: it acts as an anti-coagulant so it must not be given after surgical procedures (including tooth extraction); it can cause stomach ulcers; it should be avoided in asthmatic people; and must not be prescribed to children under 16 years of age because of the rare complication of **Reye's syndrome** (an often fatal brain disease).

# 7 Infection Control and Sterilisation

As discussed in Chapter 6, the mouth is full of micro-organisms, some of which are harmful. Consequently instruments and equipment used in dental treatment become contaminated with these micro-organisms whenever they are used. If no action were taken, infection from this contamination would be passed on from patient to patient, from patient to dental staff, and from staff to patient. The transfer of infection from person to person is called **direct cross-infection**, and from person to equipment and onto a second person is called **indirect cross-infection**. In order to prevent cross-infection it is essential to kill all the micro-organisms on contaminated instruments. This process is known as **sterilisation** and can be defined as 'the process of killing all micro-organisms and spores to produce asepsis'. The process usually involves the use of high temperatures and pressure, or industrial irradiation. **Asepsis** means the absence of all living pathogenic micro-organisms.

Countless numbers of micro-organisms live on the skin and in the mouth, nose and throat. Normally they do no harm to their host as they are living on an external surface and not among delicate internal cells. However, they may become harmful if they are introduced inside the body tissues, or are transferred from one person's mouth to another. This can occur when the tissues are penetrated by a contaminated forceps blade, a scaler or a syringe needle, and may give rise to a harmful reaction. It is imperative then that all re-useable dental instruments and equipment are sterilised before being used on another patient.

For equipment that is not used within the patient's mouth but may be exposed to a milder form of contamination just by being in the dental surgery, such as the dental chair and light and work surfaces, a process called **disinfection** is used to clean them. Disinfection can be defined as 'the destruction of bacteria and fungi, but not spores nor some viruses', and it usually involves the use of chemicals. A third method of cleaning used in dental practices is referred to as **social cleaning** which can be defined as 'clean to a socially acceptable standard, but not disinfected nor sterilised', and this describes the level of cleanliness expected of the non-clinical areas of the practice.

## Sterilisation

Instruments and dressings requiring sterilisation are made of different materials: some cannot be heated, some go rusty, and others must remain dry to be of any use. To meet these differences there are various methods of sterilisation, each suitable for certain instruments or materials. Manufacturers of dental equipment and materials are legally required to provide instructions for their sterilisation or disinfection. In dental practice, items are sterilised for re-use by being placed in an **autoclave** (Figure 7.1), which heats water to create steam under pressure and this kills all the micro-organisms.

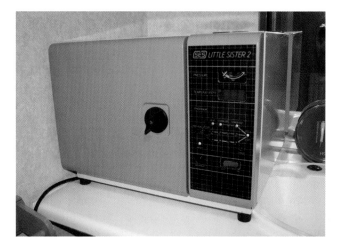

Figure 7.1  An autoclave.

There are two types of autoclave available: the older 'N' type and the newer 'S' type. Their details are as follows:

The 'N' type:

- Heats to 134°C and holds for three minutes at 2.2 bar pressure
- Steam displaces air downwards in the chamber so that it contacts all items
- Cycle lasts for 15–20 minutes, depending on its make and how often it has been in use previously
- Is suitable for unwrapped solid items laid in a single layer on perforated trays
- Machine can hold several trays at a time (Figure 7.2), cutting the number of cycles required
- Cycle can be set to dry instruments before they are removed from the autoclave
- Door cannot be opened during operation until the cycle is completed

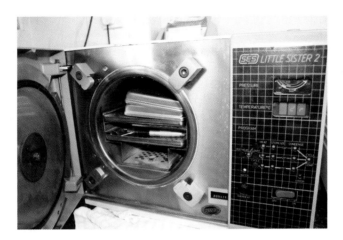

Figure 7.2  A loaded autoclave.

The 'S' type:

■ Heats to 134°C and holds for three minutes at 2.2 bar pressure
■ Air is sucked out of the chamber to create a vacuum so that steam contacts all the items present
■ Cycle lasts for 15–20 minutes, depending on its make and how often it has been in use previously
■ Is suitable for wrapped items and those with a hollow lumen, such as handpieces
■ Often have a printer incorporated so that the operating parameters for each cycle are recorded and can be checked
■ Machine can hold several trays at a time, cutting the number of cycles required
■ Cycle can be set to dry instruments before they are removed from the autoclave
■ Door cannot be opened during operation until the cycle has been completed
■ More expensive than the 'N' type autoclave

However, neither type of autoclave will sterilise items thoroughly unless they have been suitably prepared beforehand, and this is one of the most important duties for the dental nurse to complete on a daily basis. As the items are contaminated with a patient's body fluids (both saliva and blood), it is very important that any staff handling them should be wearing appropriate **personal protective equipment** (PPE). This includes:

■ Thick rubber gloves to prevent hand injuries from sharp items
■ Safety glasses or visor to prevent splashes into the eyes
■ Uniform or plastic apron to prevent contamination of clothing
■ Mask to prevent splashes onto face if very contaminated items are being cleaned

Wearing the PPE, the dirty instruments are taken to a designated instrument cleaning sink where they are scrubbed by the dental nurse, using soapy water and a brush. This is to remove all visible traces of debris which would protect underlying micro-organisms from the sterilising process. The items are then placed in either an **ultrasonic bath** or a **washer–disinfector machine**, in which less visible debris is shaken loose and removed. Both use a detergent-based cleaning agent to disinfect the items, but neither should be overloaded nor set for too short a cycle otherwise disinfection cannot occur. Once disinfected, the items can be loaded into the autoclave for sterilisation.

Once sterilised, the items are removed from the autoclave and stored appropriately, with the minimum amount of handling by the dental nurse. Ideally, instruments will have been laid out correctly on trays beforehand so that lids can be placed once sterilised, and then the whole tray is stored ready for future use. Surgical items will require bagging before storage if an 'N' type autoclave is used, or they can be sterilised in their bags in an 'S' type autoclave. Handpieces may require oiling after sterilisation, depending on the manufacturer's instructions, and then stored standing upright to allow excess oil to drain out. Any hot items can be removed safely using a pair of **Cheatle's forceps** (Figure 7.3) if necessary.

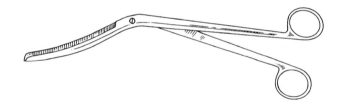

Figure 7.3 Cheatle's forceps.

As discussed, autoclaves use pressure to ensure sterilisation of the contained items, and this means that they have to comply with various Health and Safety legalities because of the potential danger they pose to staff and patients if they malfunction. The Health and Safety policy in all dental surgeries must contain written requirements for the correct use of autoclaves, as they are considered to be **pressure vessels**. The requirements are given below.

■ Daily test carried out on each autoclave, recording the temperature, pressure, and time interval for a full cycle – these details must be kept as a written record in a dated log book.
■ Only purified water should be used within the autoclave, never tap water.
■ Water should be drained from the reservoir and replaced daily.
■ Door seal and safety devices used to prevent door opening during the cycle must be visually checked on a weekly basis by designated staff.
■ Authorized engineer must carry out an annual inspection to ensure each autoclave operates correctly, and issue a certificate saying so.

- Each autoclave must also be checked for its conformation with the Pressure Systems Safety Regulations on a regular basis.
- Practice insurance policy must include third party liability cover for the use of autoclaves, in case of their explosion and resulting injury to any staff or patients.
- Any serious accident involving an autoclave, including its explosion, must be reported to the Health and Safety Executive under the **Reporting of Injuries, Diseases and Dangerous Occurrences Regulations (RIDDOR)**.

Sterilisation is the required method of cleaning for all of the following:

- Metal hand instruments
- Handpieces
- Burs
- Some rubbers and plastics
- Cotton products, and paper points

However, methods other than autoclaves, such as hot air ovens and ultraviolet lights, are no longer accepted techniques for medical and dental items.

Some single-use products are provided by manufacturers as pre-packaged sterile items, such as syringes and needles, local anaesthetic cartridges, scalpel blades, swabs and other cotton products, gutta percha and paper points used in endodontic treatments, and more recently the endodontic hand instruments themselves. These are sterilised after production by exposure to **gamma rays**, a type of radiation similar to X-rays. As gamma radiation is highly dangerous it must be used under strict regulation and in specialised control zones, so it is not suitable for use in dental practice.

## Disinfection

As stated above, disinfection involves the use of chemicals to kill all bacteria and fungi, but only some viruses and no spores. Many products are available for use in dental practice, but the commonest and best contain a chlorine-releasing agent, such as **sodium hypochlorite** (bleach), or one of the **aldehyde-based** agents, both of which have some viricidal action. **Isopropyl alcohol** (IPA) is also available for surgery use but has a more limited action than bleach and aldehyde, being a solvent rather than a true disinfectant. Because of their limited range of action, the use of disinfectants in dental practice is confined to those items that have to be re-used but which cannot be autoclaved. These include the dental chair and light, the bracket table and all piping, the curing light, the surgery work surfaces, and other exposed surgery surfaces, all of which may become contaminated by micro-organisms through aerosol spray and liquid spatter during dental treatment.

However, sodium hypochlorite products corrode metal over time, so all metallic surfaces have to be cleaned with the aldehyde alternative. Most of these products are sold as very convenient sprays or as pre-soaked wipes, but bleach products have to be made up on a daily basis as a 10% fresh solution. This is because the chlorine content is lost over the day so that the resulting solution becomes weaker, and cannot then be assumed to be strong enough to act as a viricide. Bleach also has to be used with caution on any fabrics as it will remove the colour, and it has an unpleasant smell and taste. Indeed, if ingested it is a strong chemical irritant to the digestive soft tissues, and will cause them corrosive damage. Bleach-based disinfectants are used as follows:

- 10% fresh solution to disinfect all non-metallic, non-fabric surfaces within the surgery
- 10% fresh solution to disinfect impressions and removable prostheses before transferring between the patient and the laboratory
- 50% fresh solution to clean blood spillages within the surgery

As all disinfectants are poisonous if ingested, their manufacture and usage is strictly controlled by the **Control of Substances Hazardous to Health (COSHH)** legislation, which is discussed in detail in Chapter 23.

## Prevention of cross-infection

Good infection control, with the aim of preventing cross-infection, is the duty of the whole dental team but especially the dental nurse who works within the surgery, as the potential for cross-infection is greatest in this area of the practice. As discussed in Chapter 1, all dental practices must comply with clinical governance regulations by having an **infection control policy** in place, to ensure that cross-infection does not occur. This will vary from practice to practice, as well as from community clinics to hospital departments, but the basics that must be covered by all are summarised below.

### Cleaning of hands

This is the most important method of preventing cross-infection. Nails should be kept short, and any skin wounds should be covered with a waterproof plaster to reduce the potential number of areas available for contamination by pathogenic micro-organisms. Similarly, the minimum amount of hand jewellery should be worn when working at the chairside.

The correct hand cleaning procedure is described below.

1   Turn on the tap using the foot or elbow control, to prevent contaminating the tap.
2   Wet the hands under running water of a suitable temperature.
3   Apply a chlorhexidine-based liquid soap from the elbow operated dispenser, and wash all areas of the hands thoroughly.

4   Nail brushes should not be used unless they are autoclaveable, as they will become contaminated by repeated usage.
5   Rinse hands under the running water, holding them downwards.
6   Dry the hands thoroughly using disposable, single-use paper towels.
7   Wear heavy duty rubber gloves whenever dirty instruments are being cleaned, to prevent sharps injuries to the hands.
8   Clinical gloves must be worn whenever patients are being treated and discarded safely after use with one patient, and fresh ones used for the next patient.

## Use of protective wear

Personal protective equipment (PPE) is worn to prevent staff from coming into contact with blood and other body fluids, such as saliva or vomit. It is a legal requirement for dental employers to provide such protective clothing for their staff. Full PPE should include:

- Clinical and heavy duty rubber gloves, as discussed above
- Uniform of a high temperature wash material, to be worn in the workplace only
- Disposable plastic apron to be worn over the uniform when soiling may occur, during cleaning procedures or dental treatment such as surgical cases
- Safety glasses, goggles or face visors to prevent contaminated debris or aerosol spray from entering the eyes
- Face masks of surgical quality, to be worn whenever dental handpieces or ultrasonic equipment is used to prevent the inhalation of aerosol contamination

## Cleaning of the clinical environment

All areas of the dental practice should be cleaned to a standard of social cleanliness, but clinical areas must be cleaned to a far higher standard still, because they are the areas where the highest possibility of cross-infection may occur. The practice should always be kept clean, dry and well ventilated.

Each surgery should have a written protocol to be followed by all staff with regard to its cleaning, which lays out the procedure to be followed in a logical manner, and with details of how all items should be dealt with. The following points should be included.

- All work surfaces should have the minimum number of items of equipment out for each procedure only, those not required being stored in drawers or cupboards to prevent aerosol contamination.
- A system of **zoning** should be used, where designated clean and dirty zones are allocated for instruments before and after their use, so that the clean area never becomes contaminated with dirty instruments.
- Work surfaces should be cleaned after each session with a suitable viricidal disinfectant or detergent solution.

- Static equipment, such as the dental chair, should have the control panels covered with impervious plastic sheets (such as 'cling film') so that they are not contaminated during use – these can be disinfected after use, or changed completely between patients.
- Dental aspirators and suction units should exhaust external to the clinical area to reduce the risk of aerosol contamination, and they should be flushed through daily with a recommended non-foaming disinfectant.
- All non-metallic equipment should be wiped down with a bleach-based disinfectant each day.
- All metallic equipment should be wiped down with a suitable alternative disinfectant.
- All intra-oral radiographs should be wiped over with IPA solution before being handled with clean gloves and taken for processing.
- Clinical records and pens should not be handled while gloves are being worn.
- Computer keyboards should be covered with an impervious plastic sheet that can be disinfected or changed after each use.

## Cleaning of equipment, handpieces and instruments

Intra-oral items are obviously the most potentially infective items of all, as they will have come into contact with the patient's oral tissues.

- Wherever possible, single-use disposable items should be used, as this prevents any occurrence of indirect cross-infection.
- All re-useable items (hand instruments and handpieces) must be sterilised in an autoclave after each use.
- Wearing suitable PPE, instruments should be scrubbed to remove visible debris, then placed in either an ultrasonic bath or a washer-disinfector to remove non-visible debris.
- Items should be rinsed in water to remove the disinfectant, then loaded correctly into the autoclave and sterilised.
- Handpieces must not be immersed in an ultrasonic bath, and the manufacturer's instructions should be followed with regard to bur removal and oiling before or after sterilisation, as they tend to vary between makes.
- If an 'S' type autoclave is in use, items may be bagged before loading.
- Sterilised items should be stored in lidded trays within the surgery cupboards, or loaded into bags after sterilisation (if necessary) until they are next used.
- All hazardous surgery waste should be disposed of correctly, as discussed later.

## Occupational hazards

There are three major occupational hazards in dentistry: radiation, mercury poisoning and cross-infection. All three concern dental nurses, and they must be trained to be aware of the dangers and know how to avoid them. The former two are described in later chapters, but cross-infection is covered here as its prevention is the purpose of infection control.

The most serious diseases which can be contracted from cross-infection are **hepatitis B**, **hepatitis C** and **acquired immune deficiency syndrome (AIDS)**, which are spread by contact with blood containing these viruses. Patients infected with hepatitis or AIDS viruses are usually unaware of their condition until symptoms arise, but their blood contains the virus nonetheless.

Dental practice often involves the shedding of blood, and even the most minute blood-stained droplets may contain viruses. Furthermore, such blood-borne viruses can be sprayed over a wide area of the surgery when using high-speed handpieces and ultrasonic scalers, as an aerosol, and by three-in-one syringes as spatter. Thus, not only instruments, but work surfaces, surgery equipment and surgery staff are exposed to contamination in this way.

Hepatitis and AIDS are covered in detail later in the chapter but less serious viral infections are conveniently discussed here. Special care should be taken if child patients have been in contact with virus infections such as **measles**, **mumps** and **rubella** (German measles). The virus is present in saliva before any signs of illness are apparent, and surgery staff may become infected in this way from an apparently fit child. If there is any evidence of contact, appropriate questioning of parents will allow the dentist to assess the risk of infection and decide whether to postpone treatment. Although such infections are usually trivial in children, they can cause serious complications in susceptible adults.

If rubella occurs in the first three months of pregnancy it can affect the unborn child – and this may happen before pregnancy is confirmed. Such a child is likely to have serious physical defects; in such cases there are strong medical grounds for advising termination of the pregnancy.

Men are most at risk from mumps as it may cause sterility. All surgical staff should, therefore, check their own medical history and vaccination records. They should be immune from common childhood infections previously contracted and are only at risk from any which are not included in these records.

Cold sores on the lips are another condition commonly met in the surgery. They are caused by the **herpes simplex type I** virus and can transmit the infection to people with no immunity to this virus. This is just one of the reasons why clinical staff are required to wear new gloves for every patient. Dental staff should accordingly take great care to avoid direct skin contact with cold sores, as they can result in a very painful herpetic *whitlow* if operating gloves are not worn.

Even such a trivial viral infection as the common cold is infectious. If surgery staff or their patients have a cold, transmission to others can be prevented by wearing protective clothing. Although the effects of a cold are not serious, they often necessitate time off work with the resultant inconvenience caused by staff shortage.

Bearing in mind that it will rarely be known if a patient is infectious or carrying a dangerous virus, and very likely that the patient is unaware of it too, or unwilling to admit it, the *only* safe approach to the problem of cross-infection is to assume that *every* patient is infectious, and to treat them all accordingly, by following a strict infection control policy. This is the basis of what is termed **Universal Precautions** and is best practice in all areas of medicine and dentistry.

Fortunately, vaccination is available against measles, mumps and rubella (MMR), hepatitis B, poliomyelitis, diphtheria, pertussis (whooping cough), tuberculosis, tetanus, meningitis, chickenpox and influenza. All practice staff must be protected in this way, and keep written records of their immunisation status, including booster dates and evidence of hepatitis B seroconversion after their initial vaccination course. This gives evidence of their immunity to these diseases.

## Hepatitis B

Hepatitis B is an inflammation of the liver caused by a virus. Its effect varies from a mild attack of jaundice to a severe or fatal illness. Over 50% of cases are undiagnosed as their symptoms are too mild to indicate the disease. On the other hand, 80% of primary liver cancers are as a result of hepatitis B.

The hepatitis B virus (HBV) is always present in the blood of people suffering from the disease. It may also be present in people who have no symptoms of the disease. Such people are called **carriers**; they may or may not have had any symptoms before and most of them are unaware that they are carriers. About one person in every thousand of the population is an HBV carrier. Thus all dentists are likely to treat patients who are carriers.

### Infectivity

Hepatitis B is highly infective. As mentioned in Chapter 6, HBV is very resistant to destruction. It can survive boiling for up to half an hour, immersion in chlorhexidine (Hibitane), and can live outside the body for some weeks. Disinfectants capable of killing HBV include hypochlorites.

HBV has been found in all body fluids, including blood, saliva and breast milk. It is transmitted by people suffering from the disease, and by carriers who have no symptoms at all and are unaware of their condition. Diagnosis is by blood test. In dental practices, the main source of infection is by direct contact with blood containing HBV. This is most likely to occur from a needlestick injury, i.e. accidentally pricking oneself with a syringe needle used on an HBV carrier; one in three of such accidents results in HBV infection.

Staff are also at risk from the use of high-speed equipment, such as an air turbine handpiece with water spray, an ultrasonic scaler or a three-in-one syringe. These release a cloud of water and saliva particles into the air which, if contaminated with a carrier's blood, may infect the dentist or dental nurse via the nose, eyes or skin abrasions. Furthermore, adjacent working surfaces become infected too, while inadequate sterilisation procedures may cause infection of other patients. Infection of staff from non-sharp causes may be prevented by protective clothing, as described previously.

Although the risks may seem alarming, all dental nurses and other chairside staff are required to be vaccinated against HBV and are thereby immune from danger.

*High-risk groups*

Among the general population the main modes of transmission of HBV are during childbirth, the sharing of needles by drug users, and sexual contact. Thus certain groups of people are much more likely to be carriers. They include:

- Drug users
- Sexually promiscuous people
- Those who have received long-term regular blood transfusions (such as haemophiliac patients, patients on dialysis and transplant patients)
- Special needs patients living in institutions, and staff in close contact with them
- Those working or living in institutions (such as prisons or rehabilitation centres for drug users and alcoholics)
- Partners and close relatives of carriers, not necessarily through sexual contact

*Prevention*

As the majority of HBV carriers are unaware of their condition, it has been estimated that 400 carriers are treated daily in dental practice. But provided that the sterilisation and surgery hygiene procedures in this chapter are adopted, there need be no cause for alarm. However, the existence of high-risk groups emphasises the importance of obtaining an adequate medical history before treatment.

Fortunately all dental staff can obtain protection against hepatitis B by vaccination. This will also protect their patients against HBV infection from dental staff. Vaccination is available under the NHS. It involves a series of three injections, followed by a blood test to check its success. A booster injection may be needed three to five years later. As vaccination is a requirement for chairside employment, documentary evidence of successful immunisation must be kept. Although vaccination is completely safe, special arrangements are necessary for staff who are pregnant, or become pregnant, during the course of injections.

*Treatment of known carriers*

The basic principle of preventing infection with HBV is to avoid contact with the patient's blood. In addition to the sterilisation and surgery hygiene procedures already detailed, the following extra precautions have been recommended for general practice.

- For operations involving extensive loss of blood, such as multiple extractions and minor oral surgery, or if the disease is in an active state, refer the patient to hospital – where full sterile surgical facilities are available.
- Reserve the last appointment of the day for treatment of known carriers. This allows more time for infection control procedures before any more patients are seen, but does not excuse non-compliance with the full infection control procedures at other times.

- Move all unnecessary equipment and materials away from the chairside. Protect essential working surfaces and equipment controls, such as switches, operating light handle and three-in-one syringe, with plastic bags or cling film.
- Take great care to avoid inoculation injuries.
- Regard steel burs and matrix bands as disposable. After treatment, flush aspirator with hypochlorite and leave the solution in a collection jar overnight.
- Items which cannot be sterilised by heat or hypochlorite should be immersed in a suitable disinfectant for the manufacturer's recommended time.
- Launder linen and towelling in a hot wash of 90°C for 10 minutes.
- Pregnant staff or those who have not been vaccinated against HBV should not be involved in the treatment of known carriers.

## Hepatitis C

This disease is similar to hepatitis B in the way it is contracted, transmitted and diagnosed. However, it is a far more dangerous disease with a much higher mortality rate, and there is no vaccine for it. In the past cases were caused by blood transfusion, but this has not happened since 1993, when screening of donors began.

Nowadays the main sources of infection are drug addiction, tattooing, body piercing and other modes of infected blood-to-blood contact, but sexual transmission is uncommon. The causal microbe is the hepatitis C virus (HCV).

The greatest risk to dental staff is from an inoculation injury, but provided that the safety precautions to prevent this are followed, there is no danger of HCV infection. However, it should be understood that if such a situation does arise, there is a 1 in 30 chance of transmission of the disease.

## AIDS

AIDS is the abbreviation for **acquired immune deficiency syndrome**. This means that the body's natural defence mechanism (Chapter 6) against infection is seriously impaired. Consequently AIDS patients succumb to infections which are not usually serious or which are not usually experienced. The outcome of AIDS is usually fatal as there is no cure, no vaccination and no resistance to infection. However, progress of the disease can be delayed, and life prolonged, by use of anti-viral drugs and others which boost the immune system. The apparent success of these treatments is, unfortunately, having the perverse effect of increasing the number of people contracting the disease. The reason for this is that many people are now ignoring the safety measures that were followed in the past, when AIDS was rapidly fatal.

AIDS is caused by infection with a virus called the **human immuno-deficiency virus (HIV)**. There are no particular symptoms of AIDS as they depend solely upon whichever chance infection affects the sufferer. Like hepatitis B the AIDS virus has been found in most body fluids but is transmitted mainly by contact with blood containing the virus. HIV is present in the blood of all infected persons but it usually takes years before they suffer any effects. Furthermore, as there are no specific symptoms, many of those infected with HIV are unaware that they have AIDS. Diagnosis is by blood test.

*Infectivity*

Unlike HBV, the AIDS virus is not very infective and is not resistant to heat or disinfectants. Although every infected person is potentially infectious, repeated exposure to HIV in blood or body fluids is usually required for transmission of AIDS. Among the general population the usual modes of transmission are sexual promiscuity, the sharing of needles by drug users, during childbirth and repeated transfusions with contaminated blood.

In dental practice the main hazard is needlestick injury, but the infectivity of HIV is so low that a single such accident would only result in a 1 in 300 chance of contracting AIDS. However, no chances can be taken as AIDS is a fatal disease for which there is no cure and no vaccine.

*High-risk groups*

From the modes of transmission of HIV just described, those most at risk of being carriers are:

- Sexually promiscuous people
- Drug users
- Haemophiliac patients and other patients who have received long-term regular blood transfusions
- Sexual partners of the above groups
- Infants born to infected mothers

*Prevention*

Although no preventive treatment by drugs or vaccination is possible, AIDS is easily avoided. All that is required as far as the general population is concerned is to avoid any form of sexual promiscuity, or the sharing of needles with drug addicts.

In dental practice, prevention is the same as for hepatitis B: by correct sterilisation and surgery hygiene procedures.

Dentists may be the first healthcare workers to see the early signs of AIDS as some very unusual mouth conditions may occur for no apparent reason. As in the case of oral cancer (page 68) early referral to a specialist may be a life-saving measure.

*Treatment of known carriers*

This is the same as for hepatitis carriers. Fortunately HIV has a very low infectivity and is easily destroyed by routine sterilisation procedures. Nevertheless, no chances can be taken as AIDS is fatal and no vaccination is available.

Known carriers of HIV and hepatitis viruses are those who are aware of their condition and have informed the dentist when their medical history is taken. The requirement of confidentiality mentioned in Chapter 2 is of paramount import-ance in such cases. Most carriers are either unaware of their condition, or unwill-ing to disclose it in case their condition is revealed to unauthorised people. Some are also afraid of being denied dental treatment if they admit to being carriers. When any medical history is taken, it is ethically and legally essential to ensure that it cannot be overheard anywhere else in the practice, and under conditions that give patients the confidence to provide a complete relevant history without embarrassment.

As only a minority of carriers are known to be such, most are treated without the dentist being aware of their condition. This emphasises the importance of strict adherence, by all practice staff, to correct procedures for the prevention of cross-infection.

## New variant Creutzfeldt–Jakob disease

New variant Creutzfeldt–Jakob disease (vCJD) is one of a group of rare, but fatal, related diseases (similar to 'mad cow disease') caused by infection with a unique non-microbial source of disease called a **prion protein**. Its importance is entirely due to the fact that prions cannot be destroyed by normal methods of sterilisation.

Consequently, current recommendations are to consider all endodontic instru-ments that come into contact with the tooth pulp as single use items, to prevent the transmission of the disease by indirect cross-infection, although the risk is considered to be only theoretical.

## Sharps injury

Also known as an inoculation or needlestick injury, this is a very real potentially serious accident that may occur in the dental surgery, to any dental staff but particularly to dental nurses while assisting at the chairside or while cleaning instruments. Nearly all dental procedures involve the use of sharp items – these include local anaesthetic needles, sharp instruments, or scalpel blades. All must be handled with great care by staff to avoid a sharps injury, as carriers of serious diseases are often unaware of their condition. Every dental practice must have a policy in place to avoid a sharps injury, and it should ideally include all of the following points.

- The dentist using a local anaesthetic needle should be responsible for its re-sheathing and safe placement in a sharps bin, so that injury to others does not occur as there is no transference of the sharp item from one person to another.
- Needle guards should be used when re-sheathing needles, so that they can be placed within their plastic sheath without being held in the fingers.
- Heavy-duty rubber gloves and full PPE should be worn by any staff respons-ible for instrument cleaning and debridement before sterilisation.

Although a sharps injury from a sterile, unused instrument may be momentarily painful, it is of no consequence save to reconsider the level of care taken by the staff member involved. However, in the unfortunate event of a contaminated sharps injury occurring, the following actions form the ideal 'sharps injury policy' and should be undertaken.

1 Stop treatment immediately and attend to the wound.
2 Squeeze the wound from above the puncture site to encourage bleeding, but do not suck the area.
3 Wash the area with soap and water, dry it, and cover with a waterproof dressing.
4 Check the medical history of the source patient to determine the likely risk of contamination.
5 If they are a known or suspected carrier of HIV, contact the consultant microbiologist at the local hospital immediately so that the necessary antiviral treatment can commence within the hour.
6 Their emergency number must be included in the 'sharps injury policy' of the dental practice.
7 Complete the practice accident book, detailing how the injury occurred and the actions taken.
8 Report the incident to the senior dentist, and to the local Occupational Health contact.

## Waste disposal in dental practice

Besides the **domestic waste** that all dental practices produce, in the form of office waste and record cards, they are also classed as producers of **non-domestic waste** by the Environment Agency, the government body responsible for the environment and for the safe disposal of all potentially harmful waste products created by all people and businesses. Non-domestic waste produced by dental practices can be segregated into two categories:

- **Hazardous waste**
- **Special waste**

### Hazardous waste

This is any waste produced within the dental surgery itself, which could potentially be contaminated by a patient's body fluids, and which poses a real risk of indirect cross-infection to any person in contact with it, including waste disposal personnel. It includes all of the following:

- Disposable surgery items contaminated, or potentially contaminated, by blood, saliva, or other body fluids

- All items used to clean the clinical environments on the premises
- All disposable covers used to prevent cross-infection during treatment
- All **sharps** items, including those contaminated by blood, saliva, or other body fluids
- All extracted teeth that do not contain amalgam restorations

All of the non-sharp items listed must be collected from each surgery and placed in a **yellow hazardous waste sack** (national and international variations apply). This must be sealed and tied with an identifying tag issued specifically for each practice, so that the source of the hazardous waste can be identified if necessary. The yellow bags must then be stored safely on the premises, away from public access, until they are collected by an authorised collection agency and taken away for incineration. All of the sharps items must be handled differently, as by definition they are capable of causing a contaminated sharps injury to both practice staff and waste disposal personnel. Consequently, they must all be carefully placed in a rigid, puncture proof, yellow sharps box (national and international variations apply; Figure 7.4), which has a snap-shut lid that cannot be reopened once closed. The boxes must never be more than three-quarters full before being sealed. Once sealed, they must be stored away from the public until collected and incinerated by an authorised waste disposal collector. The items that may be placed in a sharps box are as follows:

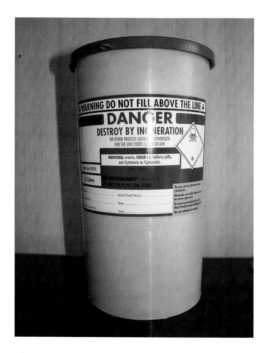

Figure 7.4  A sharps box.

- Scalpel blades
- All needles
- Empty local anaesthetic cartridges
- Empty emergency drugs vials
- Metal matrix bands
- Orthodontic wires
- Endodontic instruments

The safe disposal of hazardous waste is regulated and legally governed by the following Act and regulations.

- **Environmental Protection Act 1990** – the duty of care is on the dentist to store all hazardous waste safely and securely, and to arrange for its correct disposal by incineration.
- **Environmental Protection Regulations 1991** – the hazardous waste collector must have a certificate of registration, and supply transfer notes to be signed by both parties. Repeat collections can be covered by one note per year, but they must be kept by the practice for two years.
- **Carriage of Dangerous Goods Regulations 1996 updated in 2002** – so that the yellow sacks must be stored and transported in United Nations (UN)-approved rigid containers, and sharps boxes must comply with BS 7320 standards.

## Special waste

Special waste is so categorised because it cannot be disposed of by simple incineration due to its dangerous nature, or needs to be handled with special care because of its potential for causing serious harm to the waste disposal personnel or to the environment if not disposed of in the correct manner. It includes all of the following waste products that are routinely produced by all dental practices:

- **Waste amalgam** – contains mercury, which is toxic
- **Waste amalgam capsules** – contain traces of residual mercury
- **Radiograph fixer and developer solutions** – are both toxic and irritant to the skin and respiratory system
- **Lead foil from x-ray film packets** – is toxic and carcinogenic (causes cancer)
- **Partially empty local anaesthetic cartridges** – contain prescribed medicine
- **Out-of-date emergency drugs** – contain prescribed medicine

As stated, each is either toxic, irritant, a carcinogen, or can have adverse effects on the body tissues if they come into contact with anyone. They are all especially harmful to the public and the environment if not disposed of correctly, and additional legislation is therefore in place to ensure their correct handling. If they are incorrectly disposed of, the waste producers are able to be traced and prosecuted if necessary. The extra legislation is as follows:

- **Consignment notes** must be used and signed at each stage of the disposal process
- These notes must be kept by the dental practice for three years after issue
- The dentist has to pay **additional charges** for the safe disposal of the special waste, as it cannot be simply incinerated
- Radiograph processing solutions can no longer be disposed of via the sewers without the written permission of the appropriate water company
- **Waste amalgam** can no longer be posted to scrap metal companies, but has to be collected from the premises by a certified waste collector, with the relevant consignment and transfer notes issued

All staff have a duty of care to behave sensibly and act in accordance with the health and safety policy of their employer with regard to hazardous and special waste production and collection. With the General Dental Council (GDC) registration of dental nurses now in operation, they become personally liable for any omissions on their part with regard to the relevant legislation, if it is shown that the employer had all the correct procedures in place. This could result in a serious professional misconduct hearing, and possible removal from the GDC register.

# 8  Head and Neck Anatomy

The anatomy of the head and neck region of the human body is of relevance to the dental nurse in providing the underpinning knowledge required to understand dental nursing in total. Qualified dental nurses are often asked for information and advice from patients with regard to their oral health, and within the bounds of their profession, they will be able to give more accurate and useful information when it is based on the head and neck area in full, rather than just on teeth. For instance, a full understanding of the subject of local anaesthesia requires knowledge of skull and oral anatomy, as well as of the drugs used.

## Anatomy of the skull

The skull can be divided into three regions as follows:

- **Cranium** – enclosing the brain
- **Face** – surrounding and supporting the eyes and the nose
- **Jaws** – the upper and lower jaws, supporting the teeth and the tongue, and providing the openings for the respiratory tract and the digestive tract

Like most bones in the body, the skull develops in the fetus as cartilage, which is gradually converted to bone during the growth of the body into adulthood. The outer layer of bone is called **compact bone**, and is perforated by many natural bony openings (**foramina**) to allow the passage of nerve and blood vessels throughout. The inner layer is called **cancellous bone** and is quite sponge-like in appearance, as a solid structure throughout would make the bone too heavy for the muscles to be able to lift.

### Cranium

The cranium is made up of relatively thin plates of bone surrounding the brain. At birth, these plates are widely separated to allow growth of the brain as the baby grows, and the gaps between them are called **fontanelles**. During growth, the spaces gradually become filled with bone and close together to provide a protective helmet to surround the brain. The bony plates join together like a jigsaw puzzle at the **coronoid sutures** (Figure 8.1). The bony plates are as follows:

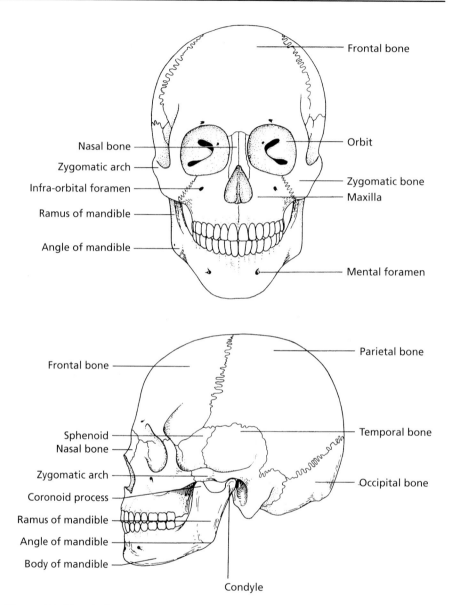

Figure 8.1 The skull.
Source: *Clinical Anatomy*, 11th edn, H. Ellis, 2006, Blackwell Publishing, Oxford.

- **Frontal bone** – one plate forming the forehead
- **Temporal bones** – one plate on either side of the skull at the temples; they form part of the **temporo-mandibular joint** (**TMJ**) of the lower jaw, and provide muscle attachments for jaw closing

- **Parietal bones** – two plates joined along the top of the skull and forming the majority of its sides and back
- **Occipital bone** – one plate forming the base of the skull, and through which the spinal cord passes into the vertebral column of the back, via a natural bony opening called the **foramen magnum**

There are many natural openings through bone in the base of the skull to allow the passage of all of the nerves that branch off directly from the brain itself and which supply the head and neck region only. They are called the **cranial nerves**, there are 12 pairs of them and those supplying the oral region are of relevance to the dental nurse. The blood vessels that supply the brain also pass through similar natural openings, each of which is called a **foramen** and has its own specific anatomical name, but these are not relevant to the dental nurse.

The nerves that supply the rest of the body all branch off the spinal cord at various points down the spinal column, and are referred to as the **spinal nerves**. They are not relevant to the dental nurse.

## Face

The face is made up of several pairs of bones, and the three pairs that are relevant to the dental nurse are as follows:

- **Zygomatic bones** – this pair of bones connect the cranium to the immovable upper jaw – the **maxilla** – at the temporal bones, and form part of the eye sockets
- **Zygomatic arches** – these are the cheekbones, which provide muscle attachments for jaw closing
- **Nasal bones** – these are joined together centrally and to the frontal bone above, to form the bridge of the nose

The inner surface of the nasal cavity is separated by the nasal septum and each half has several tube-like **turbinate bones** present whose soft tissue linings help to warm and filter inspired air as it passes over their extensive capillary beds.

## Jaws

The upper jaw is called the **maxilla** and is fixed solidly to the cranium, while the lower jaw – the **mandible** – is able to move in a hinge-like action around its jointed connection to the temporal bone at the **TMJ**.

## Maxilla

The maxilla is made up of two bones which are separated above by the nasal cavity. They join together below the nose as the **hard palate**, which forms the floor of the nose and the roof of the oral cavity, or mouth. Each side of the maxilla forms part of the eye socket, the nose and the front of the cheekbone. The two bones themselves are hollow within, as if they were solid bones they would be too heavy to allow the head to be lifted up. Each hollow space is called the **maxillary antrum** or **sinus**, and lies just above the root apices of the upper molars and premolars (Figure 8.2). The space can be easily perforated during the extraction of these teeth, causing an unwanted connection between the mouth and the antrum, called an **oro-antral fistula**. When suffering from the common cold, patients may experience inflammation of the maxillary antra (sinusitis) which causes toothache in the upper posterior teeth. A natural connection between the nasal cavity and the antra exists, to allow drainage of the sinuses and to give resonance to the voice.

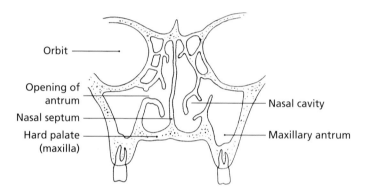

**Figure 8.2** Facial bones and air spaces in cross-section.
Source: *Basic Anatomy and Physiology for Radiographers*, 3rd edn, M.R.E. Dean & T.E.T. West, Blackwell Science Ltd, Oxford.

A horseshoe-shaped ridge of bone called the **alveolar process** runs around the hard palate and supports the upper teeth. The back end of each side of this process is called the **maxillary tuberosity**, and can be fractured during difficult upper wisdom tooth extractions (Figure 8.3).

The maxilla is perforated by several foramina to allow the passage of the nerves and blood vessels supplying the upper teeth and their surrounding soft tissues. The three main ones are:

- **Infra-orbital foramen** – beneath the eye sockets, through which the nerves supplying the upper teeth and their labial soft tissues pass
- **Greater palatine foramen** – at the back of the hard palate, through which the nerves supplying the palatal soft tissues of the upper posterior teeth pass
- **Incisive foramen** – at the front centre of the hard palate, through which the nerves supplying the palatal soft tissues of the upper anterior teeth pass

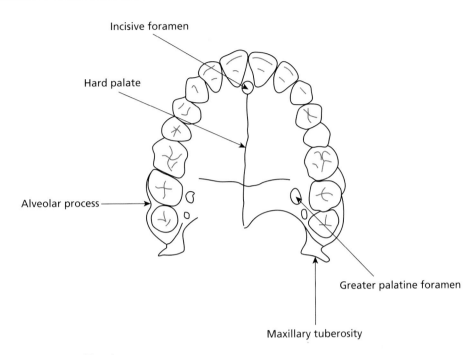

Incisive foramen

Hard palate

Alveolar process

Greater palatine foramen

Maxillary tuberosity

**Figure 8.3** Alveolar process.

*Mandible*

The mandible is also made up of two bones, joined together in the midline at the **mental symphysis** to create a horseshoe-shaped structure, with its two back ends bent upwards vertical to the horseshoe. The vertical section is called the **ramus of the mandible**, and the horizontal section is called the **body of the mandible**, and the point at which they join is the **angle of the mandible** (Figure 8.4).

The mandible's only connection with the rest of the skull is at the two **TMJs**, where the bone is able to move as a hinge joint, allowing the mouth to open and close. The point at which the mandible connects with the temporal bone at the TMJ is the **head of condyle** (Figure 8.5). The muscles of mastication, which allow jaw closing, all connect between the cranium and various points on the mandible, as discussed later.

The mandible also has an **alveolar process** running around it, which supports all of the lower teeth. Below this process, on the inner side of the body of the mandible lies a ridge of bone called the **mylohyoid ridge**, where the mylohyoid muscle attaches to form the floor of the mouth. A bony ridge also lies on the outer surface of the ramus of the mandible, called the **external oblique ridge**, which marks the base of the alveolar process in this area.

The front edge of the ramus rises up to the **coronoid process**, and the dip between it and the head of condyle at the back of the ramus is called the **sigmoid notch.** When the mouth is closed the coronoid process slots under the zygomatic arch of the face.

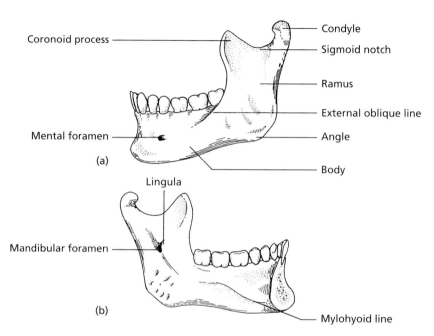

Figure 8.4  The mandible. (a) Outer side. (b) Inner side.
Source: *Clinical Anatomy*, 11th edn. H. Ellis, 2006, Blackwell Publishing, Oxford.

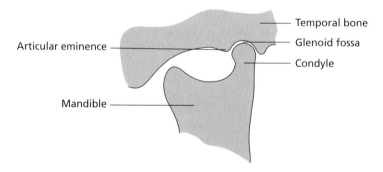

Figure 8.5  Temporo-mandibular joint.

The two foramina in the mandible which are of interest to the dental nurse are:

- **Mandibular foramen** – half way up the inner surface of the ramus, through which the nerve supplying the lower teeth and some of their surrounding soft tissues enters the mandible
- **Mental foramen** – on the outer surface of the body of the mandible, between the premolars, through which the nerve with the same name exits the mandible

## Movements of the jaws

The only jaw which can move is the mandible. The first movement involved in eating is a hinge-like opening of the mandible to separate the incisors. The mandible then moves forwards until the incisors can grasp the food between their cutting edges. The mandible then moves backwards and closes. This produces a shearing action of the incisors, which thereby cut the food into smaller pieces ready for chewing. It is similar to the cutting action of a pair of scissors.

Chewing is brought about by rotary movement of the mandible which swings from side to side, crushing food between the cusps of opposing molars and premolars.

### Temporo-mandibular joint

This joint is formed between the condyle of the mandible and the temporal bone at the base of the skull. When the mouth is shut the condyle rests in a hollow in the temporal bone called the **glenoid fossa**. The front edge of the glenoid fossa is formed into a ridge called the **articular eminence**.

Thus the mandibular surface of the joint consists of the condyle, and the temporal surface consists of the glenoid fossa and articular eminence. Between these two surfaces there is a disc of fibrous tissue, called the **meniscus**, which prevents the two bones from grating against each other during jaw movements. When the meniscus slips in front or behind its normal position during opening and closing of the mouth, the patient experiences 'jaw clicking'.

As already described, the first stage of opening the mouth is a hinge-like opening of the mandible to separate the incisors. The condyle remains in the glenoid fossa during this stage. As the mouth opens further, the condyle slides downwards and forwards from the glenoid fossa along the slope of the articular eminence. When the condyle reaches the crest of the articular eminence, the mouth is open to its fullest extent and the incisors can grasp food between their cutting edges. For the closing movement, which produces the shearing action of the incisors, the condyle returns to its rest position in the glenoid fossa.

Sometimes the condyle slips too far forwards and gets stuck in front of the articular eminence. When this happens it cannot move back and the joint is said to be **dislocated**. It is manifested by an inability to close the mouth. The problem can be resolved by pressing down on the lower molars to force the condyle downwards and backwards into the glenoid fossa, but sedation or a general anaesthetic may be necessary to allow the muscles of mastication to relax fully and allow treatment to be carried out.

The rotary movements of chewing involve alternate forwards and backwards movements of each condyle as the mandible swings from side to side. When the mandible swings to the right, the *left* condyle moves forwards and the right stays put. For the return movement to the left, the *right* condyle moves forwards while the left returns backwards into the glenoid fossa. These movements of the condyle can be felt by placing a finger in front of the ear while opening and closing the mandible. They are all produced by the muscles of mastication.

## Muscles of mastication

Four pairs of muscles connect the mandible to the base of the skull or face and act to allow chewing movements and mouth closing. They are:

- **Temporalis**
- **Masseter**
- **Lateral pterygoid**
- **Medial pterygoid**

All the muscles of mastication receive nerve impulses from the fifth cranial nerve which cause them to contract so that the length of the muscle shortens. This then causes the various movements of the mandible associated with mouth closing, jaw clenching, and chewing, as described later. The muscles of mastication **do not cause mouth opening**, this is controlled by a different group of muscles called the **suprahyoid muscles**. They are attached to the body of the mandible just below the chin, and run downwards to connect to the **hyoid bone** that lies embedded in the soft tissues of the throat, just above the larynx (Figure 8.6).

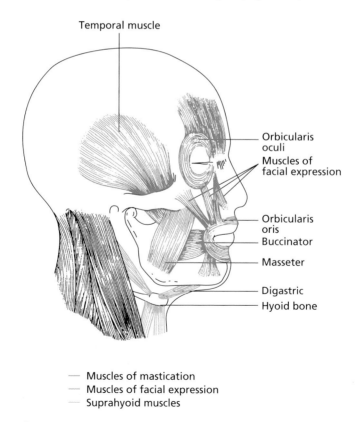

Temporal muscle

Orbicularis oculi

Muscles of facial expression

Orbicularis oris

Buccinator

Masseter

Digastric

Hyoid bone

— Muscles of mastication
— Muscles of facial expression
— Suprahyoid muscles

**Figure 8.6** Oral musculature.

Each set of the muscles of mastication is connected to the skull or the face at one end – called their **point of origin** – and at their other end to the mandible – called their **point of insertion**. The contraction of individual sets of muscles, or of just one of the lateral pterygoid muscles alone, shortens their length between these two points. As the mandible is the only moveable bone of the TMJ, this muscle shortening causes the movement of the mandible into various positions to allow closing and chewing actions to occur. They are summarised below:

### Temporalis

- Point of origin – **temporal bone** of the skull
- Point of insertion – **coronoid process** of the mandible, passing under the zygomatic arch
- Action – **pulls the mandible backwards to close the mouth**

### Masseter

- Point of origin – outer surface of **zygomatic arch**
- Point of insertion – outer surface of **mandibular ramus and angle**
- Action – **closes the mouth**

### Lateral pterygoid

- Point of origin – **lateral pterygoid plate** at the base of the cranium
- Point of insertion – **head of the mandibular condyle** and into the TMJ meniscus
- Action – **both contracting brings the mandible forwards** to bite the anterior teeth tip to tip, **one contracting pulls the mandible to the opposite side**

### Medial pterygoid

- Point of origin – **medial pterygoid plate** at the base of the cranium
- Point of insertion – inner surface of **mandibular ramus and angle**
- Action – **closes the mouth**

When the teeth are clenched, the temporal and masseter muscles can be felt by placing a hand on the side of the head and face, respectively. They form the superficial layer of the muscles of mastication, while the medial and lateral pterygoid muscles form the deep layer.

Acute inflammatory conditions sometimes result in a protective spasm of the muscles of mastication. This condition is called **trismus** and its effect is an inability to open the mouth. It occurs most often in acute inflammation of the gum surrounding an erupting lower wisdom tooth (pericoronitis), after surgical removal of these teeth, and in acute inflammation of the parotid gland (mumps). Its purpose is to rest the inflamed part and prevent pain.

## Temporo-mandibular disorders

The TMJ and muscles of mastication may be subjected to excessive strain from seemingly trivial causes. These can produce a variety of effects ranging from spasm of the muscles of mastication to degenerative changes in the joint. They result in a wide range of symptoms but the commonest are pain or tenderness over the joint, clicking noises and restricted movement of the mandible.

The symptoms are most common in young women and people under emotional stress. It often affects people who habitually grind or clench their teeth. Tooth-grinding activity is called **bruxism** and often occurs during sleep. It can be recognised by excessive wear facets on the teeth.

Treatment of these disorders depends on the symptoms and may include tranquillisers, physiotherapy, an occlusal splint to prop open the occlusion, or even TMJ surgery in severe cases.

## Muscles of facial expression

These are the muscles lying within the soft tissues of the face, that are responsible for a huge variety of facial movements and expressions: smiling, frowning, winking the eye, pursing the lips, and so on. For the sake of simplicity, they can be divided into three groups:

- Muscles of the eyes
- Muscles of the mouth
- Cheek muscles

The main muscle of the eye is a ring of tissue called **orbicularis oculi** and that of the mouth is called **orbicularis oris**. Thin straps of muscle run between these rings and into the surrounding tissues, to allow movement of the eyelids, lips, mouth and nostrils.

The cheek muscle is called **buccinator**, and is attached above and below to the outer surface of the alveolar process of each jaw. It connects to the muscular wall of the throat behind, and to orbicularis oris in front. Buccinator helps with chewing movements by helping to keep ingested food within the confines of the teeth, while the jaws' actions cause the teeth to cut and shred the food before swallowing.

## Soft tissues of the mouth

The *skin* of the mouth, i.e. the red tissue covering the cheeks, floor of the mouth, palate and tongue, etc., is called **mucous membrane**. It contains many tiny glands which contribute to the lubricating and cleansing functions of saliva. The space between the teeth and the mucous membrane lining the cheeks is called the **buccal sulcus**, and that between the teeth and lips is the **labial sulcus**.

## Soft palate

The soft palate is a flap of soft tissue attached to the back of the hard palate. Its function is to seal off the oral cavity from the nasal cavity during swallowing to prevent food passing up into the nose. The free edge of the soft palate has a central prolongation called the **uvula**. You can see this for yourself by looking in a mirror with your mouth wide open. To either side of this area at the back of the mouth, called the **oropharynx**, lie the tonsils which appear as small ball-like structures with a pitted surface. They are most noticeable when inflamed during a 'throat infection', as in **tonsillitis**.

## Tongue

The floor of the mouth lies within the arch of the mandible and is occupied by the tongue, which is composed of many bands of muscle lying in various directions to allow the organ its wide range of movements. It is attached to the floor of the mouth by a thin band of fibrous tissue called the **lingual frenum**. Where excess of this fibrous tissue occurs, the tongue is held more rigidly than normal so that its movements are restricted, and the person affected is described as 'short tongued' due to the lisp created as they speak. The upper lip is attached to the gum above the central incisors by a similar frenum, and when this attachment is thicker than usual there is often a space created between the two incisor teeth, called a **median diastema**. The muscles of the tongue are covered by a thick layer of mucous membrane above, and a thinner layer below.

The functions of the tongue are as follows:

- **Speech** – by allowing certain sounds to be created by touching the tongue to the upper anterior teeth or palate (such as 's', 't', 'n', 'the', and so on)
- **Taste** – the tongue is covered by different types of taste buds (including **filiform papillae**, **fungiform papillae**, and **vallate papillae**) that allow the recognition of the four basic tastes – sweet, sour, salt and bitter
- **Aids mastication** – by packaging ingested food into a parcel, or **bolus**, for easier chewing before swallowing
- **Aids swallowing** – by guiding the bolus to the back of the mouth
- **Cleansing** – by moving around the oral cavity and the smooth surfaces of the teeth to dislodge food particles

The lower layer of mucous membrane covering the underside of the tongue is so thin that it can very rapidly absorb drugs placed under it. Patients given glyceryl trinitrate tablets or spray for the treatment of angina pectoris use their medication in this way.

## Swallowing

Swallowing is a complex muscular action which aims to direct the food bolus into the oesophagus while also preventing it from entering the nasal cavity or the larynx. The bolus is mixed with saliva to lubricate it, and then propelled by the tongue from the mouth to the oropharynx, and then into the oesophagus. The sequence of events in the swallowing process is given below.

1    The lubricated ball of food is propelled to the oropharynx by the tongue.
2    The soft palate rises up and seals off the nasopharynx from the oropharynx to prevent the bolus from passing into the nose.
3    At the same time, the larynx lifts up and is sealed by the epiglottis to prevent the bolus passing into the trachea and being inhaled into the lungs.
4    The bolus is propelled downwards from the oropharynx to the oesophagus by the throat muscles.
5    Oesophageal muscles then move the bolus downwards by peristalsis into the stomach.

Soreness and inflammation of the tongue, called glossitis, can occur in conditions such as anaemia, vitamin B deficiency and hormonal disturbances. It is associated with a thin, smooth glazed appearance of the normally thick layer of mucous membrane on its upper surface.

## Salivary glands

The functions of saliva are covered in Chapter 11. It is produced by the minor mucous membrane glands lining the oral cavity, and by the three pairs of major salivary glands, which are situated close to the mandible. Saliva passes through tubes, called ducts, from these salivary glands into the mouth, so they are described as **exocrine glands**, because they do not secrete their contents directly into the bloodstream. Glands that do so are described as **endocrine glands**, and include organs such as the liver and the adrenal glands that lie over the kidneys.
The three pairs of major salivary glands are (Figure 8.7):

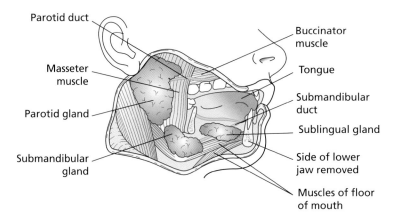

Figure 8.7  Salivary glands.

- Parotid salivary glands
- Submandibular salivary glands
- Sublingual salivary glands

The **parotid gland** lies partly over the outside and partly behind the ramus of the mandible, in front of the ear. It is the largest of the three major salivary glands, and the only one to be affected by the viral infection **mumps,** which is caused by a paramyxovirus. The tube connecting the gland to the oral cavity, **Stensen's duct,** passes forwards across the surface of the masseter muscle, and then inwards through the cheek to open into the buccal sulcus opposite the upper second molar. The parotid gland is the commonest salivary gland to be associated with both benign and malignant tumours.

The **submandibular gland** lies in the posterior region of the floor of the mouth below the mylohyoid line, against the inner and lower surface of the body of the mandible and near the angle. The submandibular duct (**Wharton's duct**) passes forwards in the floor of the mouth to open at the midline, beside the lingual frenum. It is the longest of the ducts, and the most likely to become blocked by salivary stones (calculi).

The **sublingual gland** also lies in the floor of the mouth, but above the mylohyoid line and much further forward than the submandibular gland. There are several sublingual ducts and these open into the floor of the mouth just behind the orifice of the submandibular duct (Figure 8.8).

The locations of the salivary ducts against the upper second molars and the lower incisors allows dental calculus to build up easily in these areas, as can be seen in patients attending for scaling.

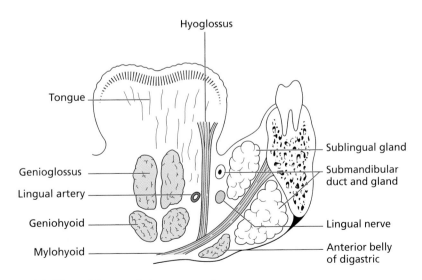

**Figure 8.8** Floor of the mouth in cross-section.
Source: *Clinical Anatomy*, 11th edn, H. Ellis, 2006, Blackwell Publishing, Oxford.

# Nerve supply of the head

The head is supplied by 12 pairs of **cranial nerves**. They all branch off from the brain, one from each pair supplying the left side, while the other supplies the right.

The nerves which make muscles and glands work are called **motor** nerves, and they carry electrical impulses from the brain to effect contraction of the muscles or secretion from the glands. Those nerves which convey pain and other sensation are called **sensory** nerves, and they carry electrical stimulation from the body tissues (including teeth) to the brain. Cranial nerves are either motor or sensory, or a combination of the two, and those relevant to dental nurses are as follows:

- **Trigeminal nerve** – the fifth cranial nerve; supplies the teeth and surrounding soft tissues, and the muscles of mastication
- **Facial nerve** – the seventh cranial nerve; supplies some taste sensations, some salivary glands, and the muscles of facial expression
- **Glossopharyngeal nerve** – the ninth cranial nerve; supplies some taste sensations, the parotid salivary glands, and the muscles of the pharynx
- **Hypoglossal nerve** – the twelfth cranial nerve; supplies the muscles of the tongue

## Trigeminal nerve

The name of this nerve indicates that it splits into three divisions, each of which has several branches. The three divisions are:

- **Ophthalmic division** – sensory supply of the soft tissues around the eye and the upper face
- **Maxillary division** – sensory supply of the upper teeth, the maxilla and the middle area of the face
- **Mandibular division** – sensory supply of the lower teeth, the mandible and the lower area of the face, and motor supply to the muscles of mastication

This cranial nerve is the most relevant to dental nurses, as its branches and areas of supply dictate the correct use of local anaesthetics by the dentist. It is discussed in detail in Chapter 9.

## Facial nerve

This is a combination nerve, carrying both sensory and motor fibres. Its sensory component carries taste sensation from the anterior two-thirds (front part) of the tongue, while its motor components supply the muscles of facial expression, and the secretions of both the submandibular and sublingual salivary glands. Temporary paralysis of this nerve (left or right) gives rise to **Bell's palsy**.

### Glossopharyngeal nerve

Again, this is a combination nerve. Its sensory component carries taste sensation from the posterior one third of the tongue, while its motor component supplies the muscles of the pharynx and the parotid salivary gland.

### Hypoglossal nerve

This nerve has a motor component only, and supplies the tongue muscles to effect its complicated movements during speech, mastication, swallowing and so on.

As with all the cranial nerves, the electrical transmissions of these four can be affected by many disorders affecting the brain, including tumours. Altered taste sensations or sudden loss of facial sensations with no obvious cause require neurological investigation to rule out any sinister causes. The dental team has a significant role in detecting these aberrations, and referring patients for more specialist investigation and diagnosis.

## Blood supply

The face, teeth and jaws are supplied by branches of the **external carotid artery**. This vessel is responsible for the pulse that is able to be felt to either side of the neck. Veins draining these parts eventually join the superior vena cava and enter the right side of the heart, where deoxygenated blood will be pumped to the lungs for reoxygenation.

All of the blood vessels run as neurovascular bundles alongside the nerves supplying the area.

# 9 Nerve Supply of the Teeth and Local Anaesthesia

As mentioned in Chapter 8, the teeth, jaws and face are supplied by the **trigeminal nerve,** the fifth cranial nerve, which splits into its three divisions of the **ophthalmic**, the **maxillary**, and the **mandibular**. The nomenclature used to name the various nerves follows that used in other areas of anatomy, so **anterior** and **posterior** refer to front and back, respectively, and **superior** and **inferior** refer to upper and lower, respectively. The areas of supply in relation to the teeth and their surrounding soft tissues follows the dental terminology used in naming tooth surfaces, as explained in Chapter 10.

## Maxillary nerve

The maxillary division of the trigeminal nerve further splits into five branches, all of which are sensory. By definition then, they transmit sensations (such as heat, cold and pain) from the area to the brain, including from the upper teeth (Figure 9.1). It is these branches that have to be anaesthetised before painless dental treatment can be carried out on the upper teeth. The five branches and their general anatomical paths are described below.

- **Anterior superior dental nerve** – supplies sensation from the upper incisors and canines, and their labial gingivae. In addition, it supplies sensation from the soft tissues of the upper lip and around the nostrils.
- **Middle superior dental nerve** – supplies sensation from the upper premolars and the anterior half of the upper first molars, and their buccal gingivae.
- **Posterior superior dental nerve** – supplies sensation from the posterior half of the upper first molars and the second and third molars, and their buccal gingivae.
- **Greater palatine nerve** – supplies sensation from the palatal gingivae of the upper molars, premolars and posterior half of the canines.
- **Naso-palatine nerve** – previously called the **long spheno-palatine nerve**, supplies sensation from the palatal gingivae of the upper incisors and anterior half of the canine teeth.

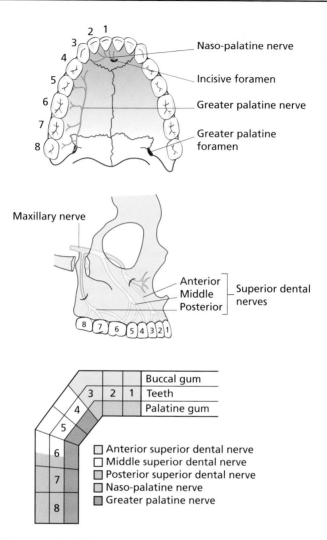

**Figure 9.1** Nerve supply of the upper teeth.

The maxillary nerve emerges from the base of the skull and passes forward through the floor of the orbit. Before entering the orbit it gives off its posterior superior dental and palatine branches. Within the orbit it gives off the middle and anterior superior dental nerves. It emerges from the orbit through the **infra-orbital foramen** at the front of the maxilla to supply the skin and mucous membrane of the lower eyelid, cheek and upper lip.

The posterior superior dental nerve enters the back of the maxilla to reach its destination, while the greater palatine nerve also passes through the back of the maxilla and reaches the surface of the hard palate through the **greater palatine foramen**, opposite the third molar.

The naso-palatine nerve passes through the floor of the nasal cavity to reach the surface of the palate through the **incisive foramen** behind the central incisors, and the anterior and middle superior dental nerves branch off from the maxillary nerve in the floor of the orbit. They pass down inside the maxilla, in the walls of the maxillary sinus, to reach the teeth.

## Mandibular nerve

The mandibular division of the trigeminal nerve splits into four branches: one motor and three sensory (Figure 9.2). The sensory branches of this nerve require anaesthetising before painless dental treatment can be carried out on the lower teeth. The four branches and their general anatomical paths are described below.

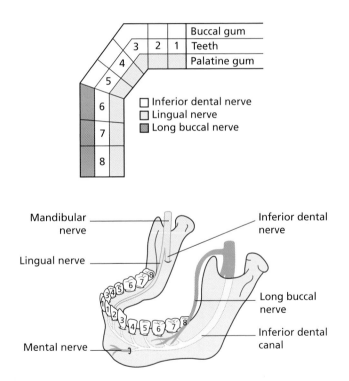

Figure 9.2 Nerve supply of the lower teeth.

■ **Inferior dental nerve** – supplies sensation from all of the lower teeth, and from the buccal or labial gingivae of all **except** the molar teeth. In addition, it supplies sensation from the soft tissues of the lower lip and the chin.

- **Lingual nerve** – supplies sensation from the lingual gingivae of all of the lower teeth, the floor of the mouth, and touch sensation from the anterior two-thirds of the tongue.
- **Long buccal nerve** – supplies sensation from the buccal gingivae of the lower molar teeth.
- **Motor branch** – supplies stimulation to the muscles of mastication, to effect jaw closing and chewing movements.

The mandibular nerve passes down from the base of the skull on the inner side of the ramus of the mandible, between the medial and lateral pterygoid muscles, and divides into the above branches.

The **inferior dental nerve** supplies all the lower teeth and enters the mandible through the **mandibular foramen**. This is situated at the centre of the inner surface of the ramus and is guarded on its front edge by a small bony projection called the **lingula**. After entering the mandibular foramen, the nerve passes through a canal running inside the mandible, below the apices of the teeth. A branch of the inferior dental nerve emerges on the outer surface of the mandible through the **mental foramen**, which is situated below the apices of the premolars. It is called the **mental nerve** and supplies the buccal gum of incisors, canine and premolars, plus the lower lip and chin.

The **long buccal nerve** supplies the buccal gum of the molars. It passes into the gum on the outer surface of the mandible, over the external oblique ridge. The **lingual nerve** supplies the lingual gum of all lower teeth. It passes along the floor of the mouth on the inner surface of the mandible, where it also supplies the anterior two-thirds of the tongue and floor of the mouth. The distribution of the trigeminal in full is shown in Figure 9.3.

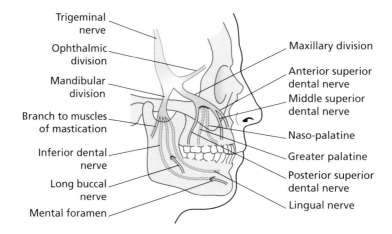

Figure 9.3 Trigeminal nerve distribution.

# Local anaesthesia

Pain messages passing along a nerve to the brain cause a sensation of pain in the area supplied by that nerve. A **local anaesthetic** injected into the vicinity of a nerve prevents the passage of such messages, thus producing a temporary local anaesthesia. All perception of pain, including stimulation by temperature changes, are lost but other sensations, such as pressure or vibration, are still felt.

**Anaesthesia** means the complete loss of feeling and **analgesia** means loss of pain only. Thus local anaesthesia (LA) should, strictly speaking, be called **local analgesia** but the former term is in such common use that it will be continued to be used here.

## Local anaesthetic drugs

Many local anaesthetics are available for use in dentistry, as shown below, and they are all supplied in glass or plastic cartridges for use in special dental syringes. The cartridges are available as either 2.2 mL or 1.8 mL, and contain the following:

- **Anaesthetic** – to block the electrical nerve transmissions to the brain so that neither pain nor temperature changes can be felt
- **Sterile water** – as a carrying solution making up the bulk of the cartridge contents
- **Buffering agents** – to maintain the contents at a neutral pH, so they are neither acidic nor alkaline
- **Preservative** – to give an adequate shelf-life to the contents
- **Vasoconstrictor** – present in some makes, to prolong the action of the anaesthetic by closing local blood vessels so that the solution is not carried away so quickly

Both the anaesthetic and any vasoconstrictor present are classed as drugs, and are therefore subject to strict regulations with regard to their safe disposal. This is covered in Chapter 7, where it is explained that the rules differ with regard to empty LA cartridges, which are classed as **hazardous waste**, and part empty cartridges, which are classed as **special waste**.

The more commonly used local anaesthetics in dentistry are:

- **Lidocaine** – 2% lidocaine hydrochloride as the LA with 1:80 000 adrenaline (epinephrine) as a vasoconstrictor (Lignospan and Xylocaine)
- **Carticaine (Articaine)** – carticaine as the LA with 1:100 000 adrenaline as a vasoconstrictor
- **Prilocaine (Citanest)** – 3% prilocaine hydrochloride as the LA with 0.03 units/mL felypressin (Octapressin) as a vasoconstrictor
- **Prilocaine (Citanest)** – 4% prilocaine hydrochloride as the LA (Citanest plain)
- **Mepivacaine** – 3% mepivacaine hydrochloride as the LA (Scandonest)

Adrenaline is the commonest vasoconstrictor used in LA, but it is a potent cardiac stimulant which acts to increase the rate and depth of a patient's heart beat generally. This explains its usefulness as an emergency drug in various situations, such as in anaphylaxis when the blood pressure falls to such low levels that the heart can stop beating. Unfortunately, it also means that LAs containing it cannot be used safely on patients with certain medical conditions, including the following:

- **Hypertension** – high blood pressure
- **Cardiac disease** – poor functioning of the heart, whether due to valve defects or acquired problems such as coronary artery disease
- **Hyperthyroidism** – an over-active thyroid gland, which tends to increase the overall metabolic rate of the patient

In addition, care should be taken with the following groups of patients or with those taking certain drugs:

- **Older patients** – as they may have complicated medical histories, be taking other drugs that could react with adrenaline, have undiagnosed diseases, or simply may not be able to excrete drugs efficiently due to their age
- **Hormone replacement therapy (HRT)** – given to women to delay the onset of the menopause, but which is often linked to hypertension
- **Thyroxine** – a drug given to patients with hypothyroidism (an under-active thyroid gland), which increases their overall metabolic rate

It is thought that patients taking certain antidepressants, including tricyclics and monoamine oxidase inhibitors (MAOIs), are also at higher risk of adverse events.

The use of LAs containing no vasoconstrictor is possible in these groups of patients, but then the action of the LA would wear off more quickly and there is more risk of haemorrhage during surgical procedures. Alternatively, they can be given 3% prilocaine (Citanest) – the only contraindication to its use being **pregnancy**, as felypressin is a potent drug used to induce labour due to its contractive action on the muscles of the uterus.

## Local anaesthetic equipment

The LA cartridge is a glass or plastic tube sealed at one end with a thin rubber diaphragm and at the other with a rubber bung. A special syringe and needle are required for use with cartridges. When a cartridge is inserted in the syringe, a double-ended needle pierces the diaphragm. Solution is injected when the syringe plunger engages the rubber bung and pushes it down the tube. As some patients are now known to have an allergy to latex, the rubber bung and diaphragm have been replaced by plastic alternatives in some types of specialised cartridges.

Various designs of LA syringe are available, some side-loading and some breech-loading (from the back) (Figure 9.4). The majority are metallic so that they can be sterilised in an autoclave after each use, but single-use disposable syringes are now also available. In addition, the head of the plunger is adapted in some syringes so that the dentist can use an **aspirating technique** when administering the LA (Figure 9.5). The technique is designed to avoid the injection of the LA

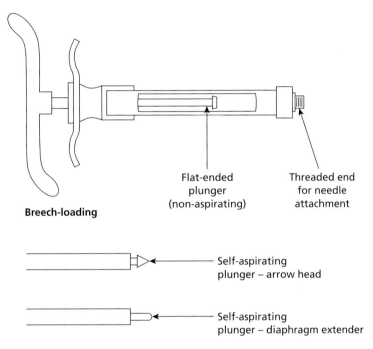

Flat-ended
plunger
(non-aspirating)

Threaded end
for needle
attachment

**Breech-loading**

Self-aspirating
plunger – arrow head

Self-aspirating
plunger – diaphragm extender

Figure 9.4  Syringe types.

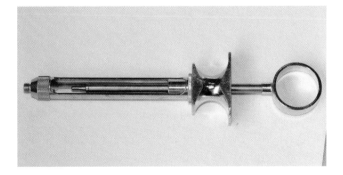

Figure 9.5  LA aspirating syringe.

solution into a blood vessel, rather than around the nerve as is the required position. Once the needle has been positioned, the plunger is drawn back before injection so that if a blood vessel has been pierced, blood will flow visibly into the LA cartridge. The needle tip can then be repositioned, the cartridge aspirated to check again, and then the contents safely injected into the correct position around the nerve.

## Surface anaesthetics

Surface anaesthetics anaesthetise the surface of mucous membrane so that a syringe needle can be inserted painlessly. They can be in the form of paste, solution or spray, which is applied to the appropriate site a few minutes before an injection is given. Commonly used surface anaesthetics are 5% lidocaine and 20% benzocaine.

Surface anaesthetics are also used to minimise the discomfort of superficial scaling and fitting of matrix bands, and for preventing sickness when taking impressions.

## Types of injection

There are four methods used to administer LAs in dentistry (Figure 9.6):

- Nerve block
- Local infiltration
- Intra-ligamentary injection
- Intra-osseous injection

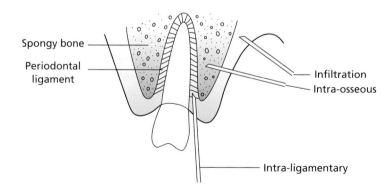

Figure 9.6 Types of injection.

## Nerve block

A nerve block is an injection which anaesthetises the nerve trunk as it runs in soft tissue, either before it enters the jaw bone or after it leaves it to reach the teeth and associated parts. Pain sensation from every part supplied by the nerve is blocked at the site of injection and cannot reach the brain. A nerve block is used when it is necessary to anaesthetise several teeth in one quadrant or where a local infiltration cannot work.

The commonest example of this type of injection is the **inferior dental block**. For this injection the anaesthetic solution is injected over the mandibular foramen. At this site the inferior dental and lingual nerves are so close to each other that both nerves are anaesthetised together. Thus it has the effect of anaesthetising all the lower teeth and lingual gum on that side, together with half the tongue as well. Furthermore it anaesthetises the lower lip and buccal gum of incisors, canine and premolars as these are supplied by the mental branch of the inferior dental nerve. So once the patient confirms the numbness of the lower lip, the dentist knows that all the lower teeth on that side are numb too.

The only part unaffected by the inferior dental block is the buccal gum of the lower molars; this area of soft tissue is supplied by the long buccal nerve, which is too far from the injection site to be affected.

Other nerve block injections are:

- **Mental nerve block** – given to anaesthetise the end portion only of the inferior dental nerve as it leaves the mandible through the mental foramen, so that only the anterior teeth and their buccal or labial soft tissues are affected
- **Posterior superior dental nerve block** – to anaesthetise this nerve before it enters the maxillary antrum, so that both the upper second and third molars are affected

The nerve block technique is useful in situations where an infection is present around a tooth requiring dental treatment, as it can be anaesthetised without risking the spread of the infection, by placing the injection at a distance from the tooth involved.

As stated previously, the nerves tend to run as neurovascular bundles and an aspirating technique should be used during injection, to prevent the inadvertent placement of the cartridge contents into a blood vessel.

## Local infiltration

A local infiltration injection is given over the apex of the tooth to be anaesthetised. The needle is inserted beneath the mucous membrane overlying the jaw. The anaesthetic soaks through pores in the bone and anaesthetises the nerves supplying the tooth and gum at the site of injection. Thus the difference between these two types of injection is that a nerve block applies the anaesthetic to the nerve trunk, whereas an infiltration applies it to nerve endings.

A local infiltration injection can only be used where the compact bone is sufficiently thin and porous to allow the anaesthetic to penetrate into spongy bone. Thus it is usually effective for all upper teeth, and for the lower incisor teeth. The compact bone overlying the mandibular premolars and molars, however, is too thick and an inferior dental block or a mental block is necessary for these, respectively. Local infiltration can also be used to anaesthetise gum only (see the section on injections for extractions).

## Intra-ligamentary injection

The intra-ligamentary injection technique tends to be used in conjunction with either infiltration or nerve block, to produce deeper anaesthesia around hypersensitive teeth. Various specialised syringes are available (Figure 9.7), which hold smaller LA cartridges within a protective plastic sheath. The force required to administer the cartridge contents is considerable, so a ratchet design of plunger is used to maintain the pressure, and the plastic sheath prevents injury if a glass cartridge shatters during use, as sometimes happens.

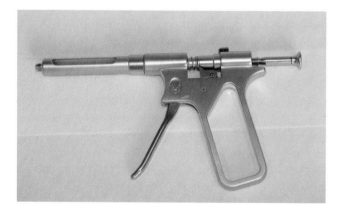

Figure 9.7 Ligmaject syringe.

The LA is administered into the periodontal ligament of the tooth, and the surrounding gingivae can be seen to blanch as it takes effect. The technique is especially useful when a nerve block has failed to produce sufficient anaesthesia of the tooth, but it cannot be used in the presence of gingival infection unless the tooth is being extracted. The force required for administration may also cause some post-operative soreness for the patient.

## Intra-osseous injection

An intra-osseous injection is given directly through the outer cortical plate of the jaw and into the spongy bone between two teeth (Figure 9.8). A few drops of anaesthetic are first injected into the overlying gum to permit painless drilling of a

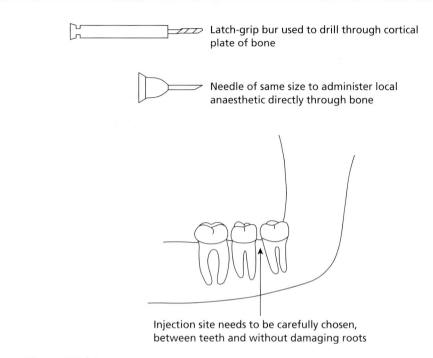

Latch-grip bur used to drill through cortical plate of bone

Needle of same size to administer local anaesthetic directly through bone

Injection site needs to be carefully chosen, between teeth and without damaging roots

**Figure 9.8** Intra-osseous system.

small hole through the compact bone, to allow a needle to be inserted directly into spongy bone.

This injection provides anaesthesia of relatively short duration, but profound depth, for the tooth and buccal and lingual gum, on either side of the injection site. However, it does not numb the cheek, lip or tongue. This makes it an excellent method for extractions. Other advantages are that it works immediately and rarely fails, thus making it useful where an infiltration or block has been unsuccessful. The disadvantages are that it cannot be used where gingival (gum) infection is present, nor should it be used in the region of the mental foramen of the mandible, as the nerve could easily be damaged.

The technique is very old but gained a new lease of life with the introduction of the Stabident kit, containing a special drill for perforating the compact bone, and a matching ultra-short needle for injecting directly into spongy bone.

## Local anaesthesia for extractions

For extraction it is necessary to anaesthetise not only the tooth, but also its surrounding gum. The injections required will be more readily understood by referring back to the nerve supply of teeth.

## Upper teeth

To anaesthetise any upper tooth for extraction a local infiltration injection is given on its buccal and palatal sides (Figure 9.9). For the second and third molars, some operators prefer to give a posterior superior dental block instead of a local infiltration on the buccal side.

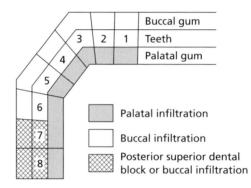

Figure 9.9 Injections for upper teeth.

## Lower teeth

An inferior dental block injection blocks the lingual as well as the inferior dental nerve. This single injection will therefore suffice for the extraction of premolars, canine and incisors. For molars, local buccal infiltration is required in addition to an inferior dental block.

The compact bone in the incisor region of the mandible is sufficiently thin to allow the use of a buccal and lingual local infiltration, and many operators prefer this to an inferior dental block for anaesthetising lower incisors (Figure 9.10).

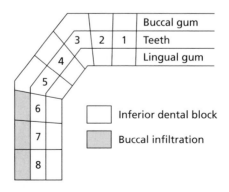

Figure 9.10 Injections for lower teeth.

## Local anaesthesia for fillings

It is unnecessary to anaesthetise the gum for fillings. Only the injection which anaesthetises the tooth is given; there is no need for a second injection.

### Upper teeth

A local buccal infiltration is enough. A posterior superior dental block is sometimes preferred for the second and third molars.

### Lower teeth

An inferior dental block will anaesthetise every lower tooth. For incisors, a local buccal infiltration will do instead.

## Preparation for local anaesthesia

All cartridges and needles are supplied by their manufacturers pre-sterilised and ready for use. Syringes are sterilised as usual in an autoclave.

A long needle of 27 gauge is used for a nerve block. For local infiltration, a short needle of 30 gauge is usually preferred. Although needles rarely break during an injection, precautions must still be taken to deal with such accidents immediately. A suitable pair of forceps (e.g. Spencer Wells) should always be available to grasp and remove the broken end.

A surface anaesthetic is applied for a few minutes while the *dentist* prepares the syringe and needle. The smaller guard at the syringe end of the needle is removed and the needle screwed on to the hub of a sterile syringe. As injection of cold solutions can be painful, cartridges should not be stored in a refrigerator but kept at room temperature. The injection site is then dried and disinfected. This is done by applying a suitable disinfectant, such as chlorhexidine or iodine, with a pledget of cotton wool for 15 seconds. The injection is now given and the needle guard refitted immediately.

The used needle is a real source of cross-infection, as it has pierced the patient's tissues and will be contaminated with blood, no matter how small the amount. Re-sheathing of the needle is the commonest cause of needlestick injuries to the dental team, and various needle guard devices have been designed to lower the incidence. Whatever the design, the needle sheath needs to be firmly held upright in a container, so that the syringe can be safely held by its back end while the needle is re-sheathed. In this way, fingers are kept away from the dirty needle and injury is unlikely. The dentist should also always take responsibility for re-sheathing the needle personally, to reduce the number of potential injured persons involved. If a needlestick injury does occur, the actions described in Chapter 7 must be followed.

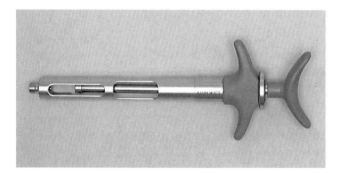

Figure 9.11 Aspirating syringe.

Nervous patients sometimes faint when a local anaesthetic is given. For this reason they must not be left alone while waiting for the injection to work. Apart from nervousness, patients are liable to faint if the anaesthetic is accidentally injected into a blood vessel. One way of preventing this is to use an **aspirating** syringe (Figure 9.11). With such a syringe, blood will be seen flowing back into the cartridge if the needle has penetrated a blood vessel. If so, it must be repositioned, whereupon the injection can be given if no more blood is seen.

## Patient advice

Patients need to be informed of the expected effects they will experience after receiving LA, especially if it is their first injection. Otherwise, they may be unduly concerned at what they feel, or even inadvertently injure themselves. The necessary advice is as follows:

- Sensation will be lost in the affected area for several hours
- During this time, do not attempt to eat, drink, or smoke as you may burn or bite yourself
- When the anaesthetic is wearing off, you will feel a 'pins and needles' sensation in the area – this is called **paraesthesia**
- Nerve block techniques may cause a localised tenderness of the soft tissues
- Intra-ligamentary techniques may cause soreness of the surrounding gingivae
- Contact the surgery if any problems persist

Finally the re-sheathed needle and cartridge are discarded in accordance with legal requirements, as discussed in Chapter 7 and summarised below.

- The sheathed needle is put in the sharps bin, together with the empty glass cartridge – both are hazardous waste.
- Empty plastic cartridges are put in the hazardous waste sack.
- Any cartridge that still contains some anaesthetic must be put in the special waste bin.

As mentioned in Chapter 7, a new needle and cartridge *must* be used for every patient to prevent cross-infection from blood containing hepatitis B or C or the human immunodeficiency (HIV) viruses or any other contaminants. Methods of sterilisation used in the surgery cannot penetrate the hollow interior of a blood-stained needle. Similarly, a partially used cartridge may also be contaminated with blood as microscopic aspiration takes place even without using aspiration methods.

# 10 Dental Anatomy

The oral cavity contains the teeth, which have the following functions:

- To cut up and masticate food into suitable sized portions before swallowing
- To expose the food surfaces to enzymes and allow digestion to occur
- To support the oral soft tissues and enable clear speech

All teeth are composed of a **crown** – the visible portion of the tooth within the mouth – and a varying number of **roots** which lie under the gingivae and anchor the teeth into their supporting structures. The four types of teeth are:

- **Incisors**
- **Canines**
- **Premolars** (in adults)
- **Molars**

The various shapes of the teeth, and their numbers of roots, is discussed later. This is called **tooth morphology**.

## Structure of the teeth

Every tooth consists of a **crown** and one or more **roots**. The crown is the part visible in the mouth and the root is the part hidden inside the jaw. The junction of crown and root is called the **neck** and the end of the root is called the **apex**. Every tooth is composed of enamel, dentine, cementum and pulp (Figure 10.1).

### Enamel

Enamel is the protective outer covering of the crown and is the hardest substance in the body. Its properties and microscopic structure are given below.

- It is made up of 96% mineral crystals (inorganic) arranged as **prisms** in an organic matrix called the **interprismatic substance**.
- The main mineral crystals are **hydroxyapatite**.

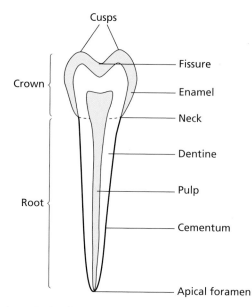

**Figure 10.1**  Structure of a tooth.

- The prisms lie at right angles to the junction with the next tooth layer, the **dentine**.
- The junction between these two layers is called the **amelodentinal junction** (ADJ).
- Enamel is formed before tooth eruption by the **ameloblast cells**, which lie at the ADJ.
- It contains no nerves or blood vessels and therefore cannot experience any sensation.
- It is a non-living tissue which cannot grow and repair itself, so progressive damage caused by injury or tooth decay is permanent.
- It can, however, remineralise its surface after an acid attack.
- The crystal structure can also be altered by the exchange of various minerals, especially **fluoride**, to form **fluorapatite crystals** – these make the enamel surface harder and more resistant to acid attack.
- The enamel layer is thickest over the biting surface of the tooth (the occlusal surface or the incisal edge), and thinnest at the neck of the tooth – the cervical margin.
- It is translucent in appearance.

## Cementum

Cementum is the protective outer covering of the root and is similar in structure to bone. It meets enamel at the neck of the tooth, and normally lies beneath the gingivae. It allows the attachment of the tooth root to the supporting structure of the periodontal ligament. The thickness of cementum may vary at different parts of the root, and changes throughout life, depending on the forces exerted on individual teeth.

## Dentine

Dentine forms the main bulk of a tooth and occupies the interior of the crown and root. It is covered by enamel in the crown of the tooth, and by cementum in the root of the tooth. Its properties and microscopic structure are given below.

- It consists of up to 80% inorganic tissue, mainly calcium.
- It is composed of **hollow tubes** which contain sensory nerve endings called **fibrils**.
- It is a living tissue and can transmit sensations of pain and thermal changes to the brain.
- Its hollow structure allows it a degree of elasticity so that it can absorb normal chewing forces without breaking.
- However, it also allows tooth decay (**caries**) to spread more rapidly through its structure.
- Dentine is formed by **odontoblast cells** and these lie along the inner edge of the pulp chamber throughout life, and can lay down more dentine as required.
- In this way, it can repair itself by laying down **secondary dentine**.
- This type of dentine is also formed as part of the natural ageing process, and its formation gradually narrows the pulp chamber.
- Dentine is a yellowish colour, and gives teeth their individual shade.

## Pulp

Unlike enamel, dentine and cementum, the pulp is purely soft tissue. It lies within the very centre of every tooth, both the crown and the root, and its properties and microscopic structure are given below.

- The pulp contains sensory nerves and blood vessels.
- It allows the tooth to feel hot, cold, touch, and pain by the stimulation of its sensory nerve endings which run as fibrils in the dentine tubules.
- These pulp tissues enter the tooth through the **apical foramen**, lying at the root apex of every tooth.
- The pulp chamber itself is lined by the odontoblast cells which form dentine.
- The chamber gradually narrows with age, so that it can become completely obliterated in older patients, making endodontic treatment very difficult.
- It can also become blocked by **pulp stones** which are formed by lumps of calcium-containing crystals.

## Supporting structures

The supporting structures are the structures lying around the roots of the teeth and hold them in their sockets (Figure 10.2). Their hold is not rigid, rather it allows the teeth to 'bounce' in their sockets so that there is some shock absorption effect when the teeth are used for chewing. This prevents fracture of the tooth under normal occlusal forces. The three supporting structures are as follows:

■ **Alveolar bone**
■ **Gingiva**
■ **Periodontal ligament**

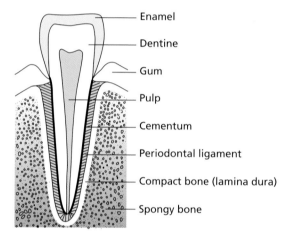

**Figure 10.2** Supporting structures of a tooth.

### Alveolar bone

The maxilla and the mandible both contain a horseshoe-shaped ridge of bone called the alveolar process. It is here that the teeth form during the growth of the fetus and then in the child, and from where they erupt into the mouth at various ages. The properties of the alveolar bone are given below.

■ It is a specialised bone found only in the jaws.
■ Its outer layer is made of hard, **compact bone** the surface of which is called the **lamina dura**.
■ The inner layer is called **cancellous bone** and is sponge-like in appearance, to allow the passage of the various nerves and blood vessels that supply the jaws, the teeth, and the surrounding oral soft tissues.
■ The sole purpose of the alveolar bone is to support the teeth, and when a tooth is extracted the bone gradually resorbs away.

- The teeth lie within individual **sockets** in the alveolar bone, each one being lined by lamina dura which shows on dental radiographs as a continuous white line – its absence indicates the presence of dental disease.
- The outer surface of the alveolar bone is covered in specialised **alveolar mucosa**, which forms the **gingivae** (gums) around the necks of the teeth.
- Destruction of the alveolar bone occurs in **periodontal disease**.

## Gingiva

This is the correct anatomical term for the gums. It is a continuous layer of specialised soft tissue found only in the oral cavity, which is firmly attached to the underlying alveolar bone as a **mucoperiosteal layer** of tissue. This layer is raised as a flap during oral surgical procedures, to expose the bone below. The properties of the gingiva are given below.

- The gingivae fit around the neck of every tooth like a tight cuff, when healthy.
- The **gingival crevice** exists as a shallow space of less than 3 mm between the tooth surface and the gingival margin.
- A natural mound of gingival tissue occurs between each tooth and is called the **interdental papilla**.
- In health, the gingivae are pink in colour with a stippled surface, like orange peel.
- Inflammation of the gingivae is called **gingivitis**, and occurs in the presence of **dental plaque**, due to poor oral hygiene control.
- Gingivitis appears as red and shiny gingivae that are swollen and bleed easily on touching.
- The gingiva can be forced to overgrow and become **hyperplastic** in patients taking various drugs, such as some anti-hypertensive drugs and some drugs used to control epilepsy.

## Periodontal ligament

The periodontal ligament is a specialised fibrous tissue which attaches the teeth to the alveolar bone and the surrounding gingivae. It acts as a shock absorber to the teeth during chewing, and its main fibres run between the alveolar bone and the cementum covering the root of the tooth. Other fibres run between the necks of the teeth, and from the cementum into the surrounding gingivae only. Its properties are given below.

- Its fibres are made up of a protein called **collagen**.
- They run in various directions, the end result being that the teeth are held in their sockets and can 'bounce' under normal chewing forces.
- This prevents tooth fracture and pain.
- When excessive occlusal forces are applied, the resultant pain experienced by the patient tends to stop further over-use from occurring.

■ Inflammation of the ligament is called **periodontitis** and occurs during periodontal disease.

## Tooth morphology

All people have two sets of teeth: the first or **deciduous teeth**, and the second or **permanent teeth**. All have different appearances or **morphology**, which depends on the set and the individual teeth themselves. Their morphology enables each tooth to be individually identified, and is determined by their shape and size, the number of cusps they have, and the number of roots present.

## Deciduous teeth

The deciduous teeth are the first set and are also known as milk, temporary or primary teeth (Figure 10.3). Their details are given below.

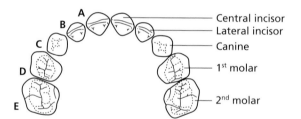

Figure 10.3  Deciduous teeth.

■ Total set of **20 teeth**, ten in each jaw.
■ They begin developing in the jaws before birth.
■ They are referred to in dentistry by letters – **A, B, C, D, and E** – starting from the midline.
■ They are **smaller** than permanent teeth, and **whiter** in colour.
■ Their roots are **resorbed** by the underlying permanent teeth, as the deciduous teeth gradually loosen and fall out – this is called **exfoliation**.
■ The roots of the deciduous molars are splayed out to accommodate the underlying permanent premolar teeth, so the roots are described as **divergent**.
■ They have a **larger pulp chamber** than the permanent teeth, with **thinner enamel**.
■ They begin erupting at around six months of age, and are usually all present by about 29 months, although individual variation does occur.

The five deciduous teeth present in each quadrant of the oral cavity are the **central and lateral incisors**, the **canine**, and the **first and second molars**. Their tooth and root morphology is summarised below.

| Tooth | Letter | Number of roots | Number of cusps (where applicable) |
|---|---|---|---|
| **Uppers** | | | |
| Central incisor | A | One | N/A |
| Lateral incisor | B | One | N/A |
| Canine | C | One | N/A |
| First molar | D | Three | Four |
| Second molar | E | Three | Five |
| **Lowers** | | | |
| Central incisor | A | One | N/A |
| Lateral incisor | B | One | N/A |
| Canine | C | One | N/A |
| First molar | D | Two | Four |
| Second molar | E | Two | Five |

The three roots of the upper molars are arranged as a tripod, with the developing permanent premolar teeth lying within this area, while the two roots of the lower molars lie one in front of the other in the alveolar bone of the mandible. The average eruption dates of the deciduous teeth, in months, are shown below.

| Tooth | Letter | Uppers (in months) | Lowers (in months) |
|---|---|---|---|
| Central incisor | A | 10 | 8 |
| Lateral incisor | B | 11 | 13 |
| Canine | C | 19 | 20 |
| First molar | D | 16 | 16 |
| Second molar | E | 29 | 27 |

The usual eruption pattern of the deciduous dentition is the lower central incisors first, followed by the other incisors, then the first molars followed by the canines, and finally the second molars.

The dentition begins changing again at about six years of age, when the permanent teeth begin to erupt by resorbing the roots of their deciduous predecessors and causing their exfoliation.

## Permanent teeth

Permanent teeth are the second and final set, and are also called the adult teeth (Figure 10.4). Their details are given below.

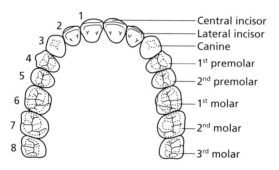

**Figure 10.4** Permanent teeth.

- Total set of **32 teeth**, 16 in each jaw.
- They begin developing in the jaws around the time of birth.
- They are referred to in dentistry by number – **1, 2, 3, 4, 5, 6, 7 and 8** – starting from the midline.
- They are of very similar morphology to the deciduous teeth, with eight extra teeth called **premolars** present, two in each quadrant.
- They are **larger** in size and **darker** in colour than deciduous teeth, with relatively **smaller pulp chambers**.
- The three permanent molars in each quadrant develop behind the deciduous teeth, using the space created as the jaws grow.
- So the **deciduous molar teeth** are succeeded by the **permanent premolar teeth**.
- It is relatively common for some adult teeth to be **congenitally missing** from the dentition, especially the third molars.
- They begin erupting at around six years of age, and all except the third molars are usually present by the age of 13 years.
- The third molars may be congenitally missing, present but unerupted due to lack of jaw space, or they may erupt from the age of 18 years onwards.

The eight permanent teeth present in each quadrant of the oral cavity are the **central and lateral incisors**, the **canine**, the **first and second premolars**, and the **first, second and third molars**. Their tooth and root morphology is summarised below.

| Tooth | Number | Number of roots | Number of cusps (where applicable) |
|---|---|---|---|
| **Uppers** | | | |
| Central incisor | 1 | One | N/A |
| Lateral incisor | 2 | One | N/A |
| Canine | 3 | One | N/A |
| First premolar | 4 | Two | Two |
| Second premolar | 5 | One | Two |
| First molar | 6 | Three | Five |
| Second molar | 7 | Three | Four |
| Third molar | 8 | Three | Four |
| **Lowers** | | | |
| Central incisor | 1 | One | N/A |
| Lateral incisor | 2 | One | N/A |
| Canine | 3 | One | N/A |
| First premolar | 4 | One | Two |
| Second premolar | 5 | One | Two |
| First molar | 6 | Two | Five |
| Second molar | 7 | Two | Four |
| Third molar | 8 | Two | Four |

Again, the three roots of the upper molars are arranged as a tripod, and the two roots of the lower molars lie one in front of the other in the alveolar bone of the mandible. The two roots of the upper first premolar teeth lie across the maxillary alveolar bone. The average eruption dates of the permanent teeth, in years, is shown below.

| Tooth | Number | Uppers (in years) | Lowers (in years) |
|---|---|---|---|
| Central incisor | 1 | 7–8 | 6–7 |
| Lateral incisor | 2 | 8–9 | 7–8 |
| Canine | 3 | 10–12 | 9–10 |
| First premolar | 4 | 9–11 | 9–11 |
| Second premolar | 5 | 10–11 | 9–11 |
| First molar | 6 | 6–7 | 6–7 |
| Second molar | 7 | 12–13 | 11–12 |
| Third molar | 8 | 18–25 | 18–25 |

Permanent teeth erupt before their roots are fully grown. About two-thirds of their root length has formed when permanent teeth erupt and the apex is still wide open. It takes another three years before root growth is complete and the apex closes. The only exceptions are canines and third molars which do not erupt until root growth is complete.

## Surfaces of the teeth

The biting surface of molars and premolars is called the **occlusal surface**. On incisors and canines it is called the **incisal edge**. The occlusal surface of molars and premolars is raised up into mounds called **cusps**. Between the cusps are crevices known as **fissures**.

The outer surface of molars and premolars – the surface facing the cheeks – is called the **buccal** surface. In the case of incisors and canines this surface is called **labial** as it faces the lips instead of the cheeks.

The inner surface of every lower tooth faces the tongue so it is called the **lingual** surface. This surface in all upper teeth is known as the **palatal** surface (Figure 10.5).

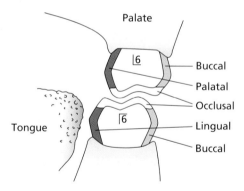

**Figure 10.5** Surfaces of the teeth – mesial aspect.

The remaining surfaces are those between adjoining teeth. These are called **proximal** surfaces: the one facing towards the front of the mouth is called **mesial** and that facing backwards is called **distal.** The point where the proximal surface of a tooth touches its neighbour is called the **contact point** (Figure 10.6).

The adjective **cervical** is used for the neck of a tooth.

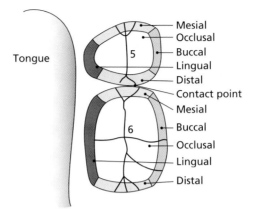

Figure 10.6 Surfaces of the teeth – occlusal aspect.

## Charting

Charting is a style of 'dental shorthand' to quickly and accurately record a patient's dentition, as it appears at the time of examination. Dental nurses are referred to the definitive 'Dental Charting Booklet' produced by the National Examining Board for Dental Nurses (NEBDN), copies of which are available on application. It describes the approved current charting notations used both for teeth and for periodontal conditions, following the three styles currently in use:

- **Palmer notation** – for tooth charting
- **International Dental Federation (FDI) notation** – for tooth charting
- **Basic Periodontal Examination (BPE)** – for periodontal charting

With tooth charting, a two-grid system is used (forensic notation) which separates the current dental status from any treatment required (Figure 10.7). So the charting grid is arranged as follows:

- **Inner grid** – shows current dental status and dental treatment already present in the mouth
- **Outer grid** – records all dental treatment that needs to be carried out

It is imperative that the dental nurse charts the dentition accurately, as otherwise not only could treatment be carried out on the wrong tooth, but in the event of a crime or the death of the patient, they could not be correctly identified. An overview of the Palmer and FDI systems is given, and an example of the accepted symbols used to chart a selection of the various treatments possible is shown (Figure 10.8). The full range of symbols is given in the NEBDN booklet.

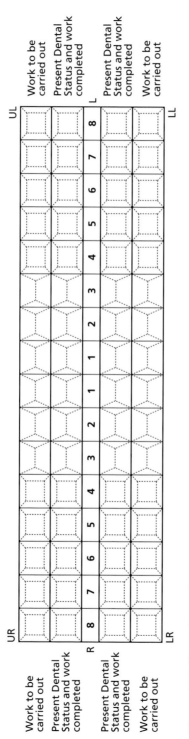

Figure 10.7  Forensic notation.

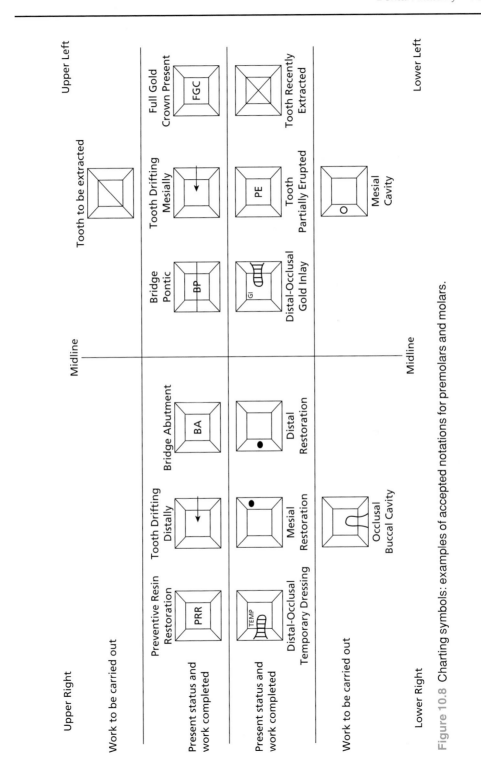

**Figure 10.8** Charting symbols: examples of accepted notations for premolars and molars.

## Palmer notation

This is based on the division of the dentition into four quadrants when looking at the patient from the front: upper left and right, and lower left and right. Using either the letters representing the deciduous dentition or the numbers representing the permanent dentition, each tooth can then be written and identified individually.

Some examples of use of this notation are given below.

| | |
|---|---|
| **Permanent second molar** | |
| upper right | 7⌋ |
| upper left | ⌊7 |
| lower left | ⌈7 |
| lower right | 7⌉ |
| | |
| **Permanent central incisor** | |
| upper left | ⌊1 |
| upper right | 1⌋ |
| lower right | 1⌉ |
| lower left | ⌈1 |
| | |
| **Deciduous first molar** | |
| lower left | ⌈D |
| lower right | D⌉ |
| upper right | D⌋ |
| upper left | ⌊D |

The system of tooth notation just described is used by the vast majority of practitioners in the UK. However, the quadrant symbols cannot readily be typed into a personal computer.

This problem is easily overcome by substituting the following notation:

- **UL** for upper left
- **UR** for upper right
- **LL** for lower left
- **LR** for lower right

Thus a notation would be typed into the computer as:

UR8 UR7 UR6 UR5 UR4 UR3 UR2 UR1 UL1 UL2 UL3 UL4 UL5 UL6 UL7 UL8 LR8 LR7 LR6 LR5 LR4 LR3 LR2 LR1 LL1 LL2 LL3 LL4 LL5 LL6 LL7 LL8

However, it is inconvenient for easy transmission of dental information in a form that can be used irrespective of the language spoken. This has led to the introduction of a two-digit system by the FDI.

This system replaces the quadrant symbol by a number: 1 for upper right; 2 for upper left; 3 for lower left; and 4 for lower right. Thus the quadrants are represented as:

| quadrant 1 | quadrant 2 |
|---|---|
| quadrant 4 | quadrant 3 |

The quadrant number forms the first digit while the second identifies an individual tooth as 1–8 in the same way as the Palmer system. Reading clockwise from the upper right third molar, all 32 teeth have their own two-digit number indicating their quadrant (first digit) and identity (second digit) as shown:

| 18 17 16 15 14 13 12 11 | 21 22 23 24 25 26 27 28 |
|---|---|
| 48 47 46 45 44 43 42 41 | 31 32 33 34 35 36 37 38 |

The lower left second premolar, for example, is written as 35 and pronounced 'three five', *not* thirty-five. Deciduous teeth are similarly treated by using quadrant numbers 5–8, and tooth numbers 1–5 as shown.

| quadrant 5 | quadrant 6 |
|---|---|
| quadrant 8 | quadrant 7 |

| 55 54 53 52 51 | 61 62 63 64 65 |
|---|---|
| 85 84 83 82 81 | 71 72 73 74 75 |

Thus the upper right deciduous first molar would be written as 54 and pronounced 'five four'.

The following examples show how the same charting is represented by the Palmer and FDI systems.

Handwritten Palmer:

| 6 E D 3 1 | C 4 7 8 |
|---|---|
| 5 3 2 A | 1 B 4 E |

Printed Palmer:

UR 6 E D 3 1   UL C 4 7 8

LR 5 3 2 A   LL 1 B 4 E

FDI:

16  55  54  13  11  63  24  27  28  75  34  72  31  81  42  43  45

## Anatomy of individual teeth

A collection of extracted teeth in good condition is a great help in learning anatomy and preparing for such items for the examination spotter and oral tests (Figure 10.9).

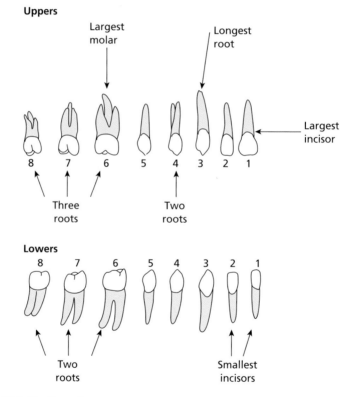

**Figure 10.9** Tooth anatomy.

### Permanent incisors

These can be identified as follows:

- They have a flattened, chisel-shaped crown
- The largest is the upper central incisor, the smallest is the lower central incisor
- All have one root

- The palatal surface of the upper incisors is often raised as a mound of enamel, called the **cingulum**
- The incisal edge is used to cut into food

## Permanent canines

These can be identified as follows:

- They have a large conical crown with a pointed incisal edge
- The upper canine is larger than the lower
- All have one root, the upper canine has the longest root of the whole dentition
- They are used to cut into and tear food

## Premolars

These can be identified as follows:

- They all have two cusps, arranged bucco-palatally or bucco-lingually across the dental arch
- The cusps are of equal size in the upper premolars, but the lingual cusp of the lowers is smaller than their buccal cusp
- The upper first premolar has two roots, one buccal and one palatal
- All other premolars have just one root
- Premolars are used to tear and chew food

## Permanent molars

These can be identified as follows:

- The upper first molar has five cusps, the small fifth one being called the **cusp of Carabelli**
- The lower first molar has five cusps, three buccal and two lingual
- All other molars have four cusps of relatively equal size
- All molars have a large occlusal surface for grinding and chewing food
- All the upper molars have three roots – a palatal, a mesiobuccal and a disto-buccal – arranged as a tripod
- All lower molars have two roots – a mesial and a distal

The deciduous teeth generally resemble their corresponding permanent teeth in morphology, but there are some differences between the two, as discussed earlier in this chapter.

## Occlusion of the teeth

When the upper and lower teeth are closed together, they are said to be in **occlusion**. The arch of the upper teeth is larger than the lower, thus upper teeth overlap the lowers on the buccal side. Lower buccal cusps accordingly bite into the fissure between upper buccal and palatal cusps (Figure 10.10).

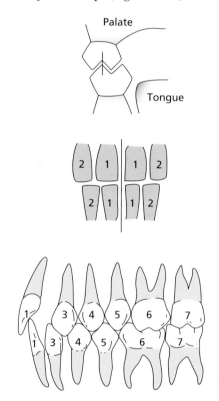

**Figure 10.10** Normal occlusion.
Source: *A Textbook of Orthodontics*, 3rd edn, T.D. Foster, Blackwell Science Ltd, Oxford.

The mesial edges of upper and lower central incisors form one straight vertical line. This is called the midline. As lower central incisors are much narrower than uppers, all the remaining lower teeth occlude with two upper teeth – their corresponding upper tooth and the one in front.

From this explanation of **normal occlusion** it is clear that:

- The mesial cusp of the upper first molar bites into the fissure between mesial and distal cusps of the lower first molar
- The lower canine bites in front of the upper canine
- The mesial edges of the upper and lower central incisors form one straight vertical midline

# 11 Dental Caries

Dental caries (tooth decay) is a bacterial disease of the mineralised tissues of the tooth, where the strong crystal structure found in both enamel and dentine is **demineralised** (dissolved) by the action of acids. This allows the softer organic component of the tooth structure to be broken down to form cavities.

The acids involved are produced as a waste product by oral bacteria, as they digest the foods we eat for their own nutrition. Although the acids are relatively weak organic ones, such as **lactic acid** or **citric acid**, they are strong enough to attack enamel and dentine. Not all of the bacteria found in the oral cavity are associated with the production of these acids. The usual ones that produce acid are:

- *Streptococcus mutans*
- *Streptococcus sanguis*
- Some **lactobacilli**

Not all of the foods that we eat can be broken down into acids either, but those foods that can easily be formed into these damaging organic acids contain carbohydrates. Foods that consist of protein or fats are not relevant to the onset of dental caries. So in summary, the relevant factors in the development of dental caries are:

- The presence of certain types of **bacteria**
- **Carbohydrate foods**
- The production of **weak organic acids** by these bacteria
- Adequate **time or frequency** for the acids to attack the tooth

The bacteria involved need to become attached to the tooth surface to be able to digest food debris and initiate dental caries, and they do this by forming themselves into a sticky layer called **bacterial plaque**.

## Bacterial plaque

Millions of bacteria live in our mouths, flourishing on the food that we eat. Some of this food sticks to our teeth and attracts colonies of bacteria to the tooth surfaces concerned. This combination of bacteria and food debris on a tooth surface forms a thin, transparent, protein-containing, soft and sticky film called **plaque**. It tends to form and stick most readily in areas where it cannot be easily dislodged, such as at the **gingival margins** of the teeth, in the **fissures** of teeth, and around the edges of **dental restorations**. These are called **stagnation areas**. The build-up of plaque at the gingival margins is directly associated with **gingivitis** and **periodontal disease** (see Chapter 12). Sticking to the tooth surfaces allows the bacteria living in the plaque to turn sugar into acid, which in turn dissolves enamel to produce **dental caries**.

The main micro-organism which initiates the process of caries is *Streptococcus mutans*. Large numbers of **lactobacilli** are then able to thrive in the acid environment, and this is put to practical use as a test for caries activity. By periodically counting the number of *Streptococcus mutans* or lactobacilli in a patient's saliva the level of caries activity and the effect of preventive measures can be monitored.

## Sugar

As mentioned in Chapter 4, all types of food are classified into three distinct groups: protein, fat and carbohydrate. Of these, only carbohydrates can be turned into acid and thereby cause caries – so they are described as **cariogenic foods** because they are capable of causing caries. The most acid-producing carbohydrates are those which are artificially added during food preparation, and which therefore tend to be based on **non-milk extrinsic sugars** (**NMEs**). As their name suggests, these types of sugar are not derived from milk and have been added artificially during the food manufacturing process, rather than being found naturally in the food product itself. The most damaging ones of all are the **refined sugars** called **sucrose** and **glucose** (also called dextrose).

Naturally occurring sugars that produce so little organic acid that they are considered harmless to teeth include the following:

- **Intrinsic sugars** – found naturally in foods, such as **fructose** in fruits
- **Milk extrinsic sugars** – especially lactose

Sugar can be instantaneously turned into acid by the bacteria concerned; it includes table sugar, sugar used in cooking, and sugar added to anything else taken by mouth, whether liquid or solid. Any food containing added sugar can cause caries. Some obvious examples are:

- Cake, biscuits, jam and sweets
- Breakfast cereals
- Pastry, desserts, canned fruit, syrups and ice cream
- Soft drinks
- Hot beverages sweetened with sugar

Sugar is widely added to many savoury foods, too, in order to flavour or preserve them, but without making its taste apparent. Such foods can include soups, sauces, canned vegetables and breakfast cereals, and are accordingly sources of **hidden sugar**. Medicines may also contain hidden sugar and be a significant cause of caries in sick children.

Sugar occurring naturally in milk, fruit and vegetables is *not* a significant cause of caries. Naturally starchy and fibrous vegetables such as potatoes, carrots, peas and beans are rich in carbohydrate but may be regarded as insignificant causes of caries as long as no sugar is added by producers or during cooking. The prime cause is refined sugar (**sucrose**) processed from sugar beet and sugar cane, and commercial **glucose**, which together constitute such a large proportion of the manufactured and sweetened food in our diet. Unfortunately, foods containing these NMEs tend to be a cheap and readily available food source in most developed countries, along with acidic drinks such as carbonated 'fizzy pops'.

## Acid formation

Sugar enters the plaque as soon as it is eaten. Within a minute or two it is turned into acid by plaque bacteria and attacks the enamel surface below the plaque. Enough acid is produced to last for about 20 minutes, and in this initial acid attack a microscopic layer of enamel is dissolved away. This phase is called **demineralisation**.

At the end of the meal or snack, when the intake of sugar is over, the acid persists for a period ranging from 20 minutes to two hours before it is neutralised by the buffering action of saliva. Saliva is the fluid bathing the oral cavity that is secreted from the salivary glands. Among its many roles, it maintains the mouth at a **neutral level**, that is neither acidic nor alkaline. The measure of acidity/alkalinity of a solution is called its **pH level,** and the neutral level maintained by saliva is **pH 7**. When the weak organic acids are produced by the oral bacteria, the pH level starts to fall and once it passes the **critical pH 5.5**, the environment is acidic enough to attack the enamel and dentine of teeth, and produce cavities.

Once neutralisation has occurred, no further demineralisation can take place until such time as more sugar is consumed. In this phase where no more sugar is present in the plaque, some natural healing takes place, mineral constituents naturally present in saliva enter demineralised enamel and restore the part lost by the initial acid attack. This healing phase is called **remineralisation**.

What happens next is entirely dependent on the frequency of sugar intake. If it is confined to mealtimes only, for example, at breakfast, midday and early evening, there will only be three acid attacks a day on the teeth. The amount of time available for remineralisation will greatly exceed that of demineralisation and the initial phase of caries will be arrested. But if a series of snacks is eaten between meals the reverse will occur. Most snacks contain some added sugar and the result is a rapid succession of acid attacks, with insufficient respite between them for saliva to neutralise the acid and allow the healing process of remineralisation to become dominant. Caries can then spread rapidly through affected teeth as described in the section on the cavity formation.

The longer the sugar stays on the teeth, the longer the duration of acid production. Thus sweet fluids, such as tea or coffee with sugar, which are rapidly washed off the teeth by saliva, are not a major cause of caries, whereas the much more frequent consumption of very sweet soft drinks by children is far more serious. But, overall, the most dangerous sources of sugar are those which have a sticky consistency when chewed. The adherent nature of such foods allows them to cling to the teeth for a very long time, throughout which they are supplying plaque bacteria with the raw materials for prolonged acid formation and demineralisation. Foremost among these sticky forms of sugar which lead to caries are:

- Toffee and other sweets
- Cakes, biscuits, white bread and jam
- Puddings with syrup or treacle

Our modern diet is of such a nature that added sugar is consumed nearly every time something is eaten, and the teeth are attacked by acid on each of these occasions. If snacks containing such sugar are frequently taken between meals there will be a corresponding increase in the number of acid attacks on the teeth. The delicate balance between the forces of destruction (demineralisation) and those of repair (remineralisation) will then be completely upset in favour of tooth destruction and **irreversible** damage will ensue. Thus it is evident that the prime cause of caries is the frequent and unrestricted consumption of sweet snacks *between* meals. It is not the amount of sugar eaten but the *frequency* with which it is eaten that is all-important. This fundamental fact forms the basis of personal caries prevention and dental health education.

## Sites of caries

The parts of a tooth most prone to caries are those where food tends to collect and plaque bacteria can flourish. Such sites are known as **stagnation areas**. Occlusal fissures and the spaces between the mesial and distal surfaces of adjoining teeth are the commonest stagnation areas. That is why caries occurs most often on occlusal and proximal surfaces. However, any other part where food debris can accumulate is a stagnation area where plaque will proliferate and caries is likely to occur. Such food traps are the necks of teeth covered by ill-fitting partial dentures, irregular teeth and unopposed teeth.

Minimal harm is caused by partial dentures which fit perfectly, but those which do not are a menace to dental health. They leave spaces between the necks of the teeth and plastic plate, or between clasps and teeth, which are dangerous stagnation areas.

During mastication, saliva and food which needs chewing actually help to clean teeth which are in good occlusion. This does not prevent plaque formation, but it does reduce the amount of retained food debris, which is responsible for the harmful effects of plaque. Teeth that are not in good occlusion, such as irregularly positioned and unopposed teeth, are not so exposed to this beneficial cleansing effect of mastication. Consequently food collects around these in-standing or out-standing irregular teeth. It also covers the crown of any tooth which is not opposed by a tooth in the opposite arch, that is the opposing tooth is missing and the space has not been filled by replacing the missing tooth artificially. To make the situation even worse, the sticky sweet food most likely to produce caries needs the minimum amount of mastication anyway, and therefore has a negligible cleansing effect – even on teeth in good occlusion.

## Caries and cavity formation

Unrestricted consumption of sugar produces an abundance of acid-forming bacteria in the plaque which collects in stagnation areas. The resultant series of continual acid attacks prevents remineralisation and allows acid to eat through the enamel until it reaches dentine, whereupon the caries spreads more rapidly (Figure 11.1). Microscopically, the process of cavity formation is as follows:

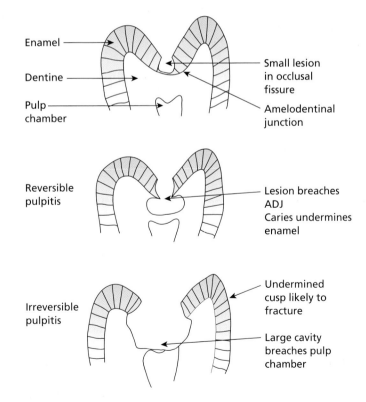

**Figure 11.1** Cavity formation. ADJ, amelodentinal junction.

1   Very early acid attacks will show as 'white spot lesions' on the enamel surface.

2   Continued and frequent acid attacks will follow the prism structure of the enamel, and eat into any exposed cementum on the tooth root.

3   **Demineralisation** occurs, followed by episodes of **remineralisation** if the acid attacks are not too frequent – these areas of repair often appear as brown lesions on the teeth, especially at contact points.

4   With frequent or prolonged acid attacks the mineral structure of the enamel is eventually destroyed and caries enters the tooth.

5   Caries extends deep into the enamel and eventually reaches the **amelodentinal junction (ADJ)**.

6   Up to this point, the patient will feel no pain as enamel contains no nerve tissue.

7   Once past the ADJ, the caries enters dentine and can spread more rapidly because of the hollow structure of this tooth layer and its lower mineral content compared with enamel.

8   This undermines the overlying enamel, and normal occlusal forces are able to fracture off pieces of the tooth surface, leaving a hole in the tooth structure – this is called a **cavity**.

9   Odontoblast cells at the ADJ react to the bacterial attack by laying down **secondary dentine** in an attempt to protect the underlying pulp tissue.

10   The nerve fibrils lying within the dentine tubules will be stimulated as the caries progresses, and the patient will begin to feel sensitivity to temperature changes and to sweet foods.

11   The pulp tissue will also become irritated and inflamed, this is called **pulpitis**.

12   At this point, the caries can be removed by the dentist and the cavity restored with a **filling** (Chapter 16), the inflamed pulp will settle and the tooth will be restored to its normal function – the inflammation is better described then as **reversible pulpitis**.

13   Otherwise, the cavity will continue to enlarge and the caries will progress towards the pulp chamber, as the production of secondary dentine is over-run by the speed of the bacterial attack.

14   The patient will be experiencing more severe pain of longer duration, and will eventually be unable to bite with the affected tooth.

15   When the carious attack reaches the immediate surroundings of the pulp chamber, the level of inflammation is too great to be resolved simply by removing the caries – this is called **irreversible pulpitis**.

16   The pain will become constant and throbbing in nature, often disturbing the patient's sleep.

17   Once the pulp chamber itself is breached by the caries, a **carious exposure** of the contents occurs and the pulp will eventually die.

18   The tooth can now only be treated by endodontics (Chapter 17) or by extraction (Chapter 20).

## Irreversible pulpitis

Pulpitis occurs when caries extends through the dentine to reach the pulp. The pulp is then said to be **cariously exposed** and the sequence of events described under inflammation (Chapter 6) follows.

1   There is an increased blood flow through the apical foramen into the pulp.
2   Swelling cannot occur, however, as the pulp is confined within the rigid walls of the root canal and pulp chamber.
3   Pressure builds up instead and causes intense pain.
4   A much more important result of this pressure, however, is the compression of blood vessels passing through the tiny apical foramen. This cuts off the blood supply and causes death of the pulp.
5   When the pulp dies, its nerves die too, and the severe toothache stops abruptly. But the respite is short as pulp death leads to another painful condition called alveolar abscess.

Pulpitis may be acute or chronic. It has many causes, apart from caries, but almost always ends in pulp death. Other causes of pulpitis are covered in Chapter 17.

## Alveolar abscess

When pulpitis occurs, the pulp eventually dies as its blood supply is cut off by inflammatory pressure. The dead pulp decomposes and infected material passes through the apical foramen to the alveolar bone at the apex of the tooth. These irritant products give rise to another inflammatory reaction in the tissues surrounding the apex. Pus formation occurs and an acute alveolar abscess develops.

- This is an extremely painful condition.
- The affected tooth becomes loose and very tender to the slightest pressure.
- There is a continual throbbing pain and the surrounding gum is red and swollen.
- Frequently the whole side of the face is involved in inflammatory swelling and the patient may have a raised temperature.
- Looseness is caused by swelling of the periodontal ligament.
- Pain is caused by the increased pressure of blood within the rigid confines of the periodontal ligament and alveolar bone. The tooth is so tender that it cannot be used for eating.
- Thus an acute alveolar abscess may show all the cardinal signs of acute inflammation:
  - Pain
  - Swelling
  - Redness

   – Heat
   – Loss of function
   – Raised body temperature.

Pulp death is sometimes followed by the development of a chronic alveolar abscess instead. This usually gives rise to very little pain and most patients are quite unaware of its presence. It may often be detected by the presence of a small hole in the gum called a **sinus**, which is a track leading from the abscess cavity in the alveolar bone to the surface of the gum. Pus drains from the abscess through the sinus into the mouth. This outlet prevents a build-up of pressure inside the bone and explains the lack of pain.

If an acute abscess is not treated it eventually turns into a chronic abscess by the drainage of pus through a sinus. This relieves the pain and the features of acute inflammation largely disappear. The relative freedom from pain does not last indefinitely, however, as a chronic alveolar abscess is liable to turn into an acute abscess at any time.

It should now be clear that pulpitis is followed by pulp death, and this eventually leads to an acute alveolar abscess, either directly or via a chronic abscess.

It was formerly taught that all carious dentine should be removed, but this is now considered unnecessary. Adequate preparation, filling and sealing of a cavity cuts it off from further plaque and acid formation, and allows a vital pulp to remineralise the deeper underlying dentine. Removal of carious dentine should therefore stop short of exposing the pulp.

## Role of saliva in oral health

The oral soft tissues in health are constantly bathed in **saliva**, the watery secretion from the three pairs of major salivary glands as well as from the numerous minor salivary glands present in the cheeks and lips. Saliva contains the following:

- **Water** – as a transport agent for all of the other constituents
- **Inorganic ions** – such as calcium and phosphate
- **Ptyalin** – a digestive enzyme which acts on carbohydrates (also called **salivary amylase**)
- **Antibodies** – as part of the defensive immune system, and known as **immunoglobulins**
- **Leucocytes** or white blood cells – also part of the body's defence system

These constituents all have important functions in the maintenance of a healthy oral environment.

- The **inorganic ions** are released as required to act as **buffering agents** to help control the pH of the oral environment, by neutralising the organic acids produced by bacteria.

- A high ion content produces thick, stringy saliva which gives the teeth good protection against caries, but allows **dental calculus** (tartar) to form easily and in large amounts.
- A low ion content produces watery saliva, which offers little protection against caries to the teeth, but prevents large amounts of calculus from forming.
- Calculus formation is associated with **periodontal disease** (Chapter 12).
- **Water** forms the carrying agent for the other salivary constituents, and allows self-cleansing of the oral environment by dislodging food debris from the teeth before being swallowed.
- The water also moistens the food bolus and the soft tissues, allowing **speech** and **swallowing** (deglutition) to occur.
- Water also **dissolves** food particles, so that the sensation of **taste** is produced – the taste buds on the tongue can only detect the taste of foods when it is in solution.
- Both **antibodies** and **leucocytes** help to protect and defend the oral environment from infection by micro-organisms.

## Reduced salivary flow

The condition of a reduced salivary flow is called **xerostomia**, or **dry mouth**. There are many reasons why a patient can suffer from this, apart from it being the result of normal age-related changes of the salivary glands themselves. These causes are:

- Low fluid intake over a period of time, or even dehydration
- Some autoimmune disorders, especially **Sjögren's syndrome** which specifically affects the salivary glands and the lacrimal glands of the eyes, which produce tears
- Several routinely prescribed drugs, including **diuretics** (to alleviate water retention), and some **anti-depressants** and **beta-blockers** (to slow down the heart rate, especially in people with angina)

Reduced salivary flow has several important consequences for the patient and for the oral health team.

- Reduced self-cleansing allows more food debris to accumulate around the teeth, increasing plaque production and the likelihood of caries and periodontal disease developing.
- It will also allow food debris to stagnate in the mouth, causing **halitosis** (bad breath).
- Reduced buffering of the oral environment allows longer and more frequent acid attacks, increasing the likelihood of caries developing.
- Poor lubrication of the oral soft tissues makes speech and swallowing more difficult.
- Reduced amount of water in the saliva affects the sensation of taste.

■ Reduced flow and amounts of saliva in the mouth will make the retention of dentures more difficult.

The opposite condition, that of excessive saliva production, is called **ptyalism**, and is often seen in patients with periodontal disease. It can also occur in Parkinson's disease and in pregnancy.

## Diagnosis of caries

Before caries is treated, it must first be detected. Early diagnosis is very important in controlling the extent of the damage, as well as the level of discomfort experienced by the patient. The earlier a cavity is detected, the better the chance of saving the tooth. This is why regular dental examinations are recommended, and the frequency of attendance should be guided by the **caries experience** of the patient – those with a high caries incidence need to be examined more frequently than others. Unfortunately, these are often the very patients who do not attend regularly for dental examination, for whatever reason.

Large cavities are obvious to the naked eye but it is easier to treat caries before cavities reach such a size. The dentist has various methods available for detecting smaller carious lesions.

■ Close visible inspection under magnification, with the help of a bright examination light and a mouth mirror to reflect it onto less visible areas (Figure 11.2).
■ The use of various **blunt dental probes** to detect any stickiness in suspicious areas – particularly a **sickle probe** or **right-angle probe** for occlusal surfaces, and a special double-ended **Briault probe** for interproximal areas (Figure 11.3).

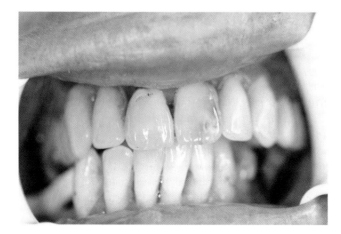

Figure 11.2 Enamel undermined by caries.

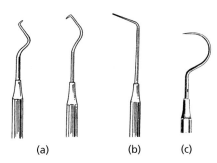

(a)                    (b)          (c)

Figure 11.3 Probes. (a) The two ends of a Briault probe. (b) Right angle probe. (c) Sickle probe.

- **Transillumination** of anterior teeth, using the curing light to shine through their contact points and viewed from behind with a mouth mirror to detect any shadowing.
- **Caries dyes** wiped into prepared cavities to stain any residual bacteria and allow their removal.
- Periodical **horizontal bitewing radiographs** (see Chapter 14) to detect interproximal caries in posterior teeth and also any **recurrent caries** beneath existing restorations, as well as early caries beneath occlusal fissures.

Although probes have traditionally been manufactured as sharp instruments, it is now recognised that they may damage the enamel in the earliest stages of caries. For early detection of occlusal caries, current advice is to thoroughly clean and dry the surface, and carefully examine it with the aid of a very bright light and magnification. Early caries will then be indicated by loss of the normal shiny enamel surface, and its transition to a dull white matt appearance. Early mesial and distal caries is detected with bitewing X-ray films, as already described.

## Prevention of caries

Caries is a breakdown of tooth structure, caused by acid produced by plaque bacteria from dietary sugar. Therefore, there are three main ways of prevention:

- **Modification of the diet** – to include less cariogenic foods and drinks, and to reduce the frequency of their intake
- **Control of bacterial plaque** – to carry out the regular and thorough removal of plaque, using good oral hygiene techniques
- **Increasing the tooth resistance to acid attack** – by incorporating fluoride into its crystal structure

All of these methods are discussed in detail in Chapter 13.

## Non-carious tooth surface loss

The enamel surface of the tooth can be lost due to causes other than dental caries, specifically by the following processes:

- **Erosion**
- **Abrasion**
- **Attrition**

**Erosion** occurs due to the action of extrinsic acid on the enamel. This is not acid that has been produced by oral bacteria, but it is dietary acid that has been ingested in foods or drinks by the patient. The usual dietary sources of acids are:

- Carbonated fizzy drinks – whether 'diet' types or not
- Acidic fruits – such as lemons, oranges, limes and grapefruit – eaten raw in large quantities
- Pure fruit juice of the above, consumed in large quantities
- Wines
- Excessive vinegar consumption

In a similar way, there are some medical conditions and eating disorders that involve the regular regurgitation, or actual vomiting of, the stomach contents into the mouth. As described in Chapter 4, the gastric juices of the stomach are very acidic, and have a similar erosive effect on the tooth enamel as extrinsic acids. Some likely causes are:

- Bulimia
- Reflux oesophagitis
- Hiatus hernia
- Stomach ulcers
- Some chemotherapy treatments for cancer

No bacteria are involved in the enamel loss caused by erosion. The tooth surface appears pitted and worn but shiny. Erosion particularly affects the labial or palatal surfaces of the upper incisors, and the occlusal surfaces of the lower molars. The teeth affected are often hypersensitive to hot, cold and sweet stimulation as the underlying dentine is exposed. This therefore mimics the symptoms of caries, but no cavity is present.

Treatment of erosion does not involve restoration, but does involve all of the following:

- Dietary and/or medical advice
- Desensitisation of the dentine
- The use of high-concentration fluoride toothpastes and mouthwashes to help to restore the pH balance

**Abrasion** occurs when patients scrub their teeth clean using excessive sawing forces, rather than brushing them. It is especially seen in smokers with significant tar staining on their teeth, who either brush with a sawing action or use abrasive smokers' toothpastes to remove the stains.

Abrasion is seen at the cervical necks of the teeth, as a deep ridge on the buccal or labial surfaces. The surface is shiny rather than carious, and sometimes the ridge is deep enough to see the pulp chamber within the tooth itself. Again, no bacteria are involved in the production of these lesions, and the patient often experiences hypersensitivity with temperature changes. As the ridges can be so deep, they are often restored with glass ionomer cements or composites (see Chapter 16). In extreme cases the pulp can be exposed, and endodontic treatment will be required to save the tooth from extraction.

**Attrition** (Figure 11.4) is the loss of enamel specifically from the biting surfaces of the teeth, and is caused by any of the following:

- Normal 'wear and tear' of chewing, especially in older patients
- Occlusion of natural teeth onto ceramic restorations, such as crowns and bridges (Chapter 18)
- **Bruxing** – the abnormal, and often subconscious, action of clenching and grinding the teeth

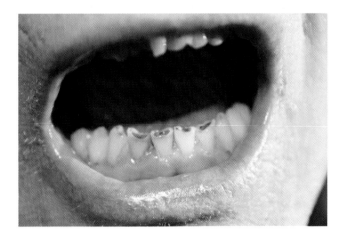

Figure 11.4 Tooth attrition.

Bruxing is a very common condition, seen in many patients but especially those under stress. It can also occur habitually while undertaking repetitive tasks, such as while exercising. Besides the obvious enamel loss and tooth fracture that occurs due to bruxing, patients often experience facial pain and disruption of the temporo-mandibular joint (TMJ). The joint and the muscles of mastication go into spasm in severe cases, and can cause jaw clicking or even jaw locking. Various muscle relaxants, anti-inflammatory drugs, and occlusal splints can be used to alleviate these symptoms, but the reason for the bruxing must also be investigated and reduced or removed.

# 12 Periodontal Disease

Periodontal disease means disease of the supporting structures of the teeth. These are the gums, periodontal ligament (formerly called periodontal membrane) and alveolar bone. The adjective relating to gums is *gingival*, and inflammation of the gum is accordingly called gingivitis.

Periodontal disease and caries are among the commonest diseases of civilisation. Caries is the major cause of tooth loss in children and young adults, while periodontal disease is the major cause of tooth loss in older people. This does not mean that periodontal disease starts much later in life – only that it takes so much longer than caries to cause tooth loss.

The earliest stage of periodontal disease is **chronic gingivitis**, which is a chronic inflammation involving the gums alone. If allowed to continue, it spreads to the underlying periodontal ligament and alveolar bone. These are gradually destroyed and the teeth become very loose as their supporting tissues are lost. The name given to this late stage of the disease is **chronic periodontitis**. There is no obvious dividing line between the two stages, as untreated chronic gingivitis usually progresses into chronic periodontitis.

## Causes of periodontal disease

Periodontal disease is an infection caused by accumulation of **plaque** at the gum margin. Plaque is a tenacious transparent film of saliva, micro-organisms and oral debris on the tooth surface. Food debris adheres to plaque and the resultant paste of saliva and food remnants attracts more micro-organisms which feed and multiply on it.

It is the same plaque as that described in Chapter 11, but whereas caries can only occur when sugar is present in plaque, the presence of sugar is not necessary for periodontal disease to occur. Any sort of food debris will allow plaque microbes to proliferate and cause periodontal disease.

Plaque can be removed by brushing, but in the absence of this counter-measure, plaque thickens as its microbial population flourishes amid a permanent food supply. Toxic products of plaque microbes then act as a continual source of bacterial irritation which causes chronic inflammation of the gum margin (chronic gingivitis). The plaque extends above and below the gum margin and wherever it is present **calculus** (tartar) can form.

Calculus is the hard rock-like deposit commonly seen on the lingual surface of lower incisors. Two factors are necessary for its formation: plaque and saliva. Their interaction allows mineralisation to occur within the plaque and produce a deposition of calculus, which may be defined as solidified plaque. It is most easily seen opposite the orifices of salivary gland ducts – on the lingual surface of lower incisors and the buccal surface of upper molars. This visible calculus on the crowns of teeth has a yellowish colour and is called **supragingival calculus** as it forms above the gum margin. However, it also occurs in plaque beneath the gum margin on all teeth and in that situation it is known as **subgingival calculus**. This is harder and darker than supragingival calculus and its surface is covered with a layer of the soft microbial plaque from which it was formed.

Calculus plays only a *passive* mechanical role in periodontal disease. Its rough surface and ledges create food traps which are inaccessible to a toothbrush and thus allow even more food debris to fertilise the plaque. The *active* role in periodontal disease belongs to plaque micro-organisms.

This description shows that supragingival plaque and calculus are associated with poor oral hygiene. If teeth are cleaned properly plaque and calculus are less able to accumulate. But if they are allowed to do so, they spread subgingivally and become inaccessible to toothbrushing.

There are also some other reasons for plaque formation which are not the patient's fault. These are caused by imperfect dentistry, and are known as **iatrogenic factors**. For example:

- Fillings or crowns which have an overhanging edge at their cervical margin
- Fillings or crowns with loose contact points
- Ill-fitting or poorly designed partial dentures

These defects are food traps which patients cannot keep clean. Plaque and calculus proliferate there and periodontal disease follows at these sites, even though the rest of the mouth may be perfectly healthy. Food stagnation also occurs on unopposed and irregular teeth, with consequent liability to periodontal disease as well as caries. The full microscopic sequence of events leading to periodontal disease will be described later in this chapter.

## Periodontal tissues in health

To be able to recognise the presence of periodontal disease, the appearance of these tissues in health must be identified. Anatomically, this is as follows:

- The tooth sits in its socket within the alveolar bone
- It is attached to the bone by the fibres of the periodontal ligament, which run from the cementum of the root into the alveolar bone
- The bone and the periodontal ligament are covered by the mucous membrane of the gingiva which lines the alveolar ridges

■ The gingiva is attached to the neck of the tooth at a specialised site called the **junctional epithelium**
■ In health, a gingival crevice of up to 3 mm deep runs as a 'gutter' around each tooth, the deepest part of which is the attachment of the junctional epithelium
■ Other periodontal ligament fibres run from the alveolar bone crest to the neck of the tooth, and from the neck of the tooth into the gingival papilla
■ Looking at the tissues in the mouth then:
  – The gingiva is pink with a stippled appearance (like orange peel).
  – There is a tight gingival cuff around each tooth, with a gingival crevice no deeper than 3 mm.
  – The interdental papillae between the teeth are sharp, with a knife-edge appearance.
  – No bleeding occurs when the gingival crevice is gently probed during the dental examination.
  – Subgingivally, the periodontal ligament and alveolar bone are intact – this will only be visible on X-ray.

## Chronic gingivitis

If plaque is allowed to accumulate around the gingival margins of the teeth, the gingiva will become inflamed and the first stage of periodontal disease, **gingivitis**, will develop. When this is a generalised condition affecting the oral cavity as a whole because of poor oral hygiene, it is called **chronic gingivitis**.

The sequence of events that occur microscopically, and which lead to chronic gingivitis are as follows:

1 The bacteria within the plaque at the gingival margins use food debris to nourish themselves, so that the colony grows in size.
2 They produce **toxins** (poisons) as a by-product during their own food digestion.
3 These toxins tend to accumulate in the gingival crevice, as they are not removed by oral hygiene measures, nor washed away by the normal cleansing action of saliva.
4 The gingiva in direct contact with the toxins becomes irritated, causing inflammation and the early signs of **chronic gingivitis**.
5 The inflamed gingiva becomes red in colour, and the swelling associated with the inflammation creates **false pockets** around the necks of the teeth.
6 These pockets allow more plaque to accumulate, as cleansing becomes even more difficult, and the plaque now begins to extend below the gingival margin.
7 In this environment, there is little oxygen available for the initial bacteria to use, and the plaque becomes colonised by specialised bacteria that are able to survive without oxygen – these are called **anaerobic bacteria**.
8 Examples of these are *Actinomyces* and *Porphyromonas gingivalis*, bacteria specifically associated with periodontal disease.

9   In the meantime, the inorganic ions within saliva are incorporated into the structure of the plaque so that it hardens and mineralises as **dental calculus** develops.

10  Calculus forming above the gingival margin is called **supragingival calculus** and is **yellow** in colour (Figure 12.1).

11  Calculus forming below the gingival margin is called **subgingival calculus** and is **brown** in colour, due to the blood pigments incorporated into it.

12  The rough surface of the calculus irritates the gingiva further, and allows more plaque to develop on it.

13  The rough calculus and the irritation of the bacterial toxins causes painless **micro-ulcers** to develop within the gingiva, so that they **bleed** on touch or gentle probing.

14  The red swollen gingiva and the presence of bleeding on probing are the classic visible signs of **chronic gingivitis**.

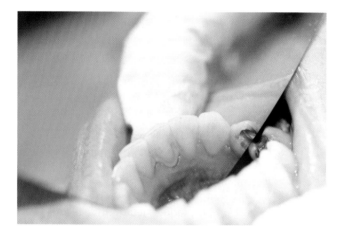

Figure 12.1 Lingual tartar.

Chronic gingivitis is fully reversible if the plaque and calculus are completely removed from above and below the gingival margins. This requires the intervention of the dental team, and then the patient must maintain a good standard of oral hygiene.

## Chronic periodontitis

If chronic gingivitis is not treated, microbial poisons from the plaque soak through the ulcers in the gingival crevice and penetrate the deeper tissues. These poisons gradually destroy the periodontal ligament and alveolar bone; while this is progressing, the gingival pocket deepens, thus further aggravating the condition.

Whereas the false pockets of chronic gingivitis are caused by inflammatory swelling of the gum, in chronic periodontitis they are **true pockets** caused by destruction of the base of the gingival crevice and its attachment to the tooth. At the same time the gingival margin may recede, exposing the root to view. This **gingival recession** is commonly known as being 'long in the tooth'. If no treatment is provided, so much bone is lost that the teeth eventually become too loose to be of any functional value (Figure 12.2).

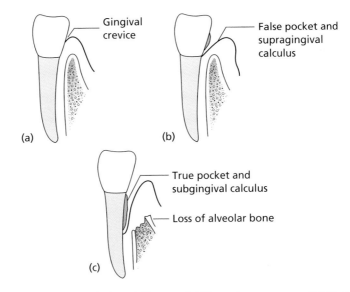

**Figure 12.2** Stages of periodontal disease. (a) Normal appearance. (b) Chronic gingivitis. (c) Chronic periodontitis.

The sequence of events that occur microscopically in the development of chronic periodontitis are as follows:

1  The bacterial toxins build up within the false pockets and eventually begin soaking into the gingival tissue itself, through the micro-ulcerated areas.
2  Here, they gradually destroy the periodontal ligament and the attachment of the tooth to its supporting tissues, and a **true pocket** forms.
3  The loss of attachment gradually moves down the tooth root, creating deeper pockets which allow more plaque and calculus to develop within them.
4  The toxins eventually begin attacking the alveolar bone itself, destroying the walls of the tooth socket so that the tooth becomes loose.
5  This is often the first indication that the patient has of the presence of their disease, as it is usually painless and often takes several years to reach this point.
6  Periodontitis also tends to have intermittent active phases where much tissue destruction occurs, interspersed with quiet phases of little bacterial activity.

This description of periodontal disease follows a slowly progressive but painless course of several years but, during that time, pus and micro-organisms in the pockets cause bad breath (**halitosis**) and may affect the general health. Once periodontal disease is actually established it can be made worse by certain other factors, which do not in themselves cause the disease. Some of these aggravating factors are:

- Smoking
- Unbalanced or excessive masticatory stress
- Natural hormonal changes such as puberty and pregnancy
- Open lip posture (mouth breathing)

Certain medical conditions and drugs may also have the same effect, such as:

- Diabetes, acquired immune deficiency syndrome (AIDS), leukaemia, and other blood disorders or diseases where resistance to infection is poor
- Epilepsy treated with phenytoin (Epanutin)
- Vitamin C deficiency
- Treatment with immunosuppressant drugs such as ciclosporin and cytotoxic agents

Dental plaque forms in everyone's mouth in a short space of time after toothbrushing, but some factors exacerbate its accumulation in certain areas and in some patients' mouths. These are called **plaque retention factors**, some of which have already been mentioned:

- Poor oral hygiene due to apathy by the patient
- Poorly aligned teeth, which increases the number of stagnation areas
- Incompetent lip seal, which allows the oral soft tissues to dry out and prevents the self-cleansing action of saliva to occur
- Small oral aperture, making effective toothbrushing difficult
- Iatrogenic causes

The rate of progress of periodontal disease depends on the balance between individual resistance and the toxic effects of plaque bacteria. Both these factors vary from time to time and in different parts of the mouth, and the predominant one determines whether the disease appears dormant or progressive.

## Diagnosis of periodontal disease

The diagnosis of periodontal disease is based on the medical history, appearance and recession of the gums, depth of gingival pockets, amount of bone loss, tooth mobility and the distribution of plaque.

Periodontal disease affects the vast majority of the population, but most people are otherwise healthy and curable if they exercise adequate plaque control. However, patients with certain conditions are more at risk of severe periodontal disease and less likely to respond so favourably to treatment.

A regularly updated medical history is an essential feature of all patients' records, whatever their reason for attendance or the treatment required. As far as periodontal disease is concerned, the dentist will be particularly interested in:

- Past and present illnesses
- Drugs prescribed
- Hormonal changes, e.g. pregnancy
- Smoking habits

Relevant illnesses are those where resistance is low, such as:

- Diabetes, leukaemia, and other blood disorders
- Vitamin deficiencies
- AIDS
- Treatment with immuno-suppressant drugs, e.g. ciclosporin (Sandimmun), used for some types of cancer, and for organ transplant patients
- Patients at risk of infective endocarditis require antibiotic cover prior to scaling and periodontal surgery

Certain drugs can cause a severe enlargement of the gums, called **gingival hyperplasia**, which requires surgical correction. Such drugs include:

- Phenytoin (Epanutin) – used for epilepsy
- Nifedipine (Adalat) – used for angina pectoris and high blood pressure
- Ciclosporin – used to prevent organ rejection after transplantation

There are many clinical signs that the dentist will look for at a routine dental examination to determine the presence of periodontal disease. The signs of early-onset chronic gingivitis are as follows:

- The gingiva bleed on brushing
- They appear red and swollen
- Plaque is visible at the gingival margins of the teeth, or can be shown using disclosing solution (Chapter 13)
- The patient has halitosis

With established gingivitis, pus can be expressed from the gingival crevice. The clinical signs of chronic periodontitis are:

- Periodontal probing detects pockets greater than 3 mm
- Both supragingival and subgingival calculus present
- Some teeth may be mobile

Radiographs will show destruction of alveolar bone in long-standing cases, with associated deep periodontal pockets present.

One of the early diagnostic signs of periodontal problems is bleeding of the gingiva. The nicotine from tobacco smoking acts on the gingival blood vessels to constrict them, causing less bleeding, if any. So the presence of periodontal disease in smokers is often masked and not evident to either the patient or the dentist without other clinical signs being present. The easiest assessment carried out by the dentist is to determine the presence of periodontal pockets, by using special **periodontal probes** (Figure 12.3).

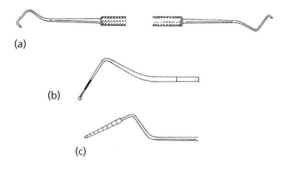

(a)

(b)

(c)

**Figure 12.3** Periodontal probes. (a) Calculus probe. (b) WHO (CPITN) probe. (c) Pocket measuring probe.

## Basic Periodontal Examination (BPE)

Normal healthy gums are firm and pink and do not bleed. They have a stippled surface, and the gingival crevice is no deeper than 3 mm. In chronic gingivitis the gums have a soft, smooth surface, are darker in colour and swollen, bleed on pressure, and have a deeper gingival crevice which may contain subgingival calculus. In chronic periodontitis these gingival changes may not be so obvious, as pockets are deeper and the active disease processes are occurring out of sight at that deeper level.

Tooth mobility and the appearance of the gums are easily checked. Detection of plaque and subgingival calculus, and assessment of pocket depth, gingival recession and bone loss require examination with periodontal probes and the use of special charts (Figure 12.4). Dental nurses are advised to study the definitive format and accepted notation of the current periodontal charts in the Examining Board for Dental Nurses (NEBDN) Charting Booklet. The **World Health Organization (WHO) probe**, also known as a CPITN (Community Periodontal Index of

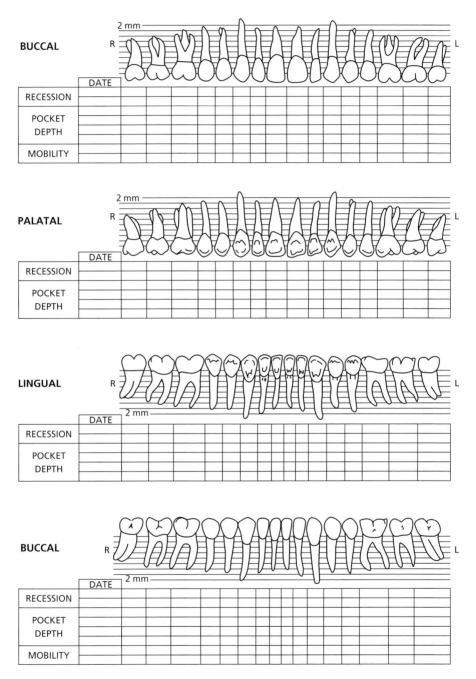

Figure 12.4 Periodontal diagnosis and treatment plan.

Treatment Needs) probe, is used for initial screening and charting. This has a coloured band which assesses pocket depth by the amount of band showing (if any) after insertion into the gingival crevice, and a tiny ball on the end which detects subgingival calculus and prevents any bleeding that might be caused by a sharp point.

A **pocket measuring probe** may also be used for charting. This has a blunt flat end (rather like that of a flat plastic instrument) with a millimetre scale marked on it. When inserted into the gingival crevice, pocket depth is read off from the scale.

Subgingival calculus is detected with a **calculus probe**. This resembles a Briault probe but has blunt ends which catch on the scales of calculus in the gingival crevice.

Bone loss can be assessed from pocket depth and dental radiographs (Chapter 14). As true pockets extend almost to the bone margin, a pocket measuring probe will indicate the amount of bone loss. X-rays show this as well, together with subgingival calculus and the cervical edges of restorations.

Plaque is normally invisible as it is a thin transparent film. However, if a red dye is painted on the teeth, supragingival plaque is stained red and shows up clearly. Dyes used for this purpose are called **disclosing agents**. This part of the examination is left until last as dyes can mask gingival colour changes.

## Charting

Whereas the mouth is divided into quarters (quadrants) for tooth charting (Chapter 10), sixths (sextants) are used for periodontal charting. The sextants are upper and lower, left and right:

- Molar sextant (876)
- Premolar and canine (543)
- Incisor (21)

A typical periodontal chart has a 2 mm interval grid to record pocket depths, and boxes for the numerical scores of pocket depth, gingival recession, bone loss, tooth mobility, plaque distribution, and other factors such as imperfect fillings, dentures, or other sources of plaque accumulation.

A similar sextant system is used by orthodontists for descriptive purposes.

## Non-surgical treatment of periodontal disease

The prevention of periodontal disease is far more desirable than having to cure it, so good oral hygiene instruction from the dental team from an early age is the best course of action. Obviously, this is not possible for patients who are seen initially as adults, especially if they already have periodontal disease when they do attend.

Oral hygiene instruction and methods of achieving a good standard of oral hygiene are discussed in Chapter 13.

The oral health messages given by the dental team will need to be reinforced regularly if problems persist, and the advice given will vary for the different age groups. Removal of all plaque and its subsequent control by the patient will bring about a complete resolution of chronic gingivitis. Failure to achieve this will allow calculus to form, and the dental team will then have to intervene to remove it.

Accessible plaque is removed by **toothbrushing** and **flossing**. Subgingival plaque and calculus are inaccessible to patients and are removed by **scaling**. Once these aims have been achieved, and maintained, the causal sources of irritation which produce the disease are lost.

In chronic gingivitis, bleeding ceases, swollen gums return to their normal healthy condition and false pockets are thereby eliminated. The patient is then cured, but strict oral hygiene and regular dental checks are required thereafter to prevent recurrence of plaque and calculus formation.

In chronic periodontitis there is no regeneration of lost bone but mild cases can be cured in the same way as chronic gingivitis. In the advanced stages of the disease, scaling alone cannot eliminate true pockets if they are too deep to be accessible. In such cases they are treated surgically by repositioning and/or recontouring the gum margin as described later in the chapter. In this way, even advanced periodontal disease can be arrested, but a return of the condition is inevitable unless the patient follows the dentist's or hygienist's instructions on supragingival plaque control, and attends regularly to check progress and continue subgingival plaque control.

Apart from scaling and gingival surgery, appropriate treatment is given for any other conditions facilitating plaque retention: for example, unsatisfactory fillings, crowns and dentures, unopposed and irregular teeth.

As periodontal disease is an infection by plaque bacteria and other micro-organisms, a relatively new approach to treatment is the application of anti-microbial drugs directly into the gingival crevice and pockets, such as with PerioChip and Dentomycin gel. The establishment of their long-term success in the battle against periodontal disease is an ongoing and exciting area of clinical research.

## Supragingival plaque control

Supragingival calculus and any overhanging cervical margins of restorations are removed in the surgery. At home, thorough twice-daily toothbrushing by the patient will then keep accessible plaque under control. Appropriate instruction in the surgery, and the use of disclosing agents at home, will show patients how well they are performing, and indicate where improvement is required.

Parts which are inaccessible to an ordinary toothbrush are the interdental spaces above or below the contact points of adjacent teeth. They can be cleaned with dental floss, wood sticks and an interspace brush. The dentist or hygienist must give the patient special instruction in these methods as they can do more harm than good if used incorrectly or unnecessarily.

**Dental floss** is thread or tape which is worked between the teeth to keep their contact areas clean. Where recession of the gum has occurred, or gingival surgery has been performed, the resulting interdental spaces may be too large for flossing. **Wood sticks** (also called interspace sticks) are used for these large spaces. They are soft wooden sticks which are passed through the spaces to keep them clear of food debris and reduce plaque formation. An **interspace brush** (also called a **bottle brush**) is a special type of toothbrush designed to clean interdental spaces in the same way as wood sticks. It has only one tuft of bristles (Figure 12.5). Popular ones available include TePe brushes.

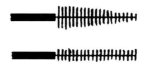

Figure 12.5 Interspace brushes.

Any calculus present cannot be removed by the patient, but instead must be treated by regular scaling. This is done by a dentist or hygienist. The patient's own efforts at supragingival plaque control are checked at the same time. Supragingival scaling removes plaque and calculus deposits from the enamel surface of the teeth down to the gingival crevice.

Scaling hand instruments are made in various designs appropriate for the removal of calculus from any part of a tooth, and those used for removing supragingival calculus include (Figure 12.6):

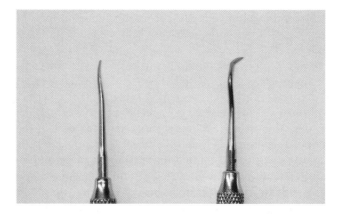

Figure 12.6 Push and Jaquette scaler tips.

- **Sickle scaler**
- **Cushing's push scaler**
- **Jaquette scaler**

Hand scaling is tiring for the operator but gives excellent tactile sensation, so specks of residual calculus are easily detectable and can be fully removed. Alternatively, an ultrasonic scaler may be used which is much faster and less tiring. However, its action depends on the water spray produced during use, and this can be uncomfortable for patients with sensitive teeth unless performed under local anaesthesia. Once scaling has been completed, the teeth are polished with prophylactic polishing paste using a rubber cup or bristle brush (Figure 12.7) in the slow handpiece. The paste is abrasive and removes any residual surface stains, leaving a smooth tooth surface that slows down the re-accumulation of plaque.

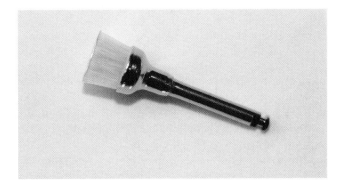

Figure 12.7 Latch grip polishing brush.

## Subgingival plaque control

With chronic periodontitis any alveolar bone loss is permanent, although research is ongoing into the use of synthetic bone in both humans and other animal species. In the meantime, however, if subgingival calculus is thoroughly and regularly removed by the dental team, and a good standard of oral hygiene is maintained by the patient, there is every chance that the periodontal ligament will reattach and any periodontal pockets will heal.

The instruments used to remove subgingival calculus have to be long enough to reach the base of any periodontal pockets, and thin enough to do so without tearing the gingival tissues. In addition, they are used to scrape the tooth root surfaces and dislodge any contaminated cementum, which is then removed from the pockets by both aspiration and irrigation. This technique is called subgingival debridement. The instruments used for subgingival scaling include (Figure 12.8):

- **Gracey curettes**
- **Other subgingival curettes**
- **Periodontal hoe**
- **Ultrasonic scaler**

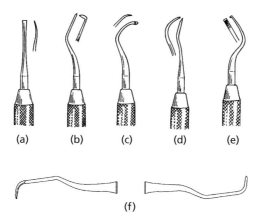

(a)      (b)      (c)      (d)      (e)

(f)

**Figure 12.8** Scaling instruments. (a) Cushing (push) scaler. (b) Jaquette scaler. (c) Periodontal curette. (d) Sickle scaler. (e) Periodontal hoe. (f) Gracey curette.

Once subgingival debridement is complete, the periodontal tissues can heal and the junctional epithelium can reattach to the tooth. In doing so, the periodontal pockets are eliminated.

Subgingival scaling entails much instrumentation within the gingival crevice and pockets. This, in addition to the gingivitis already present, produces considerable bleeding and requires the use of local anaesthesia. Antibiotic cover is also necessary for patients at risk of infective endocarditis before scaling and periodontal surgery.

Scaling with hand instruments is a tedious procedure for operator and patient, but may be done more easily and quickly with an **ultrasonic scaler**, e.g. Cavitron. This apparatus produces ultrasonic vibrations which are transmitted through a cable to a special scaling instrument. When it is applied to a tooth, the vibrations help loosen the plaque and calculus and they are flushed away by a water-cooling spray which is part of the apparatus. The scaling instrument consists of a special handpiece with a range of detachable scaling tips of various shapes. Use of a chlorhexidine mouthwash by the patient, before scaling, reduces any risk of cross-infection of staff. Patients are advised to take analgesic tablets, if required, as the area may feel rather sore for a day or two afterwards.

Scaling, as just described, cannot always remove the deepest, hardest and most adherent layer of calculus from the root surface of teeth. The additional stage of **subgingival debridement** is then carried out, using Gracey curettes. These are distinguished from other curettes by having only one cutting surface. Their planing action eliminates any residual plaque and calculus as it scrapes away some of the root cementum, to provide a smooth root surface.

Provided that the patient achieves adequate supragingival plaque control while the dentist deals with any restoration overhangs, imperfect partial dentures or other hindrances to plaque removal, and the hygienist or dentist can maintain subgingival plaque control, most cases of straightforward chronic periodontitis can be cured. Continued periodontal health is dependent to a large degree on the co-operation and motivation of the patient to maintain a consistently good standard of oral hygiene. Of all the exacerbating factors that can worsen the situation, smoking plays a large part in the failure of periodontal treatment and the ultimate loss of teeth by the patient. Also, there will be some cases in which non-surgical periodontal treatment alone cannot succeed. Patients with very deep pockets, especially pockets involving multi-rooted teeth, may present a problem of inaccessible subgingival plaque and calculus which can only be removed by surgical procedures to gain and maintain access to it.

## Surgical treatment of periodontal disease

Periodontal conditions which do not respond to plaque control procedures, such as meticulous oral hygiene by the patient and subgingival scaling by a dental operator, may require treatment by minor oral surgery procedures. These treatments are performed under local anaesthesia and may be undertaken by the patient's own dentist or a periodontal specialist.

### Flap operations

Flap operations use techniques and instruments similar to some of those described in Chapter 20 for the removal of an unerupted tooth. They cover a variety of procedures to remove inaccessible subgingival plaque and facilitate subsequent plaque control. Teeth with irregular gingival pocketing, a complex and uneven pattern of bone loss, or involvement of the **furcation** (the branching of roots of multi-rooted teeth) are those most likely to need such operations (Figure 12.9).

1   A gingival flap is reflected to expose the underlying bone, root surface and all the hidden subgingival calculus.
2   Alveolar bone surfaces may then be trimmed and contoured to eliminate bony pockets.
3   All subgingival plaque and calculus are removed.
4   In addition, all contaminated cementum and any toxin-impregnated granulation tissue are removed.

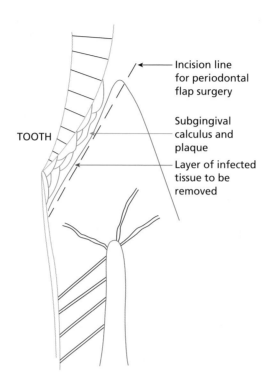

Incision line
for periodontal
flap surgery

Subgingival
calculus and
plaque

TOOTH

Layer of infected
tissue to be
removed

**Figure 12.9** Flap incision.

5   Local delivery antibiotic systems such as PerioChip may then be placed in these inaccessible areas, to help the healing process.
6   The flap is then sutured back into place.
7   There is no removal of gum but the gingival margin may be repositioned more apically, and thus permanently expose more of the root.
8   A vast range of special instruments is available, based on smaller versions of the scalpels, curettes, bone files and chisels illustrated in Chapter 20.
9   Ultrasonic scalers may also be used instead of hand instruments.

## Gingivectomy

Sometimes, successful treatment of periodontal disease is hindered by the failure of established false pockets to be eliminated. They can be surgically removed by gingivectomy. This is the removal of a strip of gingival margin level with the point of the epithelial attachment (Figure 12.10). It is mainly confined to cases with excessive overgrowth of gum (**gingival hyperplasia**) caused by certain drugs used for medical conditions. The drugs involved are phenytoin, nifedipine and ciclosporin.

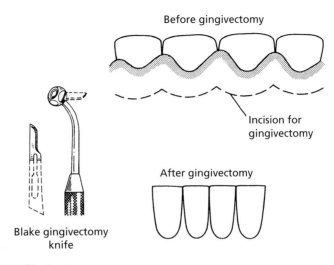

Before gingivectomy

Incision for gingivectomy

After gingivectomy

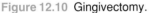

Blake gingivectomy knife

**Figure 12.10** Gingivectomy.

The excess gum is removed with a **gingivectomy knife** or one used for flap surgery. There are many different types of gingivectomy knife available with various angled handles and blades for ease of access. The strip of incised gum is removed with tweezers and the raw area covered with a **periodontal pack** to protect the gum and promote rapid painless healing. The pack is removed about a week later and thorough scaling is then performed. A modified form of zinc oxide eugenol may be used as a pack but proprietary brands (e.g. Coe-Pak, Peripac, Barricaid) are more popular and convenient. Packs are usually unnecessary for flap operations as the gum flap is sutured back into place and no raw areas are left exposed.

The procedure just described is not often necessary nowadays as there are alternative drugs to those causing gross gingival enlargement. However, a *localised* form of gingivectomy may be used for removing gum flaps over partially erupted wisdom teeth, in a procedure called an **operculectomy**. It may also be necessary for exposing more root surface prior to crown preparation, in cases where there would otherwise be insufficient retention for a crown. This procedure is called **crown lengthening**.

Surgical re-contouring of the gingiva can also be carried out once periodontal health has been established, to help the patient in their effort to thorough cleanse the area. This technique is called **gingivoplasty**, and is often carried out using an electrosurgery unit which cuts and coagulates bleeding tissues at the same time.

Following gingival surgery: patients are given or prescribed analgesic drugs to relieve after-pain; they are given an appointment for removal of sutures or pack a week later; and they are instructed to avoid smoking, eating hard food and using a toothbrush on the operative area meanwhile. A soft diet and chlorhexidine mouthwashes are advised instead.

After periodontal treatment is completed, whether by scaling and polishing alone or by surgery as well, it is then the patient's responsibility to keep teeth clean and free of plaque. They are accordingly shown how to do it, as already described, and encouraged to use disclosing agents at home to check their own performance.

It must be emphasised to patients that toothbrushing and interdental cleaning to remove supragingival plaque are of paramount importance following periodontal treatment. Failure to perform these essential tasks at least once daily will result in a reversion to the original condition of chronic periodontitis. Conservative treatment of periodontal disease by the dental team is a waste of time unless patients are prepared to co-operate by exercising rigorous supragingival plaque control. When neglect is likely, extraction is the best treatment for advanced disease.

Regular recall appointments are made to check and record the progress of plaque control and to update the periodontal charting of pocket depth and tooth mobility. Patients can then be encouraged and motivated to maintain good periodontal health, and are given further advice and treatment as required. The frequency of recalls will depend on individual response to treatment and the effectiveness of home plaque control measures.

## Other periodontal conditions

Several other interesting periodontal conditions may present in the dental surgery, although they are not as common as chronic gingivitis and periodontitis. They are summarised below.

### Sub-acute pericoronitis

This is an infection of the gingival flap that lies over a partially erupted tooth, called the **operculum**. It especially affects the lower third molars as they erupt, because these teeth are not only difficult to clean, allowing plaque bacteria to proliferate, but the operculum is often traumatised by the opposing tooth. The combination of infection and trauma produces inflammation of the operculum, which then becomes more traumatised. It is treated in a number of ways, depending on the severity of the infection and the regularity of its occurrence:

- Irrigation of any food debris from under the operculum
- Oral hygiene instruction for the area, especially the use of mouthwashes
- Antibiotics if the patient has a raised temperature
- Operculectomy if the condition reoccurs
- Alternatively, the extraction of the opposing tooth to break the cycle of trauma and inflammation

### Acute herpetic gingivitis

This condition is caused by the herpes simplex virus and most commonly affects infants. All the signs of acute inflammation are present and the rest of the oral mucous membrane may be involved too in the form of tiny blisters which leave painful ulcers (**acute herpetic gingivo-stomatitis**). The condition is short lived but uncomfortable; the patient feels unwell and may be unable to eat solids, but it resolves without treatment and the gingival condition returns to normal.

However, the virus remains dormant in the body and can be reactivated later by a common cold to produce a cold sore (**herpes labialis**) on the lip. During the acute phase or presence of a cold sore, the condition is highly infectious and treatment is best deferred until the condition has resolved.

### Acute necrotising ulcerative gingivitis

Acute necrotising ulcerative gingivitis is abbreviated to ANUG and was formerly called acute ulcerative gingivitis (AUG) or Vincent's disease. It is an acute gingivitis characterised by pain and halitosis (bad breath). The affected gum appears bright red, with a covering layer of yellow/grey membrane where the gum margin has been destroyed by bacterial action. The bacteria involved include *Bacillus fusiformis* and *Treponema vincenti*. All the features of acute inflammation are present: red, swollen, painful gums; loss of function, because it is too painful to chew hard food; and the patient often has a raised temperature.

It usually affects young adults and usually occurs in areas already affected by chronic gingivitis. In many cases stress, heavy smoking and a lowered general resistance precipitate an attack. Thus it is more common in winter when colds, influenza and other infections are rife, but more importantly in AIDS, and perhaps as its first sign. ANUG is treated as follows:

- Antibiotic treatment that is specific for anaerobic bacteria, usually **metronidazole**
- If the patient is pregnant, metronidazole cannot be used and is substituted by penicillin
- Thorough scaling and polishing once the symptoms have settled, followed by oral hygiene instruction
- Short course of chlorhexidine mouthwash

### Acute lateral periodontal abscess

This is an occasional complication of chronic periodontitis in which pus formation in a deep pocket is unable to drain through the gingival crevice. The pus accumulates instead at the base of the pocket to form an abscess. This condition must not be confused with an acute alveolar abscess (Chapter 11), which follows pulp death and occurs at the root apex. Acute lateral periodontal abscess occurs on a vital tooth at the side of the root.

Treatment depends on the depth of the pocket and the probability of curing the underlying periodontal disease. The options are:

- Drainage of the pus present
- Thorough subgingival scaling of the affected tooth
- Local administration of antibiotic, especially metronidazole
- Oral hygiene instruction
- If all else fails, extraction of the affected tooth

# 13 Assessment and Prevention of Dental Disease

The main dental diseases to be considered are as follows:

- **Gingivitis** – the inflammation of the gingival tissues at the neck of the tooth
- **Periodontitis** – the inflammation of the supporting structures of the tooth
- **Dental caries** – the bacterial infection of the mineralised tissues of the tooth

As discussed in detail in Chapters 11 and 12, the presence of **bacterial dental plaque** is a pre-requisite for the development of all three of the main dental diseases, in addition to other causative factors as described below. The causative factors of gingivitis and periodontitis are:

- **Poor oral hygiene** which allows the accumulation of **dental plaque**
- The existence of **stagnation areas**, including the gingival crevice, which allows the plaque to accumulate specifically around the necks of the teeth against the gingiva
- Failure to treat and eradicate the subsequent gingivitis allows inflammation of the periodontal supporting structures to occur, leading to periodontitis

The causative factors of dental caries are:

- A diet containing a high proportion of **non-milk extrinsic sugars** (**NMEs**)
- **Poor oral hygiene** allowing the accumulation of dental plaque and the **bacteria** it contains
- The action of the bacteria on the NMEs to produce **acid**, which demineralises the tooth structure and allows cavities to develop

## Dental plaque

The full name is **bacterial dental plaque** but, in general usage and hereafter, it is simply referred to as plaque. As it plays such an all-important part in dental disease, its origin and effects should be clearly understood by all whose work involves dental treatment or dental health education.

Plaque is a thin transparent layer of saliva, oral debris and normal mouth bacteria which sticks to the tooth surface and can only be removed by cleaning. It is then replaced within a few hours by a new deposit of plaque and may be regarded as a natural occurrence. The harm it causes comes from food debris which sticks to the plaque during meals and snacks and provides a plentiful supply of nourishment for its bacteria and other micro-organisms. They accordingly flourish, the plaque grows thicker, and caries and periodontal disease begin. Which of the two diseases predominates depends on diet, the site of plaque and age of the patient, but the plaque is the same whichever disease occurs.

Caries is mainly a disease of children and young adults whereas periodontal disease predominates in later life. The difference is caused by the rate at which the two diseases progress. Caries can cause loss of teeth within a few years whereas periodontal disease may take decades. By the time periodontal disease has reached an advanced stage, the earlier onslaught of caries has already been overcome, and is no longer a problem, as the teeth which were susceptible to caries have already been treated, by extraction, filling, fissure sealing or exposure to fluoride.

Another reason for the difference is the diet of the two age groups. Consumption of sweets and sugary food and drinks is probably far greater, and far less controlled, in children; thus their teeth are consequently much more vulnerable to caries. However, it must not be assumed that older people are immune to caries. It still occurs if childhood patterns of unrestricted, indiscriminate consumption of sweets persist. A typical example is the person who continually sucks mints after giving up smoking – and then develops rampant caries.

## The role of saliva

As discussed in Chapter 11, saliva is the watery secretion from the salivary glands that bathes the oral cavity to keep the tissues moist. It also protects against:

- Caries – by promoting remineralisation of early enamel caries
- Periodontal disease – by its cleansing and anti-bacterial properties
- Overall health of the mouth – by its lubricating and cleansing effects

People suffering from dry mouth (**xerostomia**) do not benefit from these effects and are accordingly at much greater risk of caries and periodontal disease.

## Diagnosis of dental disease

Although the patient may become aware themselves that they have a dental disease, such as having bleeding gums or a hole in a tooth, it is the dentist who usually diagnoses a dental problem. Typically this happens during a clinical assessment of the patient – either at a routine dental examination, or at an emergency appointment provided because the patient is experiencing symptoms such as pain.

For diagnosis to occur, the patient has to visit the dentist, and some patients are far more amenable to routine and regular dental examinations than others. The dentist will carry out a full clinical assessment of the patient's oral health each time that they attend, and this will cover the following areas:

- Extra-oral soft tissues
- Intra-oral soft tissues
- Deciduous and mixed dentition of children
- Permanent dentition
- Periodontal tissues

In addition, a full medical history will be taken so that the relationship between general health and oral health can be determined. This will be discussed later.

The purpose of the clinical assessment is to make an early diagnosis of any existing dental disease, so that it can be treated more easily, and also to promote the prevention of oral disease by educating the patient in oral health issues. In this way, the patient is encouraged to take responsibility for their own oral health.

The whole dental team has an important role in this assessment and prevention process.

- **Dentist** – makes the initial diagnosis, formulates a treatment plan, and carries out all treatments restricted to the dentist only.
- **Hygienist** – works under the prescription of the dentist to carry out scaling and oral hygiene instruction.
- **Therapist** – works under the prescription of the dentist to carry out suitable treatments as necessary.
- **Dental nurse** – assists the dentist during the assessment by accurately recording all the information as necessary, assists the other dental team members while treating the patient, reinforces all the oral hygiene messages given to the patient.

As the clinical assessment is so important in the process of diagnosis and prevention of dental disease, and the role of the dental nurse is so great within this process, it will be fully covered here.

## Extra-oral soft tissue assessment

This is the first area of assessment to be carried out by the dentist, usually visually although sometimes palpation of the soft tissues is necessary. The dentist checks all of the following:

- **External facial signs** – skin colour, facial symmetry, the presence of any blemishes such as moles (changes to these may indicate early skin cancer)

- **Lips** – change in colour, the presence of any blemishes, palpation to detect any lumps
- **Lymph nodes** – these lie under the mandible and in the neck, and are palpated for any swellings or other abnormality

Variations in normal skin colour do occur; some patients are naturally pale, others are naturally ruddy, and these variations are more difficult to detect in dark-skinned patients too. Sudden paleness may indicate that the patient is about to faint, while increased redness may indicate hypertension.

Normally the face appears the same on both sides – it is symmetrical. However, asymmetry may indicate the presence of inflammation or a growth, or problems with the nerve supply or muscular control of the area; all of these will require further investigation if detected. Similarly the sudden appearance of, or changes to, blemishes on the skin or lips may also indicate an abnormality. Conditions such as **herpes infection** will show as a 'cold sore' on the lips.

The lymph nodes are part of the body's immune system (see Chapters 3 and 6), so any enlargement of them indicates that the patient is fighting an infection or some other disease process. This will require further investigation if no dental source is diagnosed.

## Intra-oral soft tissue assessment

This involves inspecting all of the oral soft tissues except the gingiva, to determine the presence of any abnormalities (Figure 13.1). The dentist will assess the soft tissues in a systematic manner to avoid missing any intra-oral areas.

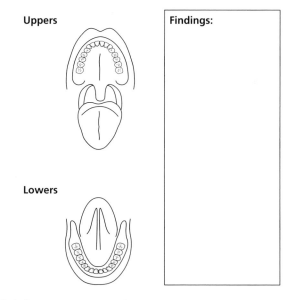

**Figure 13.1**  Soft tissue assessment sheet.

- **Labial, buccal and sulcus mucosa** – their colour and texture, their moisture levels.
- **Palatal mucosa** – the hard and soft palates, the oropharynx, and the tonsils if they are present.
- **Tongue** – its colour and texture, its symmetry and mobility, any red or white patches, or ulceration.
- **Floor of the mouth** – its colour and texture, the presence of any swellings or coloured patches.

Low moisture levels can indicate problems with the functioning of the salivary glands, such as **Sjögren's syndrome**, or **xerostomia** (dry mouth) due to age-related changes to the salivary glands or as a side effect of various medications.

Sinister lesions such as oral cancers tend to develop in the floor of the mouth or on the tongue, and especially in patients with known risk factors such as smoking. The medical history of the patient will have identified those at greater risk of serious problems, and the dentist will determine those who may need urgent further investigation when abnormalities are discovered.

## Tooth charting

Both the **Palmer** and International Federation of Dentistry (**FDI**) system of tooth charting have been covered in full in Chapter 10, along with the average **eruption dates** of both the deciduous and permanent dentition. Again, dental nurses are advised to consult the National Examination Board for Dental Nurses (NEBDN) definitive 'Charting Booklet' for the currently accepted charting information.

While examining the teeth, the dentist will record any evidence of non-carious tooth surface loss, that is **erosion, abrasion or attrition**. These conditions are covered in Chapter 11.

## Periodontal tissue assessment

Periodontal disease is the commonest dental disease found in adult patients, and can easily be missed due to its slow onset and painless nature. Although discussed in Chapter 12, the system of recording the health of the periodontal tissues in sextants – the **Basic Periodontal Examination** (**BPE**) – will be fully covered here.

Healthy periodontal tissues appear pink, firmly attached to the necks of the teeth with a gingival crevice no deeper than 3 mm, and they do not bleed when touched. Teeth are firmly held in their sockets by the periodontal supporting tissues, and no plaque is present on the tooth surfaces.

Specially designed periodontal probes are used to record the presence and depth of any periodontal pockets discovered in each sextant of the dental arches (Figure 13.2), and the coding system used is as follows:

- **Code 0** – healthy gingival tissues with no bleeding on probing
- **Code 1** – pocket no more than 3.5 mm, bleeding on probing, no calculus nor other plaque retention factor present

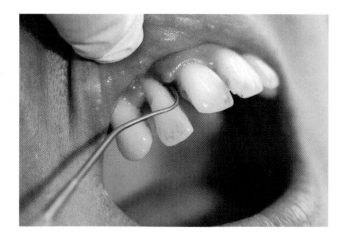

Figure 13.2  Periodontal pocket recording.

- **Code 2** – pocket no more than 3.5 mm but plaque retention factor detected
- **Code 3** – pocket present up to 5.5 mm deep
- **Code 4** – pocket present deeper than 5.5 mm
- **Code \*** – gingival recession or furcation involvement present

Higher codes therefore indicate a more serious periodontal problem (Figure 13.3). Where a code greater than 3 is recorded, a full pocket depth record will be made of each tooth in that sextant so that specific problem areas can be identified, and intensive periodontal treatment can be initiated. In addition, the sites of any plaque found will be recorded, as well as the mobility of any tooth. Tooth mobility is graded as follows:

- **Grade I** – side to side tooth movement less than 2 mm
- **Grade II** – side to side tooth movement more than 2 mm
- **Grade III** – vertical movement present

| 2 | 0 | 4 |
|---|---|---|
| 2 | 1 | 3 |

Figure 13.3  Completed BPE chart.

All of these assessments can be recorded manually, either on the patient's record card or on specific pre-printed charts, or directly into the relevant files of computerised record systems. Assessment recording accounts for a large part of a dental nurse's duties at the chairside, and the importance of accuracy and completeness cannot be over-emphasised. The relevant details of the medical and dental histories are discussed in Chapter 15.

## Methods used to carry out assessments

The dentist has many aids to assessment and diagnosis of dental disease available in the surgery, besides good eyesight and a good knowledge of the normal appearance of healthy oral tissues. The following are also invaluable aids to assessment and diagnosis:

- **Mouth mirrors** – for vision and to reflect light onto less accessible areas
- **Probes** – various designs, to detect caries and periodontal disease
- **Radiographs** – to see within the dental tissues (Chapter 14)
- **Trans-illumination** – to detect anterior caries (Chapter 11)
- **Vitality tests** – to determine the status of the tooth (Chapter 17)
- **Study models** – to record the tooth alignment and occlusion of the patient
- **Photographs** – to record the appearance of tissues at the time of assessment

**Study models** are ideal assessment tools in a variety of situations:

- Occlusal analysis in complicated fixed restorative cases
- Orthodontic assessments, taken before and after treatment
- Recording of current tooth conditions, such as non-carious tooth surface loss

Study models are produced from impressions taken of the dentition, which are then cast with a plaster-like material called **dental stone**. This is usually carried out in a laboratory.

## Prevention of dental disease

In the development of caries, the role of plaque is confined to acid formation, and this only happens in the presence of sugar. In periodontal disease there are no such limitations; it is the mere presence of plaque at the gum margin which causes the disease, no matter what kind of food is eaten.

The prevention of dental disease is therefore concerned with plaque control, but in the case of caries, additional measures such as dietary control and increasing the resistance of teeth to acid are far more important. The methods of prevention are:

- **Oral hygiene and dietary discipline** – these are the responsibility of the patient
- **Preventive dentistry** – this is the dental team's contribution
- **Oral health education** – this is the dental team's responsibility

## Prevention by good oral hygiene

Oral hygiene consists simply of keeping the teeth clean and free of food debris, thus limiting the accumulation and persistence of supragingival plaque which leads to dental disease. It can be achieved by cleaning the teeth twice daily and not eating between meals. Cleaning is best performed by brushing as this is an effective way of removing accessible plaque.

If brushing is not possible, loose food debris can be removed by using sugar-free chewing gum or finishing the meal with a **detergent food** and/or a piece of cheese. Detergent foods are raw, firm, fibrous fruits or vegetables, such as apples, pears, carrots, celery. By virtue of their tough fibrous consistency they require much chewing and stimulate salivary flow, thereby helping to scour the teeth clean of food remnants. Although plaque is unaffected by detergent foods they can remove some of the food debris which nourishes all plaque bacteria and enables some of them to produce acid. Although cheese at the end of a meal has no direct detergent effect, it stimulates salivary flow, neutralises acid and enhances remineralisation of enamel.

Toothbrushing is the most effective way of cleaning one's own teeth. When properly done it removes accessible plaque, whereas detergent food and chewing gum can only clean away loose food particles and stimulate salivary flow. Nevertheless this is a significant contribution to good oral hygiene, and an adequate alternative at the end of a meal if brushing is not possible. However, the excessive use of chewing gum should be discouraged where evidence of attrition or bruxing appears.

## Toothpaste

A wide variety of toothpastes are readily available for patients to use, from shops' own brands to specialised pastes containing a variety of ingredients, as follows:

- 95% of UK toothpastes contain **fluoride** to increase the tooth's resistance to acid attack
- This is present as **sodium monofluorophosphate** or as **sodium fluoride**
- Many contain the agent **triclosan** combined with zinc, which act together as an antiseptic plaque suppressant
- Others contain various agents designed to slow down the formation of calculus
- Some are specifically formulated to help relieve thermal sensitivity, and contain **stannous fluoride**
- Whitening toothpastes act to remove any surface tooth staining by the use of either **abrasives** or **biological enzyme systems**

*Toothbrushing*

Toothbrushing after meals can only be fully effective if it removes supragingival plaque and applies fluoride to the teeth. The object is to clean every accessible tooth surface after meals, in order to remove food debris and plaque, and leave a film of fluoride on the tooth.

- Toothbrushes with a small head and multi-tufted medium nylon bristles are probably the most effective.
- The brush is rinsed and a portion of fluoride toothpaste added.
- Each dental arch is divided into three sections: left and right sides and front.
- Side sections are subdivided into buccal, lingual and occlusal surfaces, and the front sections into labial and lingual.
- This amounts to eight groups of surfaces in each jaw, and at least five seconds should be spent on each group.
- Each jaw is done in turn and the mouth is then cleared by spitting out, but **not by rinsing**, as this removes the fluoride.
- Parents will need to perform effective toothbrushing on children up to the age of 8 years, to ensure that all plaque is removed and to teach the child how to brush correctly (Figure 13.4).
- Brushes should be washed afterwards and allowed to dry. They only have a limited life and need replacement every few months as the bristles curl up and render the brush ineffective.
- The actual method of brushing, whether by gentle scrubbing or rotary action, is not important. It is the end result – removal of plaque – that matters, not the

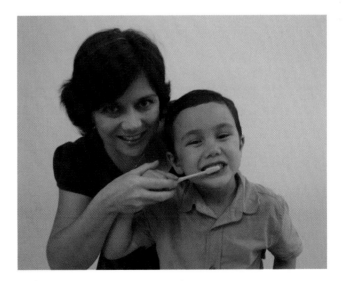

**Figure 13.4**  Parental supervision during brushing. © Joon Chai Yeoh. Reproduced with permission.

method used, although vigorous sawing styles of brushing must be discouraged, as they will result in abrasion cavities developing. By using disclosing tablets, under guidance from their dentist or hygienist, individual patients can see for themselves which method suits them best.

Effective toothbrushing requires time, knowledge and skill. Many people lack these requirements and brushing is ineffective as a plaque control measure. The whole process can be made simpler for such people by using an electric toothbrush. It cleans effectively without effort, and is particularly valuable for children and the physically handicapped. Although no better than correct manual brushing, it is probably preferable as so many people find it difficult to achieve adequate plaque removal with an ordinary toothbrush.

Many people eat an NME sugary snack at bedtime. This is the most dangerous time of all, as salivary flow is at its least effective level during sleep. Such people should be advised to undertake their second daily brushing immediately after their final snack.

## Interdental cleaning

However good the toothbrushing technique, it is still impossible to clean interdental spaces perfectly with a toothbrush alone. Consequently these mesial and distal contact areas between adjoining teeth are more prone to caries and periodontal disease. To clean them adequately, dental floss or tape, an interdental brush (Figure 13.5), or wood sticks are used. A certain amount of manual dexterity is required to use these products effectively, although the introduction of aids such as *flosettes* has helped considerably those patients who may have found interdental cleaning difficult beforehand.

Interdental cleaning methods are described in Chapter 12.

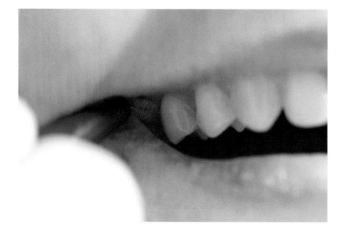

**Figure 13.5** Interproximal brushing.

## Mouthwashes

A wide range of mouthwashes are currently available, again ranging from shops' own brands to specialised products. General mouthwashes contain various ingredients including **sodium fluoride** and **triclosan**. Others are used to ease thermal sensitivity, while some contain **chlorhexidine** as an antiseptic plaque suppressant. More recently, some mouthwashes have become available for use as a general first aid measure after oral surgery or an oral infection, and contain **hydrogen peroxide** which helps to eliminate anaerobic bacteria.

## Prevention and dietary discipline

It cannot be emphasised too strongly that even if teeth are thoroughly cleaned after meals, caries will still occur if NME sugary snacks are taken between meals. This is because plaque persists in the inaccessible parts of fissures and contact points. Acid forms in this residual plaque within minutes of eating sugar, and caries will develop if frequent snacks are taken between meals. Then, as described in Chapter 11, a constant acid environment at the enamel surface allows demineralisation to proceed unchecked, and leaves insufficient time between intakes of sugar for the natural defence mechanism of remineralisation to occur. Although adequate toothbrushing and interdental cleaning twice daily may prevent supragingival periodontal disease, it cannot prevent caries unless accompanied by strict dietary discipline to eliminate NME snacks between meals.

If NME foods and acidic drinks (such as carbonated 'pops') are confined to mealtimes only, the acids involved are neutralised to some extent by the buffering action of saliva, and the extent of any demineralisation is reduced. In addition, a list of **good snacks** and **bad snacks** can be developed by the dental team, which can be passed on as dietary advice to patients. Diet sheets can also be used by the dental team to determine the presence of 'hidden sugars' in an individual patient's diet.

Good snacks include:

- Non-citrus fruit, such as apples, pears and peaches
- Fibrous raw vegetables, such as carrots and celery
- Unflavoured crisps
- Low fat cheese
- Unsweetened yoghurt

Bad snacks include:

- Sweets and other confectionery
- Biscuits and cakes
- Carbonated drinks and pure citrus fruit juices
- Tea and coffee with sugar
- Raw citrus fruits, such as lemons, limes, grapefruits, and oranges

■ Processed foods containing hidden sugars, such as ketchup, flavoured crisps, tinned products

## Preventive dentistry

Preventive dentistry includes:

■ Instruction in oral hygiene
■ Regular inspection for checking oral hygiene and ensuring early diagnosis of oral disease
■ Any necessary treatment for the prevention and removal of areas inaccessible to supragingival plaque control, and plaque retention factors
■ Specific caries prevention measures such as fissure sealing and topical fluoridation

### Instruction in oral hygiene

Dentists may delegate instruction in oral hygiene to their dental nurses provided they comply with the General Dental Council (GDC) requirements outlined in Chapter 2. Oral hygiene instruction is best given at the chairside, while posters and pamphlets in the waiting room serve as an extra reminder. Patients are told how dental disease arises and how it can be prevented. This entails an explanation of the all-important role of plaque and the effects it produces.

The most impressive way of demonstrating plaque on their own teeth is to give patients a disclosing tablet to suck. Patients can then see for themselves in a mirror whether they are cleaning their teeth properly. They are then shown how to:

■ Use a toothbrush effectively
■ Clean their interdental spaces
■ Use disclosing agents at home

They are also:

■ Advised to clean their teeth and interdental spaces twice daily
■ Warned against NME snacks between meals

However, they are not likely to heed such advice unless it is practicable. Patients must therefore be told how to care for their teeth when toothbrushing is not possible or convenient. The best substitute in such cases is to finish their meal with a detergent food such as fresh fruit or vegetables, sugar-free chewing gum, or cheese. These increase salivary flow and will leave a minimum amount of food debris on the teeth, whereas a conventional sticky sweet dessert, such as jam roll and custard, will leave the maximum amount of acid-producing debris. A sweet drink of coffee or tea after meals will do no harm if patients are encouraged to use an artificial sweetener, such as saccharin.

If supragingival plaque is thoroughly removed daily, by toothbrushing and interdental cleaning, periodontal disease may be prevented. But this is not sufficient for the prevention of caries. Acid production in residual or fresh plaque is so rapid that caries cannot be prevented if sugar is continually reintroduced by frequent snacks between meals. It must be impressed on patients and parents that caries cannot be prevented by brushing alone. It *must* be combined with dietary discipline. Sweet snacks between meals should either be stopped altogether or replaced by NME sugar-free alternatives such as fruit, nuts, low-fat cheese or crisps. Again, dietary advice must be practical if it is to be accepted. For example, parents who do not wish to deprive children of sweets can be advised to compromise by arranging for sweets to be eaten at meal times only, and not in between.

Expectant and nursing mothers are warned of the disastrous dental effects of using dummies or bottles with sweetened fruit juices. They can cause complete destruction of incisor crowns, by caries and erosion. Colour photographs of such cases may help to dissuade mothers from using them. Similar effects can arise from long-term use of medicines sweetened with sugar, and these should be replaced by sugar-free alternatives.

## Patient evaluation and motivation

Adequate communication between the patient and the dental team will determine the level of the patient's knowledge and skills in relation to their own oral health. Any existing problems that are preventing the individual from achieving and maintaining good oral health can then be identified. Some of the issues that may be encountered are:

- The level of any oral health advice given previously
- A disability that prevents adequate oral cleaning
- The level of interest they have in their oral health
- A general health problem that limits adequate oral cleaning, or that actually causes the oral health problem
- A serious general health problem (such as having cancer) that over-rides any concerns about their oral health

The information received from the patient, and their attitude to oral health issues and therefore their motivation, will vary between age groups. No matter what their age however, the patient has the right whether or not to accept and act on the help and advice offered by the dental team. In particular, some adults and older patients may feel patronised by being given oral health information from younger members of the dental team, so good communication skills are vital.

Some areas to consider when offering advice to the various age groups are given below.

*Adult patients*

- Smoking and drinking habits should be discussed in one-to-one sessions, in relation to both oral health and general health.
- Smoking cessation advice may be required, either from the dental team or a local National Health Service (NHS) centre running such advice sessions.
- Diet should be discussed in detail and linked to general health issues if necessary, using diet sheets as required.
- The oral health adviser should be attentive to the patient's concerns, and answer queries raised at the patient's level of understanding.

*Young people*

- This group often have a different outlook on life than adults, with different priorities too.
- They are likely to have little, if any, experience of oral or general health problems and often take some convincing of the existence of these problems, and of the long-term effects of poor health.
- The use of disclosing tablets and audio-visual aids is more likely to convince them that an oral health problem exists than discussions alone.
- Some may already be experimenting with alcohol and tobacco.
- More immature patients may not be willing to accept responsibility for their own oral health at the time of discussion.
- Parental influence and support will differ among patients.
- Some young people are naturally argumentative and unwilling to accept advice from others, and the dental team may have to postpone their efforts for a time.
- A friendly, patient and approachable manner is necessary at all times.

*Children*

- Children's oral health depends very much on parental influence and support, so parents should be invited into oral health discussions wherever possible.
- The vocabulary of the advice needs to be tailored to the age and understanding of the child.
- A friendly and trusting approach is required, while also trying to make the sessions fun for the patient so that their interest is maintained.
- Children have shorter attention spans than other groups, and are easily distracted.
- Interactive sessions are most likely to be successful, and especially with the use of disclosing tablets.
- A non-threatening approach is required to achieve compliance.

*Regular examination and treatment*

Prevention is better than cure, but the frequency of attendance for dental examination varies between individuals according to the following factors:

- **Caries experience** – those with a greater experience of caries will require more frequent recall for examination than those with a lesser experience
- **Periodontal experience** – similarly, those with existing periodontal problems will require more regular review and preventive treatment
- **Medical risk factors** – those suffering from conditions that directly affect their oral health will require more frequent examination (see later)
- **Controllable risk factors** – smokers, and those with high alcohol or NME sugar intake, are more likely to experience oral health problems, and should attend more regularly
- **General health** – some conditions will prevent regular attendance for examination
- **Social risk factors** – such as financial hardship, and lifestyle issues
- **Children** – during their mixed dentition stage they will require more regular examination to monitor their occlusal development

During the examination, the level of oral hygiene is checked with disclosing agents and any deficiencies shown to the patient. Encouragement and further instruction can then be given as necessary. Routine bite-wing X-rays (Chapter 14) may be taken at the same time for early diagnosis of caries and periodontal bone loss. Together with examination of the tongue and other soft tissues of the mouth, and any necessary encouragement to give up smoking, the frequency of future checks can be decided for each individual patient. These visits will detect incipient oral and dental disease which can be treated far more easily in its earliest stages than later. Such treatment may involve all branches of dentistry.

- Periodic scaling to remove inaccessible plaque and calculus can prevent the onset of periodontal disease before it reaches the stage of gingivitis.
- Early treatment of caries enables affected teeth to be conserved rather than extracted.
- If teeth have already been lost, carefully planned prosthetic treatment to restore normal occlusion and function can prevent food traps developing.
- Any unsatisfactory dental treatment which itself promotes plaque formation (such as fillings with cervical overhangs, ill-fitting or badly designed partial dentures) is rectified.
- For children, orthodontics can prevent or cure irregularities of the teeth, which might otherwise form inaccessible stagnation areas.

Dental disease, arising as it does from the accumulation of plaque, can therefore be prevented to a large extent by patients' own efforts at supragingival plaque control and avoiding NME sugar between meals. Regular dental inspection and treatment can also prevent the vicious circle of dental disease developing, by providing treatment at the very earliest stages before caries or periodontal disease have time to cause serious damage to the dentition.

## Oral health education

All of the oral health messages discussed previously, if followed, should ensure that patients can achieve and maintain a good standard of oral health. But there is one final area of help and advice that the dental team can offer, and that is the promotion of methods used to increase the **resistance** of the teeth to acid attack, thereby reducing the incidence of caries. The most successful method available is the use of **fluoride**, and it acts in the following ways.

- It can be taken into the mineral structure of enamel to form a more acid-resistant surface of **fluorapatite crystals**.
- Fluoride also has an inhibitory effect on the **feeding rate** of oral bacteria, slowing it down so that less acid is produced.

The protective effect of the fluoride on teeth is greatest after they have erupted into the mouth, and most oral hygiene products available to the public contain fluoride so that, when used on a regular basis, the teeth are being constantly strengthened against acid attack. This type of application is called **topical fluoride** because it is applied externally to the tooth. In some areas of the UK, and in some other countries, fluoride can be added to foods or the water supply so that it is taken internally by patients. This is called **systemic fluoride** but it is not welcomed by all, as the general health effects of this type of 'mass medication' are surrounded by controversy.

## Topical fluoridation

As stated, most oral hygiene products contain topical fluorides, for use at home by the patient.

- **Fluoride toothpastes** – the current recommended dose for all is 1000 parts per million (ppm), or even 1500 ppm for adults at high risk of caries.
- **Brushing** – twice daily brushing with a pea-sized amount of toothpaste achieves the maximum benefit.
- **Rinsing** – patients should not rinse the toothpaste out after brushing, but should be instructed just to spit so that the toothpaste continues its contact with the teeth.
- **Fluoride mouthwashes** – these are available for regular use during orthodontic treatment, or for those with a high caries incidence.
- **Fluoridated floss** – using this allows topical fluoride application to the interproximal areas of the teeth.

Topical application of fluoride may also be undertaken by the dentist, hygienist or therapist, but is usually confined to high-risk patients and those with special needs, such as:

- Children with rampant caries
- Patients with medical conditions, such as haemophilia and heart defects, which would make tooth extraction dangerous
- Patients with disabilities who cannot achieve adequate oral hygiene themselves

The frequency of topical fluoride application depends on the individual patient's requirements.

A popular method of application is a fluoride gel in a special applicator tray. Many such trays are available but they all provide full coverage of the entire arch; some permit both arches to be treated at the same time. These gels are pleasantly flavoured and well tolerated by patients.

The technique has two stages. First a thorough polish is done to remove plaque, after which the teeth are washed and dried. Second, the gel is applied in the special tray for a few minutes. On removal of the tray, patients are instructed not to rinse, drink or eat for half-an-hour. An alternative method is to paint the teeth with a fluoride varnish, such as Duraphat. As before, teeth must still be cleaned and dried first.

Roots exposed by gingival recession or periodontal surgery may become very sensitive to hot or cold fluids. Fluoride varnish is applied to such areas to relieve this cause of pain.

## Fissure sealing

Topical fluorides exert most of their effect on mesial and distal (proximal) surfaces. Occlusal fissures are just as vulnerable to caries but they are less well protected by fluorides. Fortunately they can receive extra, and even better, protection by the application of fissure sealants. These materials are composite fillings or glass ionomer cement, and their use is described in Chapter 16. Successful fissure sealing should make an occlusal surface safe from caries. Like topical fluoridation, it can be done by hygienists and therapists, and is therefore of major importance in preventive dentistry as it can produce a significant reduction in the commonest disease of children.

## Systemic fluoridation

This is carried out as a public health measure in some areas of the country, where fluoride is ingested and then absorbed from the digestive tract so that it can be incorporated into the enamel structure of the teeth. It is added at the **optimum concentration of 1 ppm** to drinking water, although in some areas of the world it occurs naturally.

Public health surveys have consistently proved the benefit of the use of systemic fluoride, by comparing the number of **decayed, missing and filled teeth** (**DMF count**) in various populations. In areas where systemic fluoride is present at the 1 ppm concentration, the incidence of caries is reduced by 50%. Other systemic fluorides include the following:

- **Fluoridated table salt** – not available in the UK
- **Fluoride drops and tablets** – available on prescription to children and recommended for daily use up to the age of 13 years, although the dose will vary depending on their age and the concentration of any other systemic fluorides available

## Enamel fluorosis

This condition occurs when excessive fluoride is ingested during the stage of enamel formation. The teeth erupt with **mottled white areas** within the enamel which vary in severity and can be quite unsightly. Restorative techniques, such as veneers, are able to mask the discoloured teeth, but the condition is preventable by careful advice on fluoride ingestion, especially in areas where systemic fluoride is used.

## Community health measures

### Oral health education

Dental staff can explain the causes and prevention of dental disease to individual patients in the surgery, but this only benefits regular attenders. There still remains a need for greater effort by the public health service. Expectant and nursing mothers, parents of schoolchildren, and young teenagers are the groups most in need of advice on dental care. Publicity is still necessary to warn these groups of the damage done by:

- Dummies or bottles used with sweetened fruit juices
- Unrestricted consumption of snacks between meals
- Avoiding dental examination until toothache develops

Doctors, midwives, health visitors, clinic staff and schoolteachers all have a part to play in helping the dental team to educate the public.

Nursing mothers should be encouraged to bring their babies when they have their own dental inspection. Toddlers will thereby accept the dental surgery as a place of interest and soon become regular and co-operative patients themselves, long before any treatment is necessary. The discipline of confining sweets to meal times and brushing after meals can be developed at an early age, and will establish good dental habits of lifelong value.

Parents should be warned of the danger of sugar and encouraged to restrict the consumption of sweets between meals. In school, steps should be taken to ensure that school dinners do not leave a film of sugary debris on the teeth, and the consumption of sugary snacks during breaks should be discouraged.

Young teenagers soon realise the importance of good appearance and this can be utilised in dental health education. Regular visits to the dentist can improve their appearance, health and self-confidence by means of:

■ Scaling and polishing
■ Filling cavities in front teeth
■ Orthodontic correction of crowded or protruding teeth
■ Instructions on the value of dietary discipline and oral hygiene in avoiding halitosis, caries and obesity
■ Education on the dangers of smoking

All these ways of improving appearance and health are freely available to them, but this powerful motivating factor could still be more widely communicated at national level.

Many excellent videos, films, posters and pamphlets are already available for display in clinics and schools, but these forms of dental health education are only reaching a small section of the population. To help reduce dental disease, the entire population needs to be shown how to maintain good oral health by dietary discipline, strict oral hygiene and regular dental inspection.

The message of dental health education can be condensed into four simple measures:

■ **Reduce the frequency** of consumption of food and drink containing sugar. Avoid acid drinks
■ **Oral hygiene measures**, including brushing twice daily with **fluoride** toothpaste
■ **Regular dental attendance** at least once a year
■ Do not smoke

## Effect of general health on oral health

The oral health status of a patient is not a separate issue from their general health, indeed many of the same risk factors affect both areas of the patient, such as the following:

■ Smoking and tobacco usage is linked to various cancers (including oral cancer), as well as heart disease, respiratory disease and periodontal disease
■ High sugar diets are linked to dental caries, obesity (and all of the related health issues), and heart disease
■ Excess alcohol usage is linked to oral cancer, liver disease and periodontal disease
■ Eating disorders are linked to dental erosion and general ill health
■ Diabetes is linked to general poor wound healing and periodontal disease

In addition, the following points need to be borne in mind by the dental team when assessing patients in terms of their oral health status, and in any attempts to motivate and improve this status in individual cases.

■ **Physical disabilities** may make oral hygiene control difficult for the patient.
■ **Mental disabilities** may cause difficulties in understanding oral health messages.

- Some **prescription drugs** have adverse effects on the oral soft tissues, causing hyperplasia or affecting salivary flow.
- **Social factors** affect general health, people from low socio-economic groups tend to suffer from poorer general health overall.
- **Older patients** are more likely to suffer from various illnesses, as well as being vulnerable with regard to age-related changes to their oral tissues, such as less elastic mucous membranes or brittle bones.

Overall then, the assessment of the oral health of individual patients by the dental team is a complicated task, with many factors to consider before methods of preventing dental disease can be considered. The four key issues to good oral health, shown below, apply to all patients, but all other factors have to be identified and considered in each case for any chance of success.

The key issues are:

- **Good oral hygiene**
- **Diet low in NMEs, and NMEs confined to mealtimes**
- **Use of fluoride to strengthen the teeth**
- **Regular dental examination to monitor and reinforce these messages**

# 14 Dental Radiography

Dental radiography is the taking and processing of X-ray films of the teeth and jaws. When an X-ray set is switched on, X-rays are generated and pass out of the set through a metal tube which is pointed towards the required area. To take an X-ray, the tube and X-ray film packet are placed so that the part to be X-rayed lies between them. The tube through which the X-ray beam emerges from the set is called a **collimator** and its purpose is to restrict the area of the beam and facilitate aiming the beam. In accordance with current legislation, it must be rectangular in shape to mimic that of a normal intra-oral X-ray film packet.

Although X-rays can travel unimpeded through soft tissues, such as skin and muscle, they cannot pass through hard tissues so easily and therefore project a shadow of the teeth and bone on to the film. This shadow, which forms the finished X-ray film when it is processed, varies in depth according to the thickness and density of the hard tissues, thus allowing enamel, dentine and bone to be easily recognised from each other.

## Effects of ionising radiation on tissues

The correct term for the beam of X-rays that pass from the collimator of the machine is **ionising radiation.** It is a type of electromagnetic radiation that possesses energy, in the same way as microwaves, radio waves and visible light. X-rays have enough energy to pass through body tissues to varying degrees as described above, and when they do so, one of three things may happen.

- The X-rays pass untouched through the tissues and are **unaltered**.
- The X-rays hit the tissues and are **scattered,** releasing energy.
- The X-rays hit the tissues head-on and are **absorbed,** releasing energy.

Tissues that are dense, such as enamel and bone, will absorb lots of X-rays and appear white on the radiograph – they are described as being **radiopaque**. Tissues that are thin, such as the oral soft tissues, will allow most X-rays to pass through unaltered and will appear dark on the radiograph – they are described as being **radiolucent**.

The dangerous nature of all ionising radiation is due to the energy released when the X-ray beam hits the tissues. This energy can cause cell damage or even cell death in the surrounding tissues. If the energy happens to affect the DNA-containing chromosomes of the cell, it can cause cell mutation too, which may ultimately develop into cancer. Any of these effects will happen every time that a patient is exposed to X-rays, so there can be no 'safe' level of X-ray exposure. Consequently, strict legislation is in force to minimise the risks both to patients and to the dental team. These are discussed later in the chapter but are summarised here:

- **Clinical justification** for all X-ray exposures
- **Dose** must be kept as low as reasonably achievable (ALARA)
- **Exposure** must be restricted to the patient only
- **Maintenance** of X-ray machines must be done regularly
- **Trained** staff only are to use the equipment
- **Quality assurance** procedures must be in place to maintain a consistently high standard of radiograph

## Uses of radiography

Some of the commonest uses of X-rays in dentistry are to show the following:

- Unerupted teeth, impacted teeth and retained roots
- Shape, size and number of roots of a tooth, and state of the surrounding bone, prior to extraction
- Presence of chronic alveolar abscesses on dead teeth
- Progress of endodontic treatment
- Bone loss in periodontal disease
- Early detection of caries
- Development of the teeth in children, for orthodontic purposes
- Fractures, cysts and bone disease affecting the jaws

## Radiographic changes in disease

- Chronic alveolar abscesses show up as a dark circular area at the apex of an affected tooth. This is caused by destruction of the apical lamina dura and spongy bone.
- Periodontal disease shows up as loss of the lamina dura forming the crest of the alveolar bone, loss of height of the alveolar bone, and a widening of the periodontal ligament space.
- Caries shows up as a dark area of destruction extending inwards from the enamel surface.

For examination purposes, dental nurses are not expected to interpret radiographs, but they should be able to describe normal and abnormal radiographic appearances of common dental conditions.

## X-ray film

X-ray film consists of ordinary black and white photographic film in a light-proof wrapping. There are two types of film: **intra-oral** and **extra-oral**.

### Intra-oral film

Intra-oral film is placed inside the mouth and is used to take detailed films of small areas covering a few teeth only. The standard type of film is called **periapical** (Figure 14.1). It measures 3 × 4 cm but there is a smaller size for children. A much larger size of intra-oral film is the **occlusal** film (Figure 14.2). This is 6 × 7.5 cm and is used to give a plane view of the mandible or maxilla, usually to show unerupted teeth and cysts.

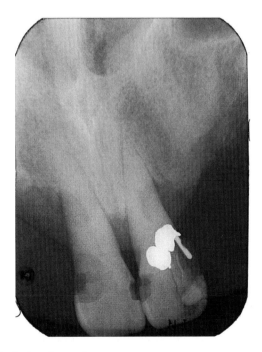

**Figure 14.1** Periapical radiograph.
Source: *Basic Guide to Dental Procedures*, C. Hollins, 2008, John Wiley & Sons Ltd, Oxford.

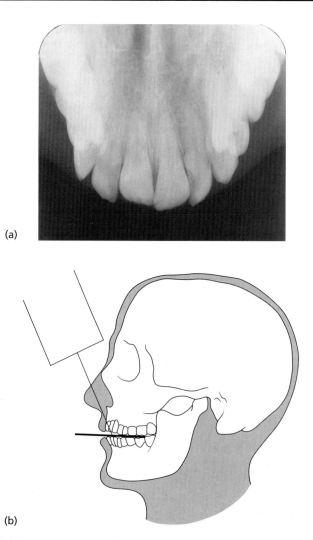

(a)

(b)

Figure 14.2  (a) Occlusal radiograph. (b) Angulation.
Source: *Dental Radiography*, 2nd edn, N.J.D. Smith, Blackwell Science Ltd, Oxford.

The contents of an intra-oral film packet are shown in Figure 14.3. When it is unwrapped for developing, the film is seen to be pale green with a mounting pimple on the side which **faces** the X-ray tube. On either side of the film is a piece of black paper to shield it from the light and prevent damage to the film. Behind the black paper, on the side **away** from the X-ray tube, is a piece of lead foil. This absorbs scattered radiation which could spoil the quality of the radiograph. All these layers are enclosed in a light-proof wrapping which has a pimple on the side **facing** the X-ray tube.

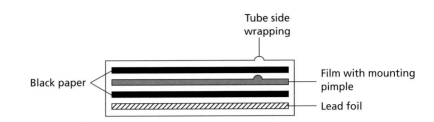

Figure 14.3  Contents of intra-oral film packet.

## Extra-oral film

One type of extra-oral film, measuring 13 × 18 cm, is used outside the mouth with ordinary dental X-ray sets. The film is placed against the face over the required area. It covers a large area of the jaws and is used to show unerupted teeth, fractures, cysts and bone diseases. The most commonly taken view is called a **lateral oblique**. Other types of extra-oral film are the **dental panoramic tomograph** (**DPT**) and the **cephalogram**. These both require the use of special X-ray machines, and are discussed later.

Extra-oral film is packed differently from intra-oral films. The latter are individually packed in light-proof wrappers but extra-oral film is not. Packets of extra-oral film only contain unwrapped film and can only be opened in a darkroom. On removal from the packet in the darkroom, a film is placed immediately in a special light-proof container called a **cassette**, which is then kept closed ready for use.

A cassette opens like a book and the film is placed in the middle. On each inside cover of the cassette there is a white plastic sheet called an **intensifying screen**, and the film is sandwiched between the two screens when the cassette is closed ready for use. The screens **fluoresce** on exposure to X-rays, creating the image on the film themselves. This allows the use of a reduced exposure time of X-rays to the patient, making the technique safer.

## Care of films

If an expiry date is given on a packet of film it should not be used beyond that date. Any remaining films should be discarded, as old film gives poor results. Films can still deteriorate before their expiry date if stored in hot or damp places, or too near an X-ray set. Film in poor condition, from any of these causes, will give a radiograph of poor quality which may have to be retaken.

## Taking intra-oral radiographs

Before any X-ray is taken, the operator is legally required to ensure that the patient is identified correctly, and the reason for the X-ray is written in the patient's notes. All the relevant legal requirements are covered later in this chapter.

The X-ray set is plugged into an electricity supply and the time switch is set to the correct exposure. This varies from 0.1 seconds to 0.5 seconds according to the tooth to be X-rayed and the type of film used. On many sets the exposures are preset according to the area to be X-rayed (Figure 14.4). The film is placed inside the mouth against the required area and the patient holds it still by biting onto the holder device being used, or by using one finger to hold the packet in place, if necessary. The X-ray tube is then positioned against the skin overlying the film, and the rectangular collimator is aligned to the film packet, then the exposure time switch is operated. The exposed film is then removed from the patient's mouth, wiped with an alcohol wipe to disinfect it, dried with a napkin, clipped on to a film hanger marked with the patient's name, and taken for processing.

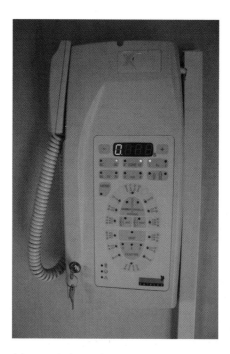

Figure 14.4  X-ray machine control panel.

Cross-infection prevention is facilitated if the film is placed in a clear plastic envelope before insertion in the mouth. The envelope is discarded on removal from the mouth. Some brands of film are supplied with envelopes already fitted.

## Angulation

The greatest difficulties in taking intra-oral radiographs are to get the patient to hold the film still in the proper place during exposure, and to angulate the tube correctly. If the tube is tilted too **far upwards** or **downwards** the radiograph may be useless as the teeth will appear **elongated** or **foreshortened**, respectively. However, these difficulties can be easily overcome by using a special X-ray beam aiming device, or holder. This consists of a bite block film holder which enables a film to be held in the mouth parallel to the teeth, when the teeth are closed together on the block, so that the X-ray beam strikes the film at right angles. In this way, no distortion of the image occurs. Patients do not have to hold the film in place; angulation is simple, irrespective of whether the patient sits upright or in a supine position, and the results are consistently good. This is called the **paralleling technique** (Figure 14.5).

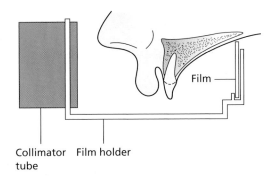

Collimator   Film holder
tube

**Figure 14.5**  Paralleling technique.
Source: *Dental Radiography*, 2nd edn, N.J.D. Smith, Blackwell Science Ltd, Oxford.

If a device such as a holder is not used, the correct way of angulating a tube is to direct it at a right angle to an imaginary line bisecting the angle between the long axis of tooth and film (Figures 14.2 and 14.6). This is called the **bisecting angle technique** and gives correct angulation in the vertical plane. In the horizontal plane the tube must be at a right angle to the film. Wrong angulation in the horizontal plane causes overlapping of teeth on the radiograph.

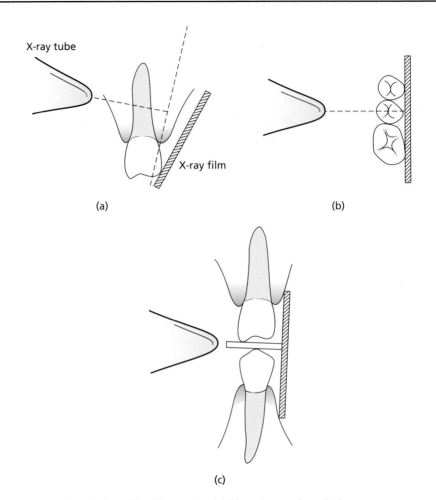

X-ray tube

X-ray film

(a)

(b)

(c)

**Figure 14.6** Angulation of the X-ray tube. (a) Bisecting angle technique. (b) Horizontal plane. (c) Bite-wing.

## Bite-wing radiographs

Bite-wing radiographs are X-ray films taken of the posterior teeth in occlusion. They show the crowns of opposing upper and lower molars and premolars on the same film and are used to detect caries at the contact points of adjacent teeth, before it can be seen by other methods (Figure 14.7).

Bite-wing film is periapical intra-oral film with a tab projecting at a right angle from its centre. This tab is bitten between the teeth and holds the film in correct position, covering the crowns of all upper and lower teeth in contact with it. There are no angulation difficulties as the tab can be felt through the cheek, and the tube is simply placed against this point at 90° to teeth and film (see Figure 14.6). Alternatively, a holder acting as an aiming device can be used with ordinary

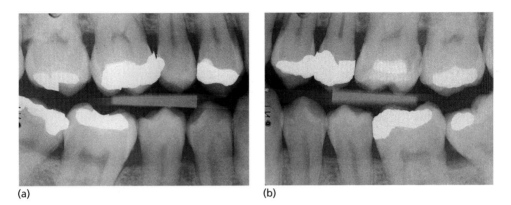

(a)                                                 (b)

**Figure 14.7** Bite-wing radiographs.
Source: *Basic Guide to Dental Procedures*, C. Hollins, 2008, John Wiley & Sons Ltd, Oxford.

periapical film packets. Again, the packet is held parallel to the teeth so that no distortion or overlap occurs.

When placed **horizontally** in the mouth, the bite-wing radiographs show the following:

- Interproximal areas of the posterior teeth, and any cavities present
- Restoration overhangs in these areas
- Recurrent caries beneath existing restorations
- Occlusal caries

When placed **vertically** in the mouth, the bite-wing radiographs show the following:

- Interproximal bone loss associated with the posterior teeth
- The presence of true periodontal pockets

## Panoramic radiography

This method of taking radiographs has been introduced into dentistry by a special X-ray set which takes panoramic films of the jaws. The film is called a **dental panoramic tomograph** (**DPT**) and it shows every single tooth, erupted or unerupted, on each side of both jaws, all on the one film (Figure 14.8). It was originally called an Orthopantomograph, and the abbreviations OPG or OPT are still in common use.

A special DPT machine is used and it takes a panoramic film by having a motor-driven X-ray tube and film cassette holder which circle round the patient's face. The patient stands or sits upright and special supports keep the head still during an exposure time of up to 15 seconds. The cassette contains intensifying screens,

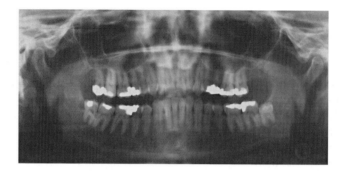

Figure 14.8 Dental panoramic tomograph.
Source: *Basic Guide to Dental Procedures*, C. Hollins, 2008, John Wiley & Sons Ltd, Oxford.

and holds an extra-oral 13 × 31 cm film which is processed in the same way as the smaller size lateral oblique film and intra-oral films.

A DPT is particularly useful for showing teeth which are otherwise difficult to X-ray, such as unerupted third molars and canines. It is also used for screening purposes to show the overall state of development of the dentition and the presence of any abnormalities. However, it is not a substitute for intra-oral films as these are still necessary for giving more detailed views of small areas, particularly the periapical region of incisors.

## Cephalometric radiography

Orthodontic diagnosis, treatment planning and recording are greatly facilitated by use of a special X-ray technique which gives standardised views of the whole skull. Side and frontal views are taken with a special machine called a **cephalostat**. The patient's head is positioned in a frame with locating posts which fit into the ear holes; the most commonly taken films are side views called **lateral skull radiographs**.

Various measurements are taken from these films to record the spatial relationships between the skull, jaws and teeth. The cephalostat allows subsequent film measurements to be accurately compared with previous ones, thus enabling jaw growth, and the progress and results of treatment to be checked and analysed. The technique is called cephalometric radiography.

Oral surgeons also use frontal and lateral skull films taken in a cephalostat for diagnosis and treatment planning, especially for cases requiring surgical alteration of the jaw relationship. They are also very useful for precise location of the position and angulation of unerupted upper canines.

This technique preceded panoramic radiography and necessitated the use of a cephalostat which could not take any other types of radiographs. However, most DPT machines can be adapted to take cephalometric films as well. Film size for these views is 20 × 25 cm with an exposure time of up to three seconds.

## Digital radiography

All the radiographic techniques described so far require the use of X-ray film which has to be chemically processed to produce a radiograph. However, digital technology now utilises computers to produce direct digital intra-oral radiographs which are viewed on a computer monitor screen at the chairside. A normal X-ray set is used but X-ray film and processing are not required. A re-usable intra-oral sensor plate is used instead of film and the radiation dose is far less than with ordinary film. It is a technique similar to the use of digital cameras to produce photographic images that can then be loaded onto the computer either from a memory card or from a scanner.

With digital radiography, the exposed sensor plate is inserted into a laser scanner which is connected to a compatible personal computer. Less than a minute later the radiograph appears on the monitor screen, and it can then be stored on disk and retrieved at will. The radiograph can be edited on the computer to give the effect of different X-ray exposures, and parts can be magnified or altered.

The advantages of this system are: elimination of film-processing; reduced radiation exposure; speed of viewing; re-usability of sensor plates; and the ability to retrieve, show and discuss radiographic findings with patients at the chairside. The disadvantages are the cost of the equipment and the theoretical possibility of legal problems arising, as the images can be easily edited and altered.

## Processing

X-ray film is ordinary photographic film and is affected by X-rays in just the same way as film inside a camera is affected by light. The processing procedure for X-ray film is just the same as that for producing an ordinary black and white film negative. After exposure, the film contains the X-ray image but it is not yet visible. The first stage of processing is to **develop** the image so that it can be seen. It cannot be used at this stage, however, as the film is still sensitive to light and would eventually darken all over if viewed in daylight. A second stage of processing is therefore necessary, to **fix** the image, and produce a usable permanent film. Processing can be carried out either manually or automatically, with the use of an automatic processor such as the Velopex machine. Both methods are described below.

### Manual processing

This is carried out in a light-tight and lockable room, referred to as the 'dark room'. The room needs to be light-tight to avoid the exposure of the unprocessed X-ray films to visible light, as this will ruin the image. It should also be lockable so that no other staff can open the door during processing, again to avoid visible light exposure. As X-ray films are most sensitive to blue light, a special **red safety light** can be used in the room during processing, which will not ruin the X-ray image and will allow the staff member to see what they are doing.

Within the dark room, a series of four tanks are present which all sit in a main water tank. The main tank is kept at the optimum processing temperature range of 18°C to 22°C with the use of an immersion heater (Figure 14.9). The four tanks are set in series, as follows:

- **Lidded developing tank** – containing the alkaline developing fluid that produces the initial **latent image**, the lid is only removed during developing as the solution will deteriorate in air
- **First wash tank** – to wash off the developing solution after the correct developing time, using tap water
- **Fixing tank** – containing the acid fixing solution which permanently fixes the image onto the celluloid film
- **Second wash tank** – to wash off the fixing solution, again using tap water

The procedure of manual processing is as follows.

1   Under ordinary light, check that all solution levels are sufficient, and that the temperature of the main water tank is in the correct range.
2   Use the chart provided to determine the correct developing time for the temperature recorded.
3   Check that the timer and a suitable hanger are available in the room.
4   Wipe all work surfaces dry to remove any previous chemical spillages, if necessary.
5   Lock the door and switch on the safety light.
6   Open the film packet or cassette, and carefully clip the film to the hanger without touching the film surface.
7   Remove the developer lid, fully immerse the film on the hanger into the developing solution, and start the timer.
8   When the timer sounds, remove the hanger and film and fully immerse them into the first wash tank, agitating the hanger so that the film is thoroughly washed.
9   Shake off excess water, then fully immerse the film and hanger into the fixing solution and start the timer.
10   While the fixing process is timing, replace the developer lid to prevent further deterioration of that solution.
11   After a minimum of one minute the timer will sound for the end of the fixing process.
12   Remove the hanger and attached radiograph and fully immerse in the second wash tank, agitating again to ensure thorough washing.
13   Switch on the ordinary light.
14   Shake off excess water and dry the radiograph, a small hairdryer is suitable for this.

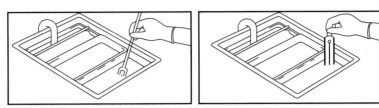

**1** Stir solutions

**2** Check temperatures of solutions

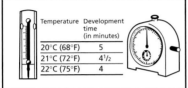

| Temperature | Development time (in minutes) |
|---|---|
| 20°C (68°F) | 5 |
| 21°C (72°F) | 4$\frac{1}{2}$ |
| 22°C (75°F) | 4 |

**3** Check development time

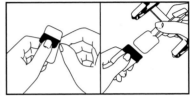

**4** Load film on hanger

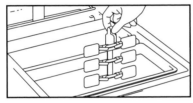

**5** Immerse films in developer and start timing

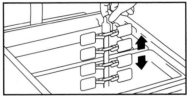

**6** Agitate films

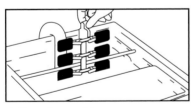

**7** Rinse thoroughly

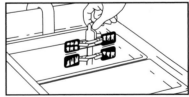

**8** Fix adequately

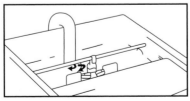

**9** Wash thoroughly

**10** Dry

**Figure 14.9** Processing.

## Automatic processing

The automatic processor follows the same principles as for manual processing, but the machine itself checks and maintains the solution temperatures, passes the exposed film through the solutions in the correct sequence and for the correct times, and then dries the film before it is ejected from the machine. The film is carried on a conveyor belt style of rollers in and out of the various tanks. The whole machine sits under a removable light-tight lid to avoid accidental exposure. The procedure of automatic processing is as follows:

1 Remove the lid and check that the solution levels are adequate.
2 Replace the lid and switch on the water supply, the machine will heat this to the correct temperature.
3 When ready, the warning lights indicating an incorrect temperature will go out and the machine is ready for use.
4 Film packets are taken into the machine through the hand ports, while cassettes are passed in through the lid.
5 The start button is activated, and the rollers begin turning.
6 The packet or cassette is opened in the usual manner and the film is carefully fed into the conveyor belt system.
7 It will be gently tugged into the machine and automatically processed.
8 Once processed and dried, the radiograph will appear at the delivery port and can be removed from the machine and viewed.
9 The refilled cassette or film packet remnants can then be removed from the machine entrance.

## Mounting

Radiographs are mounted on a transparent sheet or into preformed viewing sheets, with the patient's name and date on which they were taken. The purpose of mounting is to ensure that films do not get lost or mixed up with another patient's. Retakes are thereby avoided and the dentist has all the radiographs for one patient conveniently arranged for viewing.

In order to mount radiographs correctly, dental nurses must be able to tell whether a film is upper or lower, left or right. An elementary knowledge of dental anatomy allows a nurse to distinguish between upper and lower teeth. For example most views of upper teeth would show part of the nose or antrum air spaces, and the number of roots may also help (Figures 14.1 and 14.2). To differentiate between left and right there is a small pimple pressed into one corner of every intra-oral film. This indicates the side facing the tube (Figure 14.3). When held with the top of the convexity of the pimple facing the observer there is no difficulty in deciding which side it belongs to.

Having orientated the radiographs correctly, they are mounted as they would appear on a dental chart. Thus a radiograph of the upper left teeth is mounted at the top right of the mounting sheet, upper right teeth at the top left, lower left teeth at the bottom right, and lower right teeth at the bottom left of the mounting sheet. Extra-oral film cassettes have the letter 'L' marked into one corner, so that when placed correctly into the X-ray machine, the patient's left side is easily identifiable.

In order to avoid re-takes, it is essential that all the required information from the film can be seen properly. This requires an illuminated viewing screen with removable masking, so that only the area of the film can be seen. A magnifying glass should always be used for viewing films.

## Care of processing equipment

One of a dental nurse's many duties will be to care for all processing equipment, once trained adequately to do so. This is a vital role with regard to patient safety; poorly maintained equipment will lead to poor quality radiographs that may need to be re-taken, causing unnecessary X-ray exposure for the patient. And as stated previously, there is no 'safe level' of X-ray exposure – each one could cause cell damage. The following list summarises the points that should be included in any care and maintenance protocol.

- Ensure adequate training in processing techniques has been given.
- Always carry out the pre-processing checks correctly.
- Always wear suitable personal protective equipment (PPE) when handling all processing chemicals, as they are toxic.
- Follow the surgery policy on topping up and changing spent solutions, normally all will require full replacement on a monthly basis.
- Dispose of all waste solutions as **special waste**, under the Health and Safety policy (see Chapters 7 and 23).
- Dispose of all the lead foil from intra-oral film packets as **special waste**.
- Follow the training given, and the manufacturer's guidelines on cleaning the processing area or the automatic processor, to avoid film contamination. This is especially important with regard to the roller system in automatic machines, as films can stick to dirty rollers and be destroyed.
- Be aware of the correct functioning of the equipment, so that failures can be recognised, the equipment switched off safely, and the matter reported to the necessary person for repair.

## Causes of failure

Although many practices have abandoned manual processing in favour of automatic methods, it is still necessary for *all* dental nurses to understand what happens to a film during exposure and processing. This will help trace causes of error and prevent any need for re-takes.

Any part of a film exposed to X-rays or white light is turned black and opaque by developer. The remaining unexposed part is still sensitive to light and appears green and opaque. Fixer dissolves away the unexposed green part, leaving it completely transparent and no longer sensitive to light. Some common faults that occur during **exposure** are given in the table below.

| Fault | Reason |
| --- | --- |
| Elongation of image | Collimator angulation is too shallow, producing a long image |
| Foreshortening of image | Collimator angulation is too steep, producing a squat image |
| Coning | Collimator angulation is not central to the film, so film is partly exposed |
| Blurred image | Patient or collimator moved during exposure |
| Transparent film | Film placed the wrong way round to the collimator for exposure |
| Fogged film | Exposed to light before X-ray exposure |
| Blank film | X-ray machine not switched on, although this is unlikely to happen with modern machines, as they have exposure lights and audio signals installed |

Faults can also occur due to a poor handling technique or by poor preparation of the processing equipment – both responsibilities of the dental nurse, and both avoidable by adequate training and by following procedures accurately. Some common **handling faults** are given below.

| Faults | Reasons |
| --- | --- |
| Scratches or fingerprints | Catching the film on the tank side during immersion Not holding the film by the edges |
| Blank spots | Film splashed with fixer before developing |
| Black line across film | Film bent or folded during processing |
| Brown or green stains | Inadequate fixing due to old solution |
| Crazed pattern on film | Film dried too quickly over a strong heat source |
| Presence of crystals on film | Insufficient washing after fixing |

In addition, poor quality or unreadable radiographs will be produced if old film stock is used or if the stock has not been stored correctly. Unexposed film packets must be stored as follows:

- Away from all sources of radiation
- Away from all heat sources, ideally at room temperature
- Away from all liquids that may penetrate the packets and destroy the films before use
- In stock rotation, so that older films are used first

Poor quality radiographs can also be produced due to **equipment preparation faults**, the more common ones are given below.

| Faults | Reasons |
|---|---|
| Dark film | Developer solution too concentrated |
| | Developer solution temperature too high |
| | Over developed |
| Blank film | Film placed in fixer solution before developer solution, so the image is destroyed |
| Partly blank film | Film partially immersed in developer solution |
| Fogged film | Processing room is not light-tight |
| Faint image | Developer solution too weak |
| | Developer solution temperature too low |
| | Under developed |
| Fading image | Inadequate fixing time so image is not permanently held on the film |
| Loss of film | Film stuck in roller system due to poor cleaning and maintenance |
| Visible artefacts | Film contaminated with solution spillages, in cassettes or on work surfaces |

## Quality assurance of films

All of the faults described previously are avoidable. However, it may not be realised by the dental team that a regular problem exists unless radiographs are regularly checked for quality, and this is especially so in large, multi-dentist surgeries. A processing fault may affect the radiographs of several dentists, but unless someone is analysing the radiographs from all surgeries, it can easily be overlooked. This is the purpose of a quality assurance (QA) system – where **all** radiographs are analysed and scored according to a universal system of quality so that commonly occurring problems will be identified.

With suitable training, the running of a QA system of radiograph analysis can easily be run by the dental nurse, the aim being to reduce all faults to a minimum or to eliminate them completely. Indeed, in line with the relevant Ionising Radiation legislation and with clinical governance, the running of a QA system in dental surgeries is now a legal requirement.

When run correctly, the QA system should achieve the following:

- Involve a simple to use scoring system known by all staff
- Easily identify areas of concern
- Develop solutions to the problems identified
- Limit the number of patient exposures to the minimum required for clinical necessity, therefore, to achieve ALARA (As Low As Reasonably Achievable)

A simple to use scoring system set out in clinical governance guidelines is as follows:

- **Score 1** – excellent quality radiograph with no errors present
- **Score 2** – diagnostically acceptable quality, minimal errors present that do not prevent the radiograph from being used for diagnosis

■ **Score 3** – unacceptable quality, where errors present prevent the radiograph from being used for diagnosis

Score 1 should be at a minimum of 70% of all exposures, while score 3 should be at a maximum of 10%. The results need to be easily recorded after every exposure so that they can be analysed on a regular basis, and any problems identified.

A similar QA system can be set up to monitor other areas of dental radiography, such as equipment, working procedures, or staff training, and so on.

## Dangers of ionising radiation

X-rays cannot be seen, heard or felt, and therein lies the danger. As they cannot be perceived by any of the senses, it is easily forgotten that they are potentially dangerous to health, and it is just as easy to ignore every safety precaution. An overdose can give rise to serious effects, ranging from a mild burn to leukaemia. Special legal requirements to ensure the health and safety of persons exposed to radiation are in force for dental practice. They are described later.

In the course of dental radiography the patient never receives an overdose. It is the radiographer, not the patient, who is most at risk, as the former is continually taking X-rays and must therefore take strict precautions to avoid accidental exposure. The following precautions should be taken to protect patients and staff.

■ Radiation safety must be checked at least every three years to ensure that X-ray sets are adequately shielded to prevent stray radiation, and that processing equipment and procedure are satisfactory. All sets must have regular professional maintenance.
■ Use of the fastest film (E and F speed) will allow the shortest possible exposure time. Indeed, there is no justification for using anything but the fastest available film. Cassettes should be fitted with the fastest (rare earth) intensifying screens.
■ Plastic aiming cones on X-ray sets are no longer acceptable and must be replaced by rectangular collimator tubes to further reduce beam size to the safest level.

The combination of fastest film, shortest exposure and narrowest beam will alone reduce the amount of scattered radiation by 40%.

■ The special film-holder/beam-aiming devices, already mentioned, should be used for periapical and bite-wing radiographs, and the paralleling technique used in preference to the bisected angle method.
■ The operator must stand well clear of the X-ray beam during exposure, at the full length of the cable on the time switch; this should be not less than **2 m**. On

no account must a dental nurse hold the film in place for a patient; if a child cannot keep it still, the parent must hold it in place, and wear a protective lead apron.

- Exposure of the reproductive organs to X-rays has produced abnormalities in the offspring of laboratory animals. Similar exposure of humans may occur from scattered radiation during dental radiography. Although it is insufficient to produce such genetic changes in the case of pregnant dental patients, any possibility can be excluded by strict adherence to all the required safeguards.
- The amount of stray radiation received by staff can be checked by means of a film badge. This is an intra-oral film which is worn at waist level for up to three months. It is then processed to indicate whether an excessive dosage is being received. If so, expert advice must be sought immediately to trace and eliminate the cause. Staff working in rooms adjacent to the surgery should also wear badges as X-rays can pass through walls.

Film badges are called **personal monitoring dosimeters** and are supplied by the National Radiological Protection Board (NRPB), or a local medical physics department. They process them, notify the dosage received, and can arrange appropriate investigation if it is too high.

- Every radiograph must not only be necessary but also of diagnostic value. There should be no need for re-takes because of faulty technique or processing. Re-takes mean unnecessary additional exposure of patients and staff. To ensure perfect results the films must be in good condition, taken correctly, processed carefully and mounted properly.
- X-ray sets should be disconnected from their electricity supply when not in use.

## Legal requirements

The Health and Safety regulations governing the safe use of ionising radiation in dentistry are laid out in the following:

- **Ionising Radiation Regulations 1999 (IRR99)**
- **Ionising Radiation (Medical Exposure) Regulations 2000 (IRR(ME)2000)**

IRR99 is concerned with the protection of staff, and IRR(ME) 2000 is concerned with the protection of patients. Initially, all dental surgeries must notify the Health and Safety Executive that X-ray equipment is on the premises and is used for patient irradiation. The points of each set of regulations that are relevant to dental nurses are outlined below.

Every dental surgery must make the following formal appointments, to ensure that a named person has responsibility for the safety of staff and patients.

- **The Legal Person** – this is a designated person who has to ensure that the dental surgery and all its staff comply fully with both sets of regulations, and this is usually the senior dentist.
- **The Radiation Protection Adviser** (**RPA**) – this is a medical physicist, who is a specialist in the field of ionising radiation, and is appointed in writing to give advice on staff and public safety with regard to IRR99.
- **The Radiation Protection Supervisor** (**RPS**) – this is a designated person who can assess the risks of ionising radiation in the dental surgery and ensure that precautions are taken to minimise them, in accordance with IRR99; this is usually a senior dentist or a dental nurse with radiographic qualifications.

The role of the RPA is to give advice on the actions each surgery must take to comply with the regulations, and will include all of the following:

- The installation of all new X-ray machines
- The regular maintenance and certificated checks that are required for each X-ray machine to ensure that the minimum exposure to radiation occurs
- The **contingency plans** that need to be in place in case of a malfunction of an X-ray machine
- The investigation of any malfunction
- The designation of a **controlled area** around each X-ray machine, where no-one but the patient may be present during an exposure
- Advise on **risk assessments** with regard to restricting staff and patient exposure to ionising radiation, and review the assessments every five years
- Advise on the necessary **staff training** required so that designated duties are carried out competently and safely
- Assess staff protection with regard to the numbers of exposures carried out on the premises; if more than 150 intra-oral films or 50 DPTs are taken weekly, staff are **legally required** to wear a personal monitoring badge
- Advise on the appropriate action to take if analysis of the badges indicates excessive exposure to any staff
- Advise on the running of **QA programmes**

The Legal Person is responsible for organising a three-yearly assessment of radiation safety within the surgery, by arranging for an inspection by NRPB, or by using their X-ray machine and processing test kit to carry out the necessary checks, and then sending them to NRPB for analysis.

In addition, the Legal Person must draw up a set of **Local Rules** which have to be displayed at each X-ray machine, so that they can be referred to by all staff. The Local Rules must give all of the following information:

- The name of the designated RPS and RPA
- The identification of each controlled area to all staff and patients, to limit unauthorised entry during exposure

- Show the standard warning sign at each controlled area, indicating the use of ionising radiation – this is a black sign on a yellow background (Figure 14.10)
- A summary of the correct working instructions for each controlled area, including the designated 2 m safety zone around the X-ray machine head
- The contingency plan to be followed in the event of a machine malfunction
- The use of a red light and an audible buzzer to indicate the actual exposure time

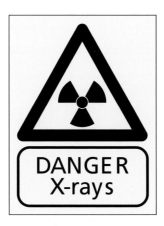

**Figure 14.10** Radiation warning sign.

## Role of the dental nurse

Following the compulsory registration of dental nurses with the General Dental Council from July 2008, no unqualified staff will be allowed to work in dental practice unless they are enrolled on an accredited dental nurse training course. These staff, and any qualified or registered dental nurses, can then be given suitable and documented 'in-house' training with regard to the use of ionising radiation so that they may carry out the following duties:

- Assist in the stock control of films and processing solutions
- Process films, and mount and store them correctly
- Clean and maintain processing equipment
- Change processing solutions as necessary, and store them safely as special waste
- Run QA programmes

Qualified and registered dental nurses may also hold the post-certificate qualification in Dental Radiography (Chapter 2), and are legally allowed to carry out the following additional duties:

- Select exposure times and doses
- Position patients and films ready for exposure
- Expose the films and patients to the X-rays
- Act as the RPS for the surgery
- Maintain and upkeep all of the necessary records with regard to ionising radiation safety in a **Radiation Protection File**

# 15 Patient Records

The purpose of dental records is to provide an up-to-date case history of each patient's condition, and includes the examination findings and treatment given on each attendance at the surgery. By referring back to previous visits the dentist can assess the results of earlier courses of treatment and thereby decide the best line of treatment on future occasions. Adequate records also facilitate the transfer of patients between dentists in the practice when absence or staff changes occur. Another dentist can then continue any previous treatment with all the required information already available.

Recording methods, and the amount of detail recorded, vary considerably from practice to practice, but patients' records consist basically of personal and clinical information. They should include all of the following:

- Patient name, address, date of birth and telephone numbers
- Doctor's details
- Full medical history
- Dental history
- Contemporaneous (date order) clinical notes of each attendance
- Tooth and periodontal chartings
- Soft tissue assessments
- Details of all appointments with other staff, such as the hygienist
- All legally required National Health Service (NHS) or private paperwork
- Consent forms
- Copies of all referral letters
- Correctly identified and mounted radiographs
- Laboratory slips
- Records of all payment transactions
- Copies of all patient correspondence

For new patients the personal details, reason for attendance, and medical and dental history are conveniently recorded by giving or sending a medical history form, such as the British Dental Association (BDA) Confidential Medical History Form, for home completion before their first visit. At that visit it would be assessed by the dentist, signed and dated, and placed in the patient's file. Clinical details of the visit, and subsequent ones, are entered on a dental chart and kept in the file.

A separate record of all attendances and treatment each day is kept in the day-book, or its computerised equivalent, and forms a valuable cross-reference system with the charts.

Apart from clinical records, those relating to practice administration are just as important. Such records concern the supply and purchase of equipment, materials and drugs used for treatment, details of despatch and receipt of work done by dental laboratories and staff personnel records.

Most practices use computers for dealing with the following:

■ Stock records and accounts
■ Patient recall systems
■ Standardised correspondence, such as account letters or appointment cancellation letters

## Importance of records

Under NHS regulations, dentists are expected to keep adequate records. In all branches of dentistry, whether NHS or private, records taken at the time are legally valid documents and serious legal difficulties may arise if they are inadequate or inaccurate. Errors or omissions in recording information may result in incorrect treatment or failure to provide necessary treatment.

Dental records are also extremely valuable as a means of establishing identity. In fatal accidents where facial features are destroyed, the teeth are usually unaffected and can be compared with dentists' records to identify a victim.

Proper records allow correct treatment planning and provide a check on details of past treatment. They form the basis on which fees are calculated and accounts rendered to patients. Failed appointments and refusals of treatment are noted and the patient's attitude to dental health assessed. Appropriate recall arrangements can then be made for each patient.

The dental nurse must accurately record information given by the patient or dictated by the dentist, ensuring that records are filed properly, made available at each appointment, and signed as necessary by patient and dentist.

Adequate records allow the practice to run with the greatest efficiency for all concerned and should be retained for at least 11 years after completion of treatment or to the age of 25 years in the case of children's records. Many difficulties concerning individual patients can be prevented altogether if complete records are available of all attendances at the practice, while no time is wasted in putting such information at the dentist's disposal. Recording and filing systems may vary considerably in different practices, but whichever method is used, records must always be accurate, legible, comprehensive and easily accessible.

The legal and ethical issues involved in good record keeping involve all of the following aspects of patient care:

- **Valid consent** (Figure 15.1)
- **Confidentiality** (Figure 15.2)
- **Data protection**
- **Patient complaints** (Figure 15.3)
- **General Dental Council (GDC) standards for professionals** (Figure 15.4)
- **Responsibilities of dental care professionals (DCPs) following registration**

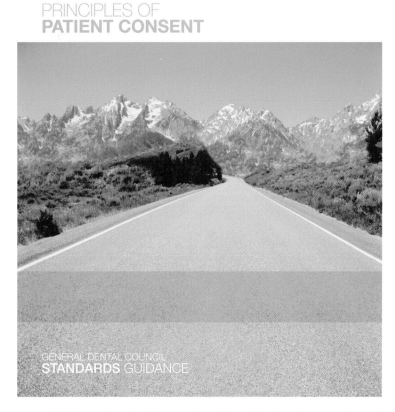

Figure 15.1 GDC Standards Guidance – Principles of Patient Consent. Reproduced with kind permission from the General Dental Council (www.gdc-uk.org).

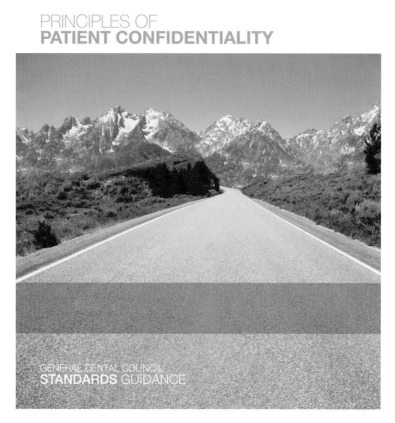

Figure 15.2 GDC Standards Guidance – Principles of Patient Confidentiality. Reproduced with kind permission from the General Dental Council (www.gdc-uk.org).

## Valid consent

The aim of good communication between the dental team and patients is to fully inform them of their proposed treatment needs, including any risks and possible complications of the proposed treatment. It should also discuss the possible consequences of not having the treatment offered, so that the patient is fully aware of all the *pros* and *cons* and can give valid consent. The issue of consent is covered by the Caldicott Report. For the patient consent to be valid it must:

- Be given voluntarily
- Be fully informed and specific to the treatment of the patient
- Be given either orally, in writing, or implied (such as by sitting in the dental chair)
- Include details of costs (whether NHS or private), and agreement to pay the costs when requested to do so
- Be specific for any necessary changes to the original treatment plan

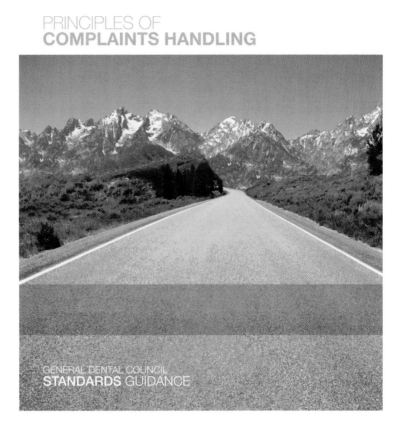

PRINCIPLES OF
**COMPLAINTS HANDLING**

GENERAL DENTAL COUNCIL
**STANDARDS** GUIDANCE

**Figure 15.3** GDC Standards Guidance – Principles of Complaints Handling.
Reproduced with kind permission from the General Dental Council
(www.gdc-uk.org).

By law, consent can be given by anyone of sound mind over the age of 16 years, or those under 16 years who are able to understand the information given. For other patients under 16 years, the written consent of a parent or guardian is required.

In the case of an incompetent adult who requires treatment, the law is quite specific on the following points.

■ The patient alone can allow the treatment to proceed, no-one can give consent on their behalf.
■ The patient must be assessed by the dentist to determine the validity of any consent given.
■ Sometimes a second professional opinion is required to determine the validity.
■ The dentist must always act in the best interests of the patient.
■ The dentist must be able to justify their actions if necessary.

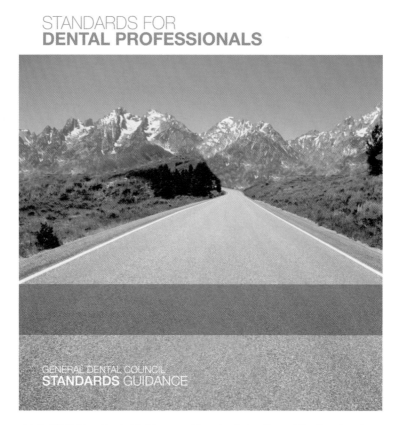

STANDARDS FOR
**DENTAL PROFESSIONALS**

GENERAL DENTAL COUNCIL
**STANDARDS** GUIDANCE

Figure 15.4 GDC Standards Guidance – Standards for Dental Professionals.
Reproduced with kind permission from the General Dental Council (www.gdc-uk.org).

In general, these patients tend to be referred for dental care to a special needs unit, where the dental team deal with these issues on a daily basis.

For all other patients seen in general practice, good communication skills must be used by the whole dental team to avoid misunderstandings. All must be able to listen to the patient, communicate at an appropriate level, avoid making incorrect assumptions, especially with regard to their social and financial status, and to always be fully open and honest with them.

## Confidentiality of patient details

Patients have a right to expect that their dental records will not be disclosed to a third party without their permission, and the whole dental team are bound by this duty of care. The specific legislation with regard to confidentiality issues is covered by the following:

- **Access to Health Records Act 1990**
- **Data Protection Act 1998**
- **Freedom of Information Act**

Before the statutory registration of DCPs began in July 2008, all dentists had vicarious liability for the acts and omissions of their staff – that meant that the dentist alone took responsibility for any mistakes made by the staff. It was the dentist's responsibility to ensure that all staff were trained in the correct practice protocols and procedures to avoid making mistakes. Since registration, DCPs are governed by the GDC and their 'Standards Guidance' documentation (Figure 15.4), as well as the 2005 Amendment Order to the Dentists Act 1984. Taken together, these quite clearly state the responsibilities of DCPs as follows:

- Work within the legislative guidelines of their profession at all times
- Always act in the best interests of the patient
- Failure to do so will render the DCP liable to prosecution, or allow the patient to take legal action against them
- If the dentist instructs the DCP to act in an inappropriate manner, they are expected to 'whistle blow' and report the matter
- They must remain up to date with all the ethical legislation governing their profession, and abide by it at all times

One of the easiest ways to fall foul of the legislation is to inadvertently breach the confidentiality of a patient, so the following issues of confidentiality must be followed at all times, by the whole dental team.

- Patients must not be discussed in front of other patients.
- Privacy must be maintained when discussing any personal matters with patients.
- Attendance at the practice is private, and cannot be revealed to other patients, to employers, nor to schools.
- All written communications with patients should be sent in sealed envelopes.
- Dental records must be kept for the correct length of time by the practice and not be destroyed beforehand, either partially or wholly.

Information about a patient can only be disclosed to a third party with the patient's written consent. However, there are some circumstances under which the dentist has a statutory obligation to disclose the necessary information:

- To assist in the identification of a driver involved in a road traffic accident, under the Road Traffic Act 1988
- When requested to do so by the Dental Practice Division of the Business Services Authority (formerly known as the Dental Practice Board)
- To provide information about a child to their parent or legal guardian

- When it is in the public's interest, such as with suspected or known criminals
- When disclosure is requested by Court Order, under the Prevention of Terrorism Act 1989 or under the Police and Criminal Evidence Act 1984

Patients also have the right of access to their own manual or computerised health records, under the Access to Health Records Act 1990 and the Data Protection Act 1998. This covers all their medical and dental records written since November 1991, with the following provisos:

- Only the dentist, as the record holder, can approve access
- The patient request must be made in writing
- The dentist must respond within 40 days
- The patient identity must be checked before releasing their records
- Once viewed, the patient can request that any inaccuracies in their records are amended
- Any dental terminology, abbreviations or jargon must be explained on request

The DCP must therefore not release any records or parts of records themselves, nor alter them in any way. They must be true, accurate and contemporaneous (as written at the time), and contain no derogatory comments. If the DCP is responsible for writing the notes, they should be written exactly as dictated by the dentist, and not altered in any way.

There are certain instances when the dentist can refuse to disclose the patient records, as follows:

- When disclosure would cause serious harm to the patient
- When a second person is mentioned by name and has not given consent for disclosure (does not include the dental team)
- When access to their records after their death has specifically been refused by the patient beforehand

## Patient complaints

The GDC requires all dental practices to have an 'in-house' patient complaint handling policy, which should aim to fully resolve any complaint received to everyone's satisfaction, and as quickly as possible. Ideally, the matter should be resolved without the need for other authorities, such as the Primary Care Trust (PCT) or the GDC, becoming involved.

Any patient complaint, if not spurious in nature, can be used by the dental team as an opportunity to review and change practice procedures if necessary, with the aim of improving the standard of service being offered to the patients. The complaint system itself must include the following:

- Patient knowledge that the system exists, by posters or leaflets as necessary
- The name of the designated staff member responsible for dealing with complaints, and their deputy
- An acknowledgement of receipt within 10 days of the complaint
- Assurance that the complaint will be handled in strict confidence

Good communication skills and an open, honest approach are important when dealing with a complaint, and a sympathetic and understanding manner will often diffuse what could be a tense situation. All complaints should be resolved at the earliest opportunity, and often all that is required by the patient is an apology. This can be given without fear of admitting liability or negligence. When a verbal complaint is received, it should be handled as follows:

- In private and away from other patients
- Listen attentively to the patient and use good body language to show that the complaint is being taken seriously
- Allow the patient to express their views without interrupting
- Take notes if necessary, so that the complaint can be summarised correctly
- If an apology is appropriate, give one immediately but without liability
- Discuss any intended action with the patient, and inform them when this has been carried out

A written complaint is often more serious, as the patient has had time to gather their thoughts and consider the matter beforehand. Each PCT issues its own guidelines on the correct protocol to follow, but generally the complaint should be handled as follows:

- Acknowledge receipt of the complaint within two working days
- Investigate the matter thoroughly
- Send a written investigation report to the patient within 10 working days
- No blame should be apportioned, nor personal comments and opinions made
- Be open and sympathetic in the response, but not defensive
- Offer an apology where appropriate, and the opportunity to discuss the matter further if the patient wishes

If the patient decides to take the matter further the PCT will become involved, or they can make a direct formal complaint to either the PCT (over NHS issues), or to the GDC (over NHS or private issues). Either body can then be requested to conciliate or order an independent review of the matter, as they see fit. As DCPs are personally liable for their own acts and omissions now, the whole dental team must have their own liability insurance in place, so that all legal costs and any compensation awards are covered financially.

## GDC standards for dental professionals

The GDC have issued a series of booklets to all registered dental professionals, which set out the standards expected of the dental team. As new team members train and become qualified, and are then entered onto the dental register by the GDC, their own copy of the standards will be issued to them. The pertinent points for the dental nurse are summarised below.

### CPD and lifelong learning

The need to constantly update the skills and knowledge required to carry out the duties of a dental nurse will ensure that the best interest of the patient is always put first. New techniques and skills will be learned, and less satisfactory issues of patient care will become obsolete. CPD and lifelong learning are covered in Chapter 2.

### Put patients' interests first

Specifically to act to protect the patient, in the following ways:

- Act in the best interests of the patient when handling questions and complaints, and respect their right to complain
- Work within the limits of your own knowledge and competence
- Make no claims that could mislead the patient
- Take action to protect the patient if you or a colleague has a health issue (Figure 15.5)

### Respect patients' dignity and choices

Respect patients' dignity and choices with regard to the following:

- Treat all patients politely and with respect, and do not discriminate against them
- Promote equal opportunities for all
- Communicate effectively with them to promote their responsibility for their own dental health
- Maintain appropriate boundaries in all relationships with patients

### Protect patient confidentiality

Protect patient confidentiality by doing the following:

- Treat all patient information as confidential
- Keep all information secure from others, and only use it for the purpose for which it was given
- Take advice if required to reveal information before doing so

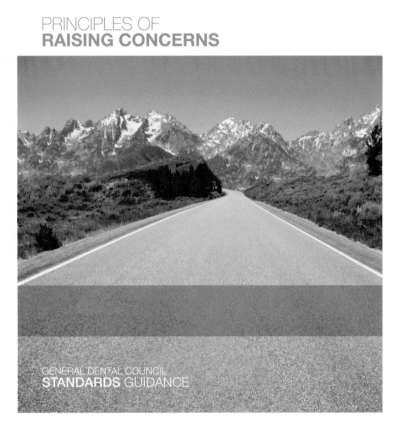

Figure 15.5 GDC Standards Guidance – Principles of Raising Concerns. Reproduced with kind permission from the General Dental Council (www.gdc-uk.org).

## Co-operate with others

Co-operate with others in the interests of the patient (Figure 15.6):

- Respect the role of others involved in patient care
- Do not discriminate against team members
- Communicate effectively with other team members

## Be trustworthy

Be trustworthy as a professional person:

- Always act honestly and fairly
- Apply all of the standards set out to all professional relationships and activities
- Maintain appropriate standards of personal behaviour at all times

PRINCIPLES OF
**DENTAL TEAM WORKING**

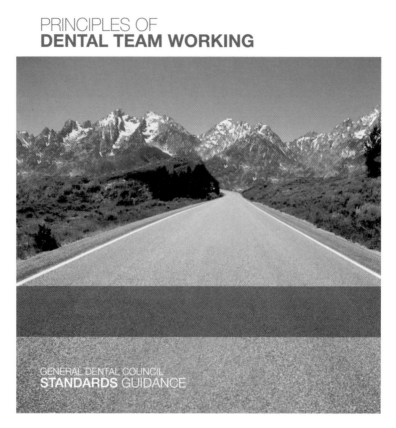

GENERAL DENTAL COUNCIL
**STANDARDS** GUIDANCE

Figure 15.6 GDC Standards Guidance – Principles of Dental Team Working.
Reproduced with kind permission from the General Dental Council (www.gdc-uk.org).

## Clinical records

Clinical records consist of the past and present appointment and day books, as well as records of each patient attending the practice. Individual patient records include the medical history, dental history, present condition, charting and treatment, consent forms, estimates, accounts and correspondence.

### Medical history and present condition

Full details of patients' past and present illnesses, and other medical issues must be regularly updated. Assessment and updating of the medical and dental significance of this history is solely the responsibility of the dentist, and should be carried out at each attendance. The patient should check any entries, and then sign and date the medical history form at each update. Medical history forms vary considerably, but the basic areas of questioning should include the following:

- Currently receiving any medical treatment
- Any history of steroid use within the past two years
- Details of any current medications, including non-prescription ones
- Any allergies, or reactions to anaesthetics
- Currently pregnant, or a nursing mother
- HIV positive status
- History of rheumatic fever, liver or kidney disorders
- History of any heart or circulatory disorders
- History of any respiratory disorders
- History of diabetes, epilepsy, or arthritis
- Details of any medical warning cards issued
- Smoking, tobacco and alcohol history

In order to ensure complete confidentiality, a medical history must be taken and discussed in private where it cannot be overheard. Patients cannot be expected to provide full details unless they are satisfied of privacy.

Many conditions or drugs may influence the dental treatment plan. Some examples are given below.

- The method of pain control (Chapter 22) may depend on the condition of the patient's heart, chest and liver, and whether drugs are being taken for medical treatment.
- If a patient has suffered from any heart conditions or rheumatic fever it may be necessary to give antibiotic cover (Chapter 6) before extractions or subgingival scaling, as a precautionary measure against infective endocarditis.
- Extractions may be inadvisable while a patient is being treated with certain drugs such as anticoagulants and corticosteroids, or after irradiation treatment of the jaws. Special care is needed for patients with bleeding disorders.
- Allergy to certain drugs may cause a severe anaphylactic reaction (Chapter 5). Patients are asked if any untoward reactions have occurred before. Penicillin and its derivatives, such as amoxicillin, are the drugs most likely to be involved in dental practice.
- Adverse reactions can occur because of an interaction between drugs being taken for medical treatment and drugs administered during dental treatment (Chapter 5).
- Patients may also be allergic to certain dental materials, such as latex rubber. A medical history of eczema and/or hay fever will alert the dentist to a potential risk of allergic reactions.
- Special care is necessary during pregnancy:
  - There must be no contact with staff or other patients who are rubella (German measles) contacts
  - Local anaesthesia is safe but general anaesthesia and drugs of any other kind should be avoided
  - In the late stages of pregnancy, patients should not be treated in the supine position

■ Patients who have been in contact with infectious diseases such as mumps and rubella should not attend the surgery while these illnesses are still active (Chapter 7).

■ Careful observation of patients will detect signs which may affect treatment: breathlessness and pallor are suggestive of anaemia, while cyanosis (blue complexion) and jaundice are indicative of heart and liver disease, respectively.

■ Special precautions are necessary for treatment of known hepatitis and human immunodeficiency virus (HIV) carriers (Chapter 7), and immunocompromised patients (Chapter 6).

The name of the patient's doctor should always be included in the records. Then, if any doubts arise, the doctor can be consulted before treatment is undertaken.

## Dental history

Diagnosis of the present condition and determination of the treatment plan may depend on details of earlier dental disorders and their treatment. Knowledge of previous difficulties such as excessive bleeding, poor response to anaesthetics, difficult extractions, allergy to dental materials, latex gloves or rubber dam, or any other complications, will help the dentist to avoid their reoccurrence.

## Present condition

The present condition of the teeth is recorded on the dental chart, and any other conditions, such as the state of existing restorations and dentures, poor oral hygiene, periodontal disease, malocclusion, close bite, discoloured teeth, etc., which may affect treatment are also noted. The dentist can then assess the patient's general attitude towards dental health and accordingly advise the most appropriate treatment.

The soft tissues of the mouth and neck are also examined for early diagnosis of oral cancer (Chapter 6) and the results noted. The periodontal condition is also noted and charted if necessary (Chapter 12). The medical history of alcohol consumption, smoking and chewing habits is directly relevant to these conditions. Habitual chewing of tobacco, pan, and use of *gutkha* or *supari* is common in Asian communities. The temporo-mandibular joint, too, is checked for clicks or pain (Chapter 8). The results of these, and any other, tests must be recorded as negative or positive in the patient's file.

## Treatment

Full details of treatment and the date on which it is given are recorded on the dental chart. These will include the results of special examinations such as:

■ X-rays, vitality tests, periodontal status, oral cancer check and orthodontic study models

- Local anaesthesia, type of filling and lining, shades of filling, artificial teeth and crowns
- Drugs and dosage, prescriptions issued
- Complications, e.g. excessive bleeding or retained roots after extractions
- Treatment plans and options, cost estimates, and the patient's choice
- Missed appointments and refusals of treatment
- Any accidents or complications, such as retained roots following extractions or breakage of an instrument, e.g. root canal file, must be explained to the patient and recorded, together with the measures and options offered, and emergency treatment arrangements

The charts and treatment notes folder will also include:

- Radiographs and clinical photographs
- Written treatment plans, cost estimates and consent forms
- Referral letters and reports
- Any other relevant documents and correspondence

As in the case of a medical history, the dentist, not the dental nurse, is responsible for obtaining consent to treatment. The issue of consent has been discussed earlier.

## NHS records

The NHS provides a large number of forms for detailing treatment plans, costs, emergency visits, orthodontic and periodontal treatment, exemption from payments, and many other aspects of NHS procedure. The most commonly used are given below:

- A standard chart (Form FP 25) for recording patient visits, and treatment required and provided, together with a folder (Form FP 25 a) to hold subsequent treatment forms and details
- Form FP17 DC/GP17DC, which is given to the patient. It outlines treatment required and the NHS charges, as well as the details and costs of any agreed private treatment
- The Dental Estimates Form FP17, which is used by practitioners to record details of treatment required, and subsequently given, and provides a form of account for payment claimed
- Form FP10D, for prescriptions

Although practitioners are not obliged to use these particular forms, they are expected to keep adequate records.

Many practices are now partially or fully computerised with regard to patient records, but all the information held must be accessible to the dental team, the authorities, and the patient, as necessary. Several software systems are available for use and the NHS records detailed above are compatible with many of them. Whichever system is used, and whether manual or computerised, the records must be written, handled, and stored in full accordance with all of the relevant legislation. A good knowledge of the use of computers and information technology is required by the modern dental nurse nowadays.

# 16 Fillings and Materials

The conservative treatment of caries, when the pulp is vital and unexposed, is by removing the caries and filling the cavity to restore the tooth. If the pulp is exposed or dead, root canal therapy (endodontic treatment) is usually necessary before the crown of the tooth is permanently filled. The aims of tooth restoration are to:

- Restore the tooth to its normal shape and prevent stagnation areas developing
- Restore the function of the tooth, for adequate mastication
- Restore the retentive shape of the tooth if it acts as a bridge abutment or denture retainer
- Restore aesthetics
- Alleviate discomfort or pain

Teeth may be restored with temporary or permanent fillings. These are described in detail in the sections on Temporary filling materials and Permanent filling materials later in the chapter.

## Classification of cavities

Cavities are classified into five different types, depending on the site of the original caries attack. This is called **Black's classification**, after the American dentist who devised it. In general usage, this classification of cavities also applies to the fillings inserted in each class of cavity.

- **Class I** cavities are those involving a **single** surface, in a pit or fissure. Thus a class I filling could be an occlusal filling or a buccal or lingual filling.
- **Class II** cavities involve at least **two** surfaces – the mesial or distal, and the occlusal surface of a **molar** or **premolar**. Thus a class II filling could be a mesial-occlusal (mo) filling in a premolar, for example, or a mesial-occlusal-distal (mod) filling in a molar.
- **Class III** cavities involve the mesial or distal surface of an **incisor** or **canine**.

- **Class IV** cavities are the same as class III but extend to involve the **incisal edge** on the affected side.
- **Class V** cavities involve the **cervical margin** of any tooth. Thus a class V filling could be a labial cervical filling in an upper incisor, or a lingual cervical filling in a lower molar.

## Cavity preparation

A permanent filling cannot be inserted directly into a carious cavity. Careful preparation of the cavity is required to ensure the following.

- All plaque and soft carious dentine is removed from the cavity margins but, as mentioned in Chapter 11, the deepest layer of dentine may be conserved to avoid exposure of the pulp.
- As much of the enamel as possible, after removal of plaque, is also conserved.
- The filling will be a permanent fixture.
- Caries will not recur at its margins.

The general principles of cavity preparation are given below.

- No plaque or caries must be left on the cavity walls. Plaque and carious dentine are removed with an **excavator** (Figure 16.1) or a large round **bur** in a low-speed **handpiece** (see Figures 16.8 and 16.10 later in the chapter).
- Undermined enamel is removed with an **enamel chisel** (Figure 16.2a–c) or a bur in a high-speed handpiece.
- The cavity is made retentive by cutting tiny grooves in the cavity walls, and the occlusal fissures are prepared for sealing if necessary. This is all done with a handpiece and fine burs.
- Burs, chisels, and **cervical margin trimmers** (Figure 16.2d) are then used to finish off the cavity according to the type of filling necessary.

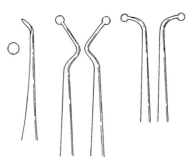

Figure 16.1 Excavators.

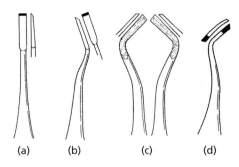

Figure 16.2 Chisels. (a) Straight. (b) Bin-angle. (c) Hatchet. (d) Cervical margin trimmer.

## Retention of fillings

Permanent fillings are meant to stay permanently and the cavity must be specially prepared to provide maximum retention. Before explaining how this is done, it is necessary to consider the types of fillings used. There are two types available: plastic and pre-constructed.

**Plastic fillings** are soft and plastic on insertion but set and harden in the cavity. They include temporary cements, amalgam, glass ionomer cement and composite fillings.

Pre-constructed restorations are called **inlays**, and these are made in the laboratory, after the teeth have been prepared, and then cemented into place.

Retention for plastic fillings is obtained by simply cutting tiny grooves in the cavity walls to make the entrance smaller than its inside dimensions (Figure 16.3). Thus a plastic filling can be packed in when soft but cannot come out once it is hardened. For fillings involving occlusal and mesial surfaces, or occlusal and distal, a **dovetail** effect is produced by grooving the cavity walls to prevent the filling coming out mesially or distally (Figure 16.3). Note that this diagram is deliberately exaggerated to show more clearly the principles of retention. In reality, sound tissue is not sacrificed for the sake of extensive undercuts. Tiny grooves in the cavity walls are sufficient.

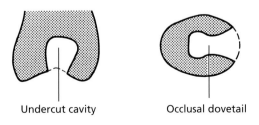

Undercut cavity          Occlusal dovetail

Figure 16.3 Cavity preparation for plastic fillings.

Sometimes it is not possible to prepare cavities which are sufficiently undercut to retain a plastic filling. In such cases they may be made retentive in other ways: by dentine pins for amalgam; acid etching for composites; and chemical bonding for glass ionomer cement. These methods are covered in the appropriate section for each filling material.

Inlays are hard and rigid when inserted into the cavity, so the dentist would not be able to place and seat them fully if undercuts were present. To prevent them coming out occlusally, they rely on parallel cavity walls and adhesive cement. As with plastic fillings, a small dovetail effect may be used to prevent mesial or distal dislodgement.

## Cavity lining

Before a permanent filling is inserted the cavity may need to be lined. A **lining** is an insulating layer of cement which has the following functions:

- Protects the pulp from temperature fluctuations through metallic materials
- Protects the pulp from chemical irritation of non-metallic materials
- Seals the pulp from any residual caries bacteria, allowing secondary dentine to be laid down

Pain, and possibly death of the tooth, may occur through failure to insert an adequate lining.

The materials used as linings are zinc oxide and eugenol cement, zinc phosphate cement, polycarboxylate cement and calcium hydroxide.

## Insertion

The technique of inserting a filling varies with the type of cavity and filling material used. This matter is therefore discussed separately under the appropriate filling material.

## Polishing

Permanent fillings may need trimming to remove any high spots or proud edges, followed by polishing to provide a clean, smooth, comfortable surface. Some fillings can be polished immediately after insertion but those with a long setting time are polished at a subsequent visit. The instruments and materials used depend on the type of filling and are detailed in the section concerned.

# Moisture control

Adequate moisture control during restorative procedures is one of the most important duties of the dental nurse. Control of moisture – from saliva, blood, or instrument cooling sprays – is necessary to:

- Protect the patient's airway from fluid inhalation
- Ensure the patient is comfortable during treatment
- Allow the dentist good visibility, therefore avoiding inadvertent patient injury
- Allow the restorative materials to set correctly, without moisture contamination
- Allow the adhesion of cements and linings to the tooth
- Avoid the uncontrolled loss of materials from the cavity during use, such as acid etchant which can burn the soft tissues

The methods used to control moisture are described below.

## Suction

Suction can be either high-speed aspiration, for fast removal of moisture, or low-speed aspiration for continual moisture control without sucking at the soft tissues. The patient holds a **saliva ejector** attached to the suction unit or **aspirator** to provide low-speed control (Figure 16.4). Many different types of ejector are used, and those with a flange to keep the tongue away are particularly helpful. The dental nurse assists in suction by holding a wide-bore aspirator tube to provide high-speed suction, or by using a retractor to keep the tongue or cheek away.

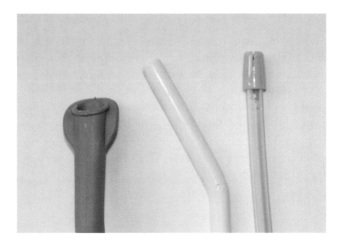

**Figure 16.4** Aspirator and ejector tips.

## Absorbent materials

Cotton wool rolls or absorbent pads are placed in the buccal or lingual sulcus to absorb saliva and to keep the soft tissues away from the teeth. Cotton wool pledgets are used to dab the actual cavity dry, while excessive saliva contamination can be prevented by placing a 'Dry guard' over the parotid salivary gland duct. These pads contain an absorbent material similar to that used in babies' nappies, and can retain considerable volumes of fluid. The cavity itself can be further dried by blowing it with compressed air from the triple syringe of the dental unit.

## Rubber dam

This is the best method of moisture control. The rubber dam is a thin sheet of rubber which is placed over a tooth to isolate it from the rest of the mouth. A **rubber dam punch** (Figure 16.5) is used to punch a small hole in the rubber sheet, which is then fitted on so that the tooth projects through the hole. The rubber dam is kept in place by a **rubber dam clamp** which is fixed on the tooth with **rubber dam clamp forceps**. Finally a **rubber dam frame** is used to support the sheet of rubber. A napkin is placed between the patient's chin and the rubber to make it more comfortable, and a saliva ejector is provided. **Dental floss** is used to work the rubber between the teeth.

Rubber dam may be applied to any number of teeth. It enables the operator to keep a tooth dry and maintain a sterile field, and prevents pieces of filling material, debris or small instruments falling into the patient's mouth. It is more comfortable for patients as it prevents water spray or irrigation fluids entering the mouth. It is also far better for the dentist, too, improving access and visibility by keeping the tongue, lips and cheek out of the way. Moreover, it helps prevent cross-infection of patients and chairside staff, by minimising the aerosol of infected debris spread by the use of compressed air and water spray.

The two main uses of rubber dam are: in root canal therapy, to maintain a sterile field and prevent inhalation or swallowing of small instruments; and during the insertion of fillings to avoid failure caused by saliva contamination. Rubber dam clamps are often used alone to hold cotton wool rolls in place, especially when filling lower molars. Ideally, rubber dam should be used for all fillings, but most operators consider it too time-consuming for routine use.

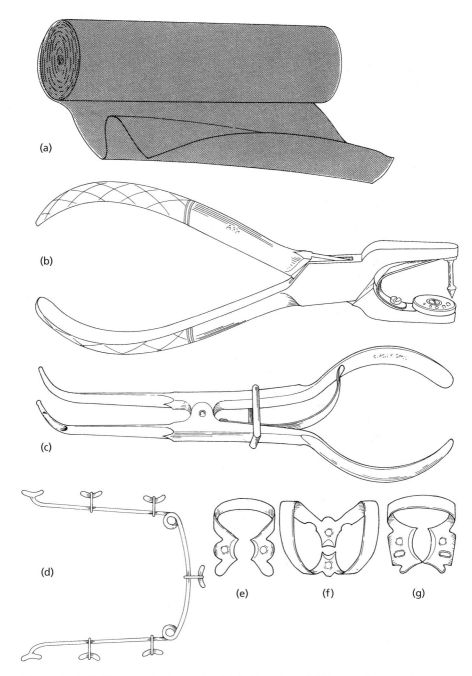

**Figure 16.5** Rubber dam instruments. (a) Rubber dam. (b) Rubber dam punch. (c) Rubber dam clamp forceps. (d) Rubber dam frame. (e) Premolar clamp. (f) Incisor (butterfly) clamp. (g) Molar clamp.

## Instruments

For each patient the instruments required are set up as a 'conservation tray'. Although each dentist will have their own preferred instruments, the basic ones are listed below.

- **Mouth mirror** – for vision, to reflect light onto the tooth, to protect and retract the soft tissues (Figure 16.6).
- **Right-angle probe** – to feel the cavity margins, to detect softened dentine, to detect overhanging restorations (Figure 16.6).
- **College tweezers** – to hold and carry various items (Figure 16.6).
- **Excavators** – small and large, to spoon out softened dentine (see Figure 16.1).
- **Amalgam plugger** – to press the plastic filling material fully into the cavity, to ensure no air spaces remain under the material, to remove excess mercury from the amalgam mix (Figure 16.7).
- **Burnisher** – ball or pear shaped, to ensure the material margins are fully adapted to the cavity walls, to prevent leakage under the restoration (Figure 16.7).
- **Plastic instruments** – especially flat plastic instruments, to adapt the plastic filling material to the cavity walls, to remove excess filling material before setting occurs, to ensure a smooth marginal contact from the restoration to the tooth (Figure 16.7).

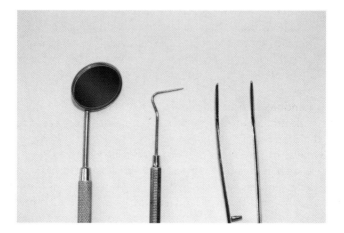

**Figure 16.6** Mirror, probe and tweezers.

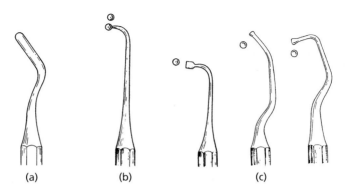

Figure 16.7 Plastic instruments. (a) Flat plastic. (b) Ball ended burnisher. (c) Pluggers.

## Handpieces

Cavities are cut with burs fitted into the head of a handpiece. The speed of cutting depends on the type of handpiece and the purpose for which it is used. The handpieces have a built-in water spray to counteract the heat generated when cutting hard tissue, and may also have fibre-optic illumination to aid cavity preparation.

Air turbine handpieces run at very high speeds of up to 500 000 revolutions a minute, and use friction grip **diamond** or **tungsten carbide burs** to cut easily through both enamel and dentine. There is a tiny air turbine motor in the head of the handpiece which is driven by compressed air. The advantages of air turbines are the ease and speed of cutting. The disadvantages are that they offer little tactile sensation to the dentist, so excessive tooth removal can occur, and their vibration may be associated with a condition called 'vibration white finger' when used over many years.

Slow handpieces run at around 40 000 revolutions per minute, and are driven by air or electric motors at the base of the handpiece. These are much more versatile in their range of speed and uses: varying from low-speed root canal treatment and removal of carious dentine to high-speed conventional cavity preparation. They use latch grip stainless steel or tungsten carbide burs when used on teeth, or friction grip stainless steel acrylic trimming burs when used on dentures. They are more 'user-friendly' for the dentist, as the tactile sensation provided is much better. Portable versions of the electric motors are particularly suitable for domiciliary treatment.

All handpieces, however driven, and of whatever age, are made in two basic designs: **contra-angle** and **straight**. A contra-angle is used most often as it provides access to every tooth. For easily accessible teeth and laboratory work a straight handpiece is used (Figure 16.8).

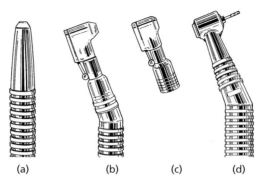

**Figure 16.8** Handpieces. (a) Straight. (b) Contra-angle. (c) Miniature. (d) Air turbine.

## Burs

Burs for low-speed procedures are made of steel. They are used for removing caries, cutting dentine, trimming dentures and other laboratory work. Burs for high-speed handpieces have **diamond** or **tungsten carbide** cutting surfaces and are used for rapid removal of enamel, dentine and old fillings.

Straight handpiece burs have a long plain shank. Burs for low-speed contra-angle handpieces are short and have a notch in the shank which fits by a **latch grip**. Short burs are also used for air turbine handpieces but they have a plain shank which gives a **friction grip** (Figure 16.9). Contra-angled low-speed handpieces with smaller heads, and using even shorter burs, are used on children. They are called **miniature** handpieces and burs.

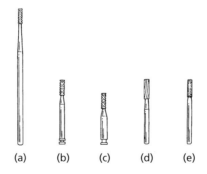

**Figure 16.9** Burs. (a) Steel for straight handpiece. (b) Steel, latch grip, for low-speed contra-angle handpiece. (c) Steel, latch grip, for miniature contra-angle handpiece. (d) Tungsten carbide, friction grip, for air turbine handpiece. (e) Diamond, friction grip, for air turbine handpiece.

The cutting ends of burs are made in many different shapes (Figure 16.10). The most commonly used burs are as follows:

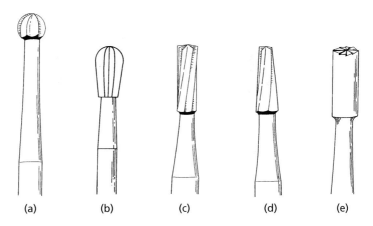

**Figure 16.10** Bur shapes. (a) Round. (b) Pear. (c) Flat fissure. (d) Tapered fissure. (e) End-cutting.

- Round – used for gaining access to cavities, and, at low speed, for removing caries
- Pear – used for shaping and smoothing cavities
- Fissure – used for shaping and outlining the cavity

## Enamel chisels

Although enamel is the hardest tissue in the body it is a brittle material; where caries has destroyed its underlying dentine, any remaining enamel which is unsupported by sound dentine can break off during mastication. Thus it is essential during cavity preparation to remove unsupported enamel. This used to be achieved by chipping it away with an enamel chisel, but these instruments are little used nowadays as burs are so much more effective. Enamel chisels have a similar blade to a carpenter's chisel and are usually single-ended (see Figure 16.2). They have tungsten carbide blades and were also used for smoothing cavity margins.

- **Straight** chisels resemble a miniature wood chisel.
- **Bin-angle** chisels have their cutting edge at right angles to the plane of the handle, just like a garden hoe.
- **Hatchet** chisels, as their name implies, have their cutting edge in the same plane as the handle.
- **Cervical margin trimmers** are modified hatchet chisels with a curved blade for removing unsupported enamel from the cervical margins of class II cavities.

## Polishing instruments

There is a great variety of polishing instruments but they generally comprise fine abrasive stones, wheels, discs and strips, finishing burs, brushes and polishing pastes. Apart from hand abrasive strips they are all used with a handpiece. Finishing burs and stones are used for smoothing cavity margins and trimming fillings. Abrasive discs and strips are used for fine trimming and polishing.

Small abrasive stones, wheels and brushes are manufactured with a shank which fits the appropriate handpiece (Figure 16.11). Larger wheels, stones and abrasive discs require an independent mounting shank called a **mandrel**. Wheels and metal discs are fitted on a Huey mandrel; sandpaper discs with a metal centre and Soflex discs use a Moore mandrel, and plain sandpaper discs a pinhead mandrel (Figure 16.11).

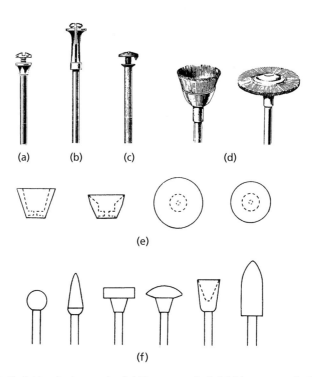

(a)         (b)         (c)                 (d)

(e)

(f)

**Figure 16.11** Polishing instruments. (a) Huey mandrel. (b) Moore mandrel. (c) Pinhead mandrel. (d) Polishing brushes. (e) Abrasive rubber cups and discs for Huey mandrel. (f) Mounted fine abrasives.

## Care of instruments

All cutting instruments must be kept sharp because blunt ones are inefficient and painful for the patient. Hand instruments such as chisels and excavators have to be sharpened regularly on a small flat oilstone (**Arkansas stone**), or with an abrasive disc in a straight handpiece. Burs are cleaned in an ultrasonic cleaner and autoclaved after use. Blunt burs are discarded into the sharps container.

All handpieces must be lubricated regularly according to the manufacturer's instructions. The manufacturer's instructions must also be followed when sterilising handpieces. (Sterilisation methods used are described in Chapter 7.)

## Air abrasion

Modern technology has allowed an old method of tooth preparation to be re-introduced into dental practice. It uses compressed air and a special handpiece to convey a jet of abrasive particles on to a tooth surface, whereupon the particle jet can remove hard tissue, soft carious tissue, surface stains, and even abrade metal or composite restorations before cementation or repairs. It is less painful than conventional cavity preparation but is not in general use as it is rather expensive.

## Temporary filling materials and cavity liners

The commonly used temporary filling materials are:

- Zinc oxide and eugenol cement
- Zinc phosphate cement
- Polycarboxylate cement

Temporary filling materials are not used as permanent fillings as they are too soft and soluble and would not remain intact for long periods. They are also used as cavity linings and, as their names imply, for cementing inlays and crowns. Although calcium hydroxide is not a temporary filling, it is an excellent cavity liner and is accordingly included in this section.

### Uses of temporary fillings

- As a first-aid measure to relieve pain
- When there is insufficient time to complete the cavity and insert a permanent filling in one visit
- For procedures requiring more than one visit, e.g. inlays, crowns and root treatment, a temporary restoration is necessary between visits to close the cavity and prevent food debris collecting
- To allow a symptomatic tooth to settle and become symptom-free, before being permanently filled

### Purpose of cavity linings

- Protection of the pulp against thermal shock, such as conduction of heat or cold through metal fillings
- Protection of the pulp against the chemical irritation of some non-metallic fillings

Zinc oxide and eugenol cement (ZOE) is made by mixing **zinc oxide** powder and a drop of **eugenol** (oil of cloves) on a glass slab with a **spatula**. It can be thickened if necessary by squeezing in a napkin. Setting takes a few hours.

- Temporary filling
- Non-irritant lining for deep cavities
- Sedative dressing for painful carious teeth and dry sockets
- Main constituent of some impression pastes, periodontal packs and root filling materials

Zinc oxide eugenol is soothing and non-irritant to the pulp and can be safely used in deep cavities.

It is too soft and slow-setting to use as a foundation for a permanent filling in one visit. But this can be overcome by using a strengthened quick-setting proprietary brand (e.g. Kalzinol). In this form it is generally regarded as a most satisfactory lining for metal fillings.

Zinc oxide eugenol is not compatible with composite fillings. The manufacturer's instructions must always be followed in selecting a suitable lining for any non-metallic fillings.

Some patients are allergic to preparations containing eugenol. Special eugenol-free alternatives are available.

Zinc phosphate cement is prepared by mixing a powder and liquid on a glass slab with a spatula. The powder consists mainly of **zinc oxide**; the liquid is **phosphoric acid**. Two different mixes are used: a thick mix of putty consistency to use as a temporary filling or a base beneath a permanent filling, and a thin creamy one to use for crown and inlay cementation. Setting takes a few minutes depending on various factors.

- A warm slab accelerates the setting while a cold slab has the opposite effect.
- A thick mix sets more quickly than a thin mix.
- A dry slab must be used as moisture accelerates setting. It is most important to screw the cap on tightly, immediately after using the bottle of liquid, to

prevent it absorbing moisture from the air. If this happens, the cement will set too quickly.

- If a long setting time is required, when cementing a bridge, for example, a cold slab is necessary. A tiny quantity of powder is mixed with the liquid a minute or so before the cement is required. The rest of the powder is then added in small quantities at a time. This ability to control its setting time is the overriding advantage of zinc phosphate cement.

Experience soon teaches a dental nurse how much powder and liquid to set out, but occasionally too little or too much powder will be put on the slab. In the former case more powder can be added from the bottle, but the mixing end of the spatula must not be used for this purpose as it will contaminate and spoil the whole bottle. Excess unused powder may only be returned to the bottle if you are certain that it has not been contaminated by any liquid or mixed cement on the slab.

A cool *thick* glass slab should be used for mixing zinc phosphate cement. Thin slabs are warmed by the dental nurse's hand and can make the cement set too quickly.

## Uses

A thick mix sets rapidly and may be used for:

- A temporary filling
- Cavity lining
- Blocking undercuts in inlay and crown preparations

A thin mix sets more slowly and is used as a **luting cement** for:

- Inlays, crowns and bridges
- Orthodontic bands

## Advantages

The advantage of this cement is that it sets very hard in a few minutes and therefore makes a sound lining for permanent fillings, and a durable temporary filling. Furthermore, its adhesive nature to dentine makes it satisfactory as a luting cement for pre-fabricated restorations.

## Disadvantages

In deep cavities it may be irritant to the pulp, and in these cases a sub-lining of calcium hydroxide is inserted before the zinc phosphate cement. Otherwise a different lining or luting cement must be used. Zinc phosphate cement is moisture sensitive and will not adhere to a damp cavity, so good moisture control is required during its use.

## Polycarboxylate cement

Polycarboxylate cement, e.g. Durelon, is prepared by mixing powder and liquid with a spatula on a glass slab or paper pad. The powder consists mainly of **zinc oxide**; the liquid is **polyacrylic acid**.

In cements using polyacrylic acid as the liquid, many manufacturers have replaced the acid with water. Polyacrylic acid, which is the normal liquid component, is dehydrated and included with the powder instead. The cement is then prepared by simply mixing the powder with water in the normal way (e.g. Poly-F Plus). The advantage of this anhydrous system is that only one bottle of material is needed; there is no liquid to deteriorate, or to be used up too soon, or left over when the powder bottle is empty. Furthermore the normal liquid is rather viscous, difficult to dispense from the bottle and difficult to mix. Mixing with water is much easier and quicker.

Polycarboxylate cement may be prepared as a thin luting mix for cementing, or a thick mix for lining. A measure is supplied by the manufacturer for dispensing correct amounts of powder. Instruments are dipped in alcohol or dry cement powder to prevent cement sticking to them. It is also easier to clean them afterwards if they are washed in water before the cement sets.

### Uses

As an alternative to zinc phosphate cement.

### Advantages

Polycarboxylate cement is less irritant than zinc phosphate cement and far more adhesive to dentine. For these reasons many operators prefer it to zinc phosphate for cementing inlays, crowns and orthodontic bands.

### Disadvantages

Polycarboxylate cement can be rather difficult to manipulate as it is adhesive to instruments. Many dentists now prefer to use glass ionomer cement for temporary fillings and as luting cements. These applications are covered later.

## Calcium hydroxide

Proprietary products, such as Dycal or Dropsin, come in the form of a powder and liquid or as pastes which are mixed together on a pad or glass slab. Non-mix light cure products are also available nowadays. If a non-setting application is required, it can be prepared by mixing calcium hydroxide powder and water into a paste on a glass slab or in a **Dappen pot**.

Uses

As calcium hydroxide is non-irritant and compatible with all filling materials, it is used as a universal cavity lining. It promotes the formation of secondary dentine and remineralisation of hard tissue. It is also used for pulp capping, pulpotomy and other root treatment procedures (Chapter 17).

### Advantages

Calcium hydroxide is the best lining material for non-metallic fillings as it has no deleterious effect on them or the pulp. Its alkalinity counteracts the acidity of zinc phosphate, and also helps to kill the bacteria present in carious lesions.

### Disadvantages

In deep cavities, with metal fillings, it can only be used as a sub-lining as it forms too thin a layer to insulate the pulp against thermal irritation. Another lining must be inserted on top of the calcium hydroxide to provide a thicker layer of insulation against the conduction of heat or cold through metal fillings. In shallow cavities, calcium hydroxide alone is a satisfactory lining for metal fillings. It is also soluble in water, unless a light cure product is used.

### Practical examination

One of the two tests in the practical examination often consists of mixing a cement, cavity lining or temporary filling material. For all these, the following procedure is recommended.

1   Before starting your mix tell the examiner that you wish to wash your hands and wear a pair of operating gloves.
2   Select correct materials and mixing instrument.
3   Dispense correct amounts of powder and liquid.
4   Replace the bottle caps immediately.
5   Ask for the manufacturer's instructions if you are unfamiliar with the brand provided.
6   Dispense liquid on to centre of the mixing slab or pad. This confines the mixing area to the centre and avoids the embarrassment of losing some of your mix over the edge.
7   Cease mixing *immediately* once the consistency is correct.
8   Collect the mix on to a clean area of the slab.
9   Wipe the mixing instrument and present your mix and the instrument to the examiner.
10   If you are dissatisfied with your mix, tell the examiner what is wrong with it and what its effect would be, for example: insufficient powder dispensed; mix too thin; would set too slowly; acidity may irritate pulp. Offer to start again.

Special requirements are necessary for the following different materials.

## Zinc oxide and eugenol cement

**Test**: Prepare a sedative lining for a deep cavity

1  Select a clean, dry glass slab and spatula, and correct bottles of powder and liquid, e.g. Kalzinol.
2  Dispense and proportion powder neatly.
3  Dispense two or three drops of liquid. Replace bottle caps.
4  Mix to a putty consistency.

## Zinc phosphate cement

**Test**: Cementing a crown

1  Select correct bottles of powder and liquid, and a clean, dry, cool, *thick* glass slab and spatula.
2  Dispense and divide powder into small portions. Replace cap.
3  Dispense two or three drops of liquid. Replace bottle cap immediately.
4  Mix sufficient portions of powder into the liquid to give a smooth creamy consistency.

**Test**: Cementing a three-unit bridge
The differences between the requirements for this mix and the previous one are:

■  A three-unit bridge contains two crowns and therefore requires more cement. Dispense double the quantity of powder and liquid
■  As bridges require more time for insertion, the cement must not set so quickly

1  Cool a *thick* glass slab under *cold* running water and dry it thoroughly.
2  Proportion the powder so that it can be mixed into the liquid in small increments.
3  Ensure slow setting by mixing one tiny portion of powder into the liquid first. Then wait a little before adding the rest of the powder by increments to achieve a smooth creamy consistency.

**Test**: Lining a cavity
The difference between this test and the previous two is that a thick mix, almost of putty consistency, is required for a cavity lining. Thus more powder is required, but otherwise the test is performed in the same way as that for cementing a single crown.

## Polycarboxylate cement

**Test**: Prepare polycarboxylate for cementing an orthodontic band

1  Select correct bottles of powder and liquid, e.g. Poly-F Plus.
2  Invert powder bottle to fluff powder before use.
3  Overfill powder scoop and remove excess with spatula to give flat surface level with edge of scoop. Do not press down on powder.
4  Dispense one scoop of powder to two drops of water on mixing pad.
5  Divide powder into two halves.
6  Add one half to liquid; as soon as wetted, add other half.
7  Mix rapidly to creamy consistency – 15 seconds.

## Calcium hydroxide

**Test**: Prepare a calcium hydroxide dressing for a deep cavity

1  Select correct materials, e.g. Dycal.
2  Dispense equal lengths of base and catalyst paste on mixing pad.
3  Mix pastes immediately by stirring with applicator until a uniform streak-free colour.
4  Take no longer than 10 seconds.
5  Wipe the applicator and present mix and applicator to the examiner.

# Permanent filling materials

Permanent filling materials are the materials used to permanently restore the tooth to its full function, and they must all have the following properties:

- Set to a hard enough degree to allow normal masticatory function to occur
- Not to dissolve in saliva over time
- To be biologically safe
- To be able to be applied to the tooth using normal conservation instruments, in a straightforward manner
- Ideally they should be aesthetically acceptable, although this limits the use of amalgam

The three commonly used materials are **amalgam**, **composite** and **glass ionomer**.

## Amalgam

Amalgam is the most widely used permanent filling for posterior teeth, as it is cheaper, more durable, and easier to use than its tooth-coloured competitors –

composite and glass ionomer. Amalgam is prepared by mixing a powdered **alloy** with **mercury**. This mixture forms a plastic mass, which is packed into the tooth cavity and sets hard in a few minutes. The main constituents of amalgam alloy are:

- **Silver** (at least 60%)
- **Copper** (up to 25%)
- **Tin** (variable quantities)
- **Zinc** (small quantities)

The alloy is supplied, together with the correct amount of **liquid mercury**, in special pre-packed disposable capsules for automatic mixing in an **amalgamator** (Figure 16.12).

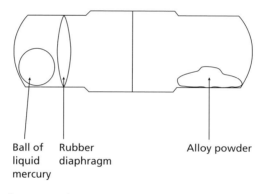

Ball of    Rubber              Alloy powder
liquid      diaphragm
mercury

Figure 16.12 Amalgam capsule.

Varying the alloy powder constituents produces an amalgam mix with different levels of marginal ditching and discoloration. Modern amalgams tend to have a 'high-copper' content to reduce these unwanted effects as much as possible. As amalgam is a plastic filling and a good conductor, cavities are made retentive and lined to insulate the pulp against thermal shock. In addition, the entire cavity may be varnished to give a good marginal seal before inserting amalgam.

Very large cavities may have too little crown structure left for adequate retention. Modern bonding agents (see later) or dentine pins are used for retention in such cases.

Recommendations for best long-term results of amalgam restorations are:

- In shallow cavities, three coats of cavity varnish suffice as a lining and marginal seal
- Medium cavities are lined with zinc oxide eugenol or glass ionomer cement, and sealed with three coats of varnish
- Calcium hydroxide is used as a sub-lining in deep cavities

The alloy and mercury are mixed together in an automatic **amalgamator** (Figure 16.13). This is a vibrator machine with a timer, which is set for the appropriate size of capsule used. Pre-packed disposable capsules are best as they contain the correct ratio of alloy to mercury and avoid spillage.

Many of these vibrator machines can also take capsules of other filling materials, such as glass ionomer (Fuji).

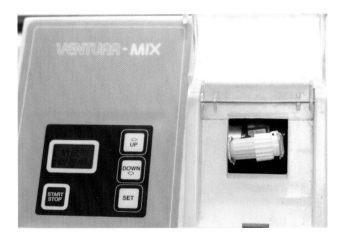

**Figure 16.13** Amalgamator machine with capsule.

Dental nurses must take great care with amalgam as mercury is poisonous. Correct preparation and attention to manufacturers' instructions are essential, as an unsatisfactory mix may cause weakness and adverse dimensional changes in the filling. This will not be apparent on completion of the filling, but results in early failure caused by leakage and recurrent caries at the margins or fracture of the amalgam restoration itself.

The precautions necessary to avoid danger to the dental nurse and ensure a satisfactory filling are listed below.

- Correct mixing time. Prolonged mixing causes **contraction** and subsequent caries. Inadequate mixing causes **expansion** and **weakness**, leading to early failure of the filling.
- Gloves must be worn when handling mercury or amalgam. Any contact with bare fingers allows mercury to be **absorbed** through the skin and may cause mercury poisoning.
- No contamination with saliva during insertion.

The cavity must be thoroughly dried and saliva kept away from the tooth by means of cotton wool rolls, absorbent pads and a saliva ejector, or better still by using rubber dam. Amalgam is introduced into the cavity by means of an **amalgam carrier** (Figure 16.14) and packed into place with hand **amalgam pluggers** (Figure 16.15) or a mechanical condenser. When packed with sufficient force, any excess mercury in the amalgam mix will rise to the surface of the restoration. A few minutes are then available before the filling sets for trimming away excess amalgam and removing excess mercury, **carving** it to the original anatomy of the tooth with plastic instruments, checking the occlusion and **burnishing** the surface.

Disposal of used capsules and other amalgam waste is covered later in this chapter.

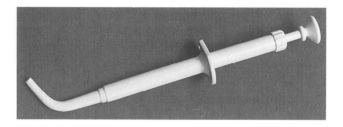

Figure 16.14  Plastic amalgam carrier. (Image from Minerva Dental Profile Issue 1.)

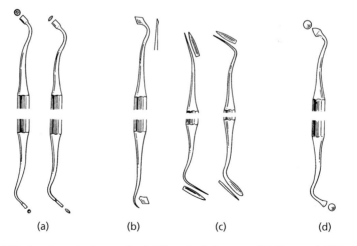

(a)          (b)          (c)          (d)

Figure 16.15  Amalgam instruments. (a) Serrated pluggers. (b) Carver. (c) Ward carvers. (d) Burnisher.

Although the initial set takes only a few minutes, it is not complete for several hours. The patient is therefore instructed to eat on the other side of the mouth for the rest of the day. If considered necessary, the filling may be polished at a subsequent visit. This is done under water spray with **finishing burs**, brushes and pumice paste. Amalgam finishing burs are made of steel for use in low-speed handpieces. They come in a variety of shapes but are recognised by having far more cutting blades than ordinary burs (Figure 16.16).

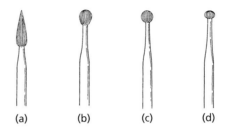

(a)        (b)        (c)        (d)

Figure 16.16 Finishing burs. (a) Flame. (b) Pear. (c) Round. (d) Oval.

Blocked amalgam carriers cause much unnecessary trouble. To avoid blockage the dental nurse must always expel any residual amalgam from the nozzle into the waste amalgam container, before it sets, and before the carrier is autoclaved. Ideally, the carriers should be dismantled to ensure all waste amalgam is removed before autoclaving.

*Matrix outfits*

Before amalgam can be inserted into a Class II cavity, such as mesial-occlusal, or distal-occlusal, a **matrix band** must be fitted round the tooth (Figure 16.17). This is to prevent amalgam escaping through the mesial or distal openings of the cavity

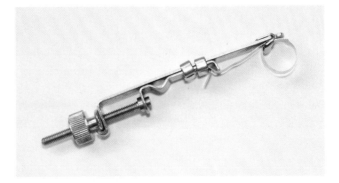

Figure 16.17 Siqveland matrix outfit.

during packing, and producing an overhang. The band is held tightly against the gum margin of the cavity by inserting a **wooden** or **plastic wedge** between the teeth. Various types of matrix outfit are available, the commonest ones being **Siqveland** (Figure 16.18) and **Tofflemire**. When packing is complete the band and wedge are removed and the band holder autoclaved, unless disposable. It is considered good practice nowadays to treat the matrix band itself as a single-use, disposable item of hazardous waste, as it is likely to be contaminated with blood. It should be safely disposed of in a sharps box.

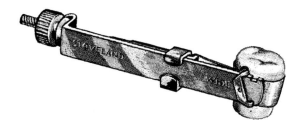

**Figure 16.18** Wide Siqveland matrix outfit.

## Advantages

- Easy to use
- Relatively cheap, compared to composites and glass ionomers
- Good set strength and easily able to withstand normal occlusal forces
- Excellent longevity, lasting many years under normal conditions in well maintained mouths

## Disadvantages

- Mercury is toxic; it can be inhaled as a vapour, absorbed through the skin, or ingested
- Undercut cavities are required for its placement, as it is not retentive to tooth tissue
- It is metallic and therefore requires varnishes, liners or bases to prevent thermal shock to the pulp
- Correct constituents and mixing times are required to produce the ideal dimensional stability of the set restoration
- Poor aesthetics, so it is limited to use in posterior teeth

## Mercury poisoning

It was formerly believed that mercury poisoning could only occur after several years of mishandling. However, it is now known that it can occur within a few months if a large quantity of mercury is spilled. Every dental nurse must accordingly understand the causes and prevention of hazards associated with the use of mercury and amalgam.

Poisoning can occur in the following ways:

- **Inhalation** of the vapours
- **Absorption** through the skin, the nail beds, the eyes, and wounds
- **Ingestion** by being swallowed

Although the possibility of skin contamination is obvious when handling mercury or amalgam, the risk of inhaling mercury vapour is not. Both mercury and amalgam release mercury vapour at ordinary **room temperature** – and the higher the temperature, the more vapour is released. Mercury vapour is odourless and invisible, so it is of the utmost importance to keep all mercury and waste amalgam in sealed containers in a cool, well-ventilated place – not near a hot steriliser or radiator, or even in sunlight.

Another source of mercury poisoning is the removal of old amalgam fillings. This releases a cloud of minute amalgam particles which can be inhaled or contaminate eyes and skin. It can be prevented by combining the use of copious water spray, and an efficient aspirator, which exhausts outside the practice. Rubber dam and eyewear are the best protection for patients.

Apart from very rare cases of allergy, there is no evidence of danger to patients from their amalgam fillings. However, it has been advised that removal or insertion of amalgam fillings in pregnant patients should be deferred, if clinically reasonable. Pregnant chairside staff involved in such procedures may also be concerned, but regular urine tests for mercury contamination of staff will show if any risk is present.

### Symptoms of mercury poisoning

The early symptoms of mercury poisoning may include headache, fatigue, irritability, nausea and diarrhoea. At this stage it is unlikely that mercury would be suspected. Later symptoms are **hand tremors** and **visual defects** such as double vision. The final stage is **kidney failure**.

### Precautions

The routine use of **personal protective equipment** (PPE) such as gloves, mask and safety glasses, or visors worn for protection against cross-infection will also provide corresponding protection against mercury hazards. Dental nurses can be reassured that no danger exists if the following precautions are taken. However, they are so important that they are covered again, together with other occupational hazards, in Chapter 23.

**To avoid absorption of mercury through the skin**

- Always wear disposable gloves when handling mercury, mixing amalgam and cleaning amalgam instruments.

- Do not wear open-toed shoes as the floor may be contaminated by spilled mercury or dropped amalgam.
- Do not wear jewellery or a wrist watch as they may harbour particles of amalgam
- Gold jewellery can be spoiled by contact with mercury or amalgam.

**To avoid pollution of the air by mercury vapour**

- Containers of mercury must be tightly sealed, and stored in a cool well-ventilated place.
- When transferring mercury from a stock bottle, great care must be taken not to spill any. It is very difficult to find and recover mercury which has dropped on the floor or working surface as it is a liquid metal and rolls away easily.
- Pre-packed disposable capsules of mercury and alloy avoid any need to keep a stock of mercury.
- For removal of old amalgam fillings, the use of a high-speed handpiece with diamond or tungsten carbide burs, water spray and efficient aspiration helps to reduce the aerosol of amalgam dust and mercury vapour; while the use of rubber dam will protect the patient. Surgery staff must wear full PPE throughout such procedures.
- All traces of amalgam must be removed from instruments before autoclaving, otherwise vapour will be released as the autoclave heats up.
- Keep the surgery well ventilated.
- Amalgamators and the capsules used therein should be checked after use as cases have been reported of mercury leakage from capsules during mixing:
  - Amalgamators must be stood on a tray lined with aluminium foil so that any droplets can be easily collected and disposed of as special waste.
  - The machines must also have a lid over the capsule holder, so that leaking capsules do not throw their dangerous contents into the surgery.
  - All premises using amalgam must have a **mercury spillage kit** so that any accidents can be dealt with swiftly and correctly.

*Surgery hygiene*

Much can be done to minimise any dangers of working with mercury by adopting the following rules.

- Smoking, eating, drinking and the application of cosmetics must not take place in the surgery. Any of these actions could permit absorption of mercury – from mercury vapour in the air or from contaminated hands.
- The storage and handling of mercury must be confined to one particular part of the surgery, away from all sources of heat, or, better still, outside the surgery.
- All handling of mercury and preparation of amalgam must be done over a drip tray (lined with kitchen foil) on a special work surface. A drip tray prevents the loss of spilled mercury and facilitates recovery. The work surface

must not allow any spilled mercury to fall on the floor or roll into inaccessible places.

- Any spillage of mercury *must* be reported to the dentist. Never be afraid to do this.
- Special kits are available for the safe recovery of spilled mercury. Vacuum cleaners must never be used for this purpose as they vaporise any mercury they pick up and discharge it back into the surgery.
- Floor coverings must not have any cracks or gaps in which mercury or amalgam can be trapped. Carpets must not be used as a surgery floor covering.
- Surgery equipment and plumbing must have easily accessible filter traps to collect particles of waste amalgam flushed through spittoons, aspirators or other suction apparatus. This waste must be collected and transferred to the surgery waste amalgam containers.
- Modern aspirators must be fitted with an amalgam trap, so that no waste material enters the drains.
- Waste amalgam must be saved in sealed tubs containing a mercury absorption chemical, and taken for collection by specialist waste contractors for recycling (Figures 16.19 and 16.20). It cannot be sent by post.
- Efficient ventilation is essential at all times of the year. Avoid high surgery temperatures.

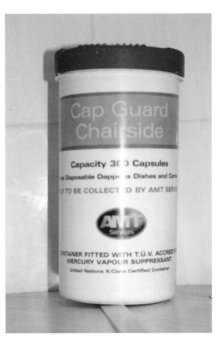

Figure 16.19 Amalgam capsule waste container.

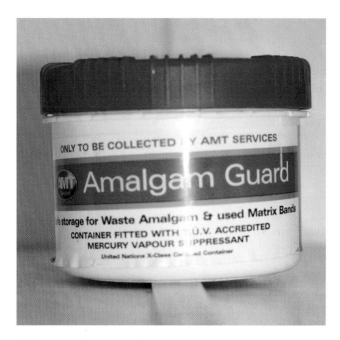

Figure 16.20  Waste amalgam container.

- If, following a spillage of mercury or inadequate mercury hygiene, it is suspected that a risk of mercury poisoning exists, the public or occupational
  health authority must be notified so that tests can be carried out.

### Disposal of waste amalgam

All amalgam waste, and extracted teeth with amalgam fillings, must only be
collected for disposal by authorised **specialist waste contractors** (Chapter 7). The
reason for this is that all other hazardous waste is incinerated, and would pollute
the air with mercury vapour if it contained any amalgam. Before collection it must
be stored in special containers, supplied by collectors, which prevent escape of
mercury vapour. They may also arrange periodic testing of the practice mercury
vapour levels, and checking of amalgamators for mercury leakage.

### Mercury spillage

Accidental spillage of mercury or waste amalgam must always be reported to the
dentist. If a spillage occurs, globules of mercury can be drawn up into a disposable
intravenous **syringe** or **bulb aspirator** and transferred to a mercury container. Small
globules can be collected by adhering to the **lead foil** from X-ray film packets.
Waste amalgam can be gathered with a **damp paper towel**. For larger spillages, the
following protocol should be followed:

- Stop work and report the incident to the dentist immediately
- Put on full PPE
- Globules of mercury or particles of amalgam must be smeared with a **mercury absorbent paste** from the mercury spillage kit
- This consists of equal parts of **calcium hydroxide** and **flowers of sulphur** mixed into a paste with **water**
- It should be left to dry and then removed with a wet disposable towel and placed in the storage container
- Larger spillages still require the evacuation of the premises, the sealing of the area, and the involvement of **Environmental Health** to remove the contamination as a specialist procedure
- The **Health and Safety Executive** will be notified, so that an investigation can be carried out to determine if the practice procedure needs to be changed to prevent a recurrence of the spillage

### Detection of mercury vapour

If a serious spillage occurs, or there are other reasons for suspecting mercury contamination in the surgery, tests are available for determining the amount of mercury vapour in the air. If such tests show an excessive concentration of mercury vapour, expert advice should be sought from Environmental Health to trace and eradicate the cause. Urine tests can also be arranged to check whether staff have absorbed dangerous amounts of mercury.

### Composite filling materials

Composite filling materials are tooth-coloured and are accordingly used for permanent fillings in front teeth. They can also be used for filling back teeth but do not wear as well as metal fillings. Consequently amalgam is still the most widely used material for back teeth.

Composite fillings consist of an **inorganic filler** in a **resin binder**. The inorganic filler, which acts as a strengthener, may consist of **powdered glass**, **quartz**, **silica**, or other **ceramic particles**. This is incorporated into the resin binder to produce a composite filling. The particle size can be varied to produce the following:

- **Microfine composites** – very small particle size, giving superior polishing for anterior restorations
- **Hybrid composites** – various size particles to give higher strength and better wear resistance for posterior restorations
- **Universal composites** – combination of microfine and hybrids, to be used for both anterior and posterior restorations

The composites used for permanent restorations contain a filler, resin binder and catalyst. When the catalyst is activated it makes the filling set. The original composites, such as Adaptic, were supplied as two pastes: one containing a resin binder and filler; the other containing a catalyst. Mixing the two together activates the catalyst and makes the filling set. This method of mixing two components to produce setting is called a **chemical-cure** (self-curing) system. However, it has been almost superseded by materials containing a catalyst which is activated by exposure to light (e.g. Tetric). This setting method is called a **light-cure** system.

## Chemical-cure system

Chemical-cure materials are supplied as two pots of paste. One pot of paste is a mixture of resin binder and inorganic filler. The other pot contains a catalyst, which acts on the resin to make the filling set.

A disposable plastic double-ended spatula is used to transfer the desired quantity of paste from one pot to a paper mixing pad. The other end of the spatula is then used to place an equal quantity of paste from the second pot on to the pad. It is essential to use different ends of the spatula for each pot; if the same end is used, the second pot will be ruined by contamination from the first. The two pastes are then mixed together with the same spatula to an even consistency. For mixing, it does not matter which end of the spatula is used but it must be discarded afterwards.

The use of chemical-cure composites for fillings has been virtually superseded by light-cured products. However, there is still a need for chemical curing in situations where metallic restorations are cemented into, or on to, prepared teeth. Light cannot penetrate metal, so a special type of **dual-cure** composite material has been developed, which can be set at the margins by a curing light and then will set chemically beneath the metallic restoration.

## Light-cure system

Unlike chemical-cure composites, which cannot set until two components are mixed together, light-cure materials (e.g. Filtek, Solitaire, Helioseal) have introduced an ideal setting system to dentistry. All they need to make them set is exposure to bright light. A single component contains the resin binder, filler and a special catalyst which is only activated when exposed to a very bright light. A special lamp is used to produce a spot of intensely bright blue light which activates the catalyst and makes the material set in less than a minute. No mixing is required.

The unique advantage of this system is that the dentist has complete control over setting. The dentist alone decides when it should set; when it is ready, all that needs to be done is to shine the curing light on it.

The single component of light-cure composites enables manufacturers to supply their product in multi-dose dispensing syringes, or single dose capsules called **compoules** (Figure 16.21) with an injector gun, thereby allowing a dentist to inject the filling directly into a prepared cavity. The dentist then has as much time as necessary to adapt, contour and trim the filling material before commanding it to set. In this way, the time-consuming removal of excess material which has set rock-hard can be avoided.

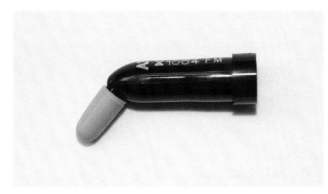

**Figure 16.21** Composite compoule.

Just a thin layer of composite is needed to fill a shallow cavity and this only requires one application of the curing light. In larger cavities this would only cure the surface layer as the light cannot penetrate layers thicker than 2 mm. In order to obtain full curing in such cases, the composite is inserted in a thin layer, then light-cured before adding another thin layer and light-curing again. This sequence is repeated **incrementally** until the cavity is completely filled with fully cured composite. One way of saving time in such cases is to partially fill a large cavity with a thick layer of lining material, followed by a surface layer of composite which can be cured in one application of the light. The usual lining material for this purpose is glass ionomer cement which is described later.

Manufacturers provide special lamps to deliver a concentrated spot of bright blue light on the tooth concerned, together with special orange glasses or shields for patients and staff safety. Halogen bulbs are used to produce the light but have the disadvantage of requiring replacement from time to time, in order to maintain their effectiveness. They are now being superseded by blue light-emitting diodes (LED) which are more durable and reliable and can be powered by low-voltage batteries. Light-cure materials are available for most uses of composites, as well as a new generation of cavity lining and bonding materials.

There are so many different brands of composite materials, and so many different types of curing lights, that it is essential to strictly follow the manufacturers' instructions for the curing time, light bulb life, and care and maintenance of this equipment. A simple test of its effectiveness is to cure a small portion of composite on a mixing pad and then check that it has set hard throughout its full thickness.

## Advantages

The advantages of composites over other permanent filling materials are as follows:

- Superior aesthetics with a wide range of shades for both dentine and enamel replacement

- Adhesive to enamel using acid etch and primers, so only small cavity under-cuts are required
- Minimal marginal leakage due to their adhesion to enamel
- Cavities can be lined with calcium hydroxide alone, or based with glass ionomer if deep
- Strength is sufficient to be used in smaller posterior restorations
- Can be used as a laboratory constructed inlay in larger restorations (Chapter 18)
- Light-cured products are set immediately

## Disadvantages

Composites have several disadvantages to consider before their use, but they are still a highly useful restorative material for the dentist.

- Their success is very technique-sensitive.
- Their use takes longer.
- They are more expensive materials, and light-cured products will only set correctly following exposure to the curing light.
- Not as strong as amalgam, so they are less useful in posterior restorations.
- Composites react with all temporary filling materials when used as bases, so glass ionomer must be used as a base in deep cavities.
- Etchants are strongly acidic and must be used with great care to prevent patient injury.
- Curing lamps will cause damage to the retina of the eyes if viewed without orange shields.

## Technique

Calcium hydroxide is a suitable lining for all these materials, although in deeper cavities a glass ionomer base is required. The correct shade of composite is then selected.

For insertion of the filling it is best to use special composite filling instruments which have ceramic non-stick tips. As composite fillings are so hard, they can abrade ordinary metal instruments and result in a filling of poor appearance caused by the incorporation of metal particles. Modern composite materials are provided for use complete with their own unfilled resin bond material, although any acid etch material can be used with all products.

Once the pulp has been protected, the enamel edges of the cavity are coated with the etchant, which is **33% phosphoric acid**. Microscopically, this roughens the enamel surface by dissolving the inter-prismatic substance and leaving the prisms projecting from the tooth surface (Chapter 10). The resin bond is then applied to this surface and cured for around 10 seconds, so that it adheres to the prisms and provides tags for the composite to stick to when placed.

The filling is manipulated with a flat plastic instrument and contoured to the tooth with a clear polyester (Mylar) or **cellulose acetate matrix strip**, held in place with a crocodile clip matrix clamp (Figure 16.22). When set, it is trimmed and polished, but special finishing agents are needed as it is so hard. Tungsten carbide, diamond finishing burs or abrasive stones are used with water spray for trimming excess material. White stones, fine abrasive discs, strips and rubber points are used for polishing (see Figure 16.11). Manufacturers recommend the best polishing procedures for their own brands and these should be followed to give optimum results.

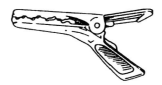

**Figure 16.22** Crocodile matrix clamp.

## Acid etching

Filling a cavity in a front tooth, as just described, is not the only use for composite materials. They are far more versatile than that. Their strength and durability allow them to be used for repair of fractured incisors and for fissure sealing. Retention for these cases is again obtained by using the **acid etch** technique.

Enamel is made retentive by applying phosphoric acid gel for up to 20 seconds. This etches the surface by attacking the enamel prisms, and produces a retentive surface which is full of microscopic pits like a honeycomb. When the filling material is applied it flows into these pits and sets into hard tags, which effectively lock it to the enamel surface.

Surgery procedure for acid etching is as follows.

- The most important requirement is a *dry* clean tooth surface.
- If a three-in-one syringe is used for drying, it is most important to check that the air is not contaminated with oil from the compressor. This can be done by holding a napkin over the syringe nozzle – whereupon any oil will show up on the napkin.
- Any exposed dentine is protected from acid by coating with a calcium hydroxide lining material or a bonding agent.
- The acid gel is applied gently with a cotton wool bud, fine paintbrush or special dispensing syringe. The gel is distinctively coloured to ensure that it is confined to the required area. Acid is caustic and must contact nothing but enamel. To achieve this, the tooth is isolated with cotton wool rolls and napkins, and full saliva control is essential. The best way is to use rubber dam. Protective glasses and a waterproof apron should be worn by supine patients. Spilt acid must be washed off with water.
- After exposure to acid, the tooth is thoroughly washed with water and carefully dried with a three-in-one syringe. It should now have a matt white frosted

appearance. If so, the enamel has been successfully etched and is ready for application of the composite, but it must remain perfectly dry and free of saliva for successful bonding.

## Restoration of fractured incisors

Before acid etching was introduced, the most satisfactory way of restoring fractured incisors was by fitting a porcelain jacket crown. Unfortunately, this is unsuitable for children as the pulp chambers of immature teeth are too large and crown preparation may cause pulp damage. This, together with the fact that incisor fractures most commonly occur during childhood, meant that some other form of temporary crown had to be used – and these were of relatively poor appearance.

Composite filling materials and acid etching have transformed the treatment of fractured incisors. Small fractures in children and adults can be permanently restored in this way. Although porcelain jacket crowns may remain the best treatment for extensive fractures, acid etched restorations provide children with a satisfactory alternative until such time as the tooth (and patient) are ready for a more suitable restoration. Other injuries to children's teeth are covered in Chapters 17 and 20.

Enamel margins are acid etched, and lined with a bonding agent. A hybrid composite filling material is applied in a clear plastic crown form, such as an Odus pella crown form. When it has set, any excess is trimmed off and the restoration is polished where necessary.

The acid etch/composite filling technique is also used for: building up malformed or mis-shapen teeth to improve their appearance; direct bonding of orthodontic brackets, porcelain veneers and small bridges (Chapter 18); and construction of temporary splints. The latter are discussed in Chapter 20, and are made by bonding a length of wire or fibreglass tape to the loose tooth and its neighbours with a light-cure composite.

## Fissure sealing

As mentioned in Chapter 11, fissure sealing is a caries prevention measure. Occlusal fissures are natural stagnation areas where caries commonly occurs. If these fissures can be filled soon after eruption, the occlusal surface should then stay free of caries.

In the past, fissure filling was done by preparing an undercut cavity and using amalgam, but, as a preventive measure, this had the disadvantage of having to cut a cavity in sound enamel. The advent of new materials, such as composites and glass ionomer cement, allows fissure sealing to be done with minimal cavity preparation.

Retention is obtained by acid etching the fissures. Whichever material is used, any existing caries is removed and the cavity is filled at the same time as the sound fissures. The sealant is introduced into the fissures and seals off these stagnation areas.

The application of fissure sealants should be done as soon as possible after eruption but requires a completely dry occlusal surface. This is difficult to achieve in young children but may be overcome by applying a fluoride varnish (e.g. Duraphat) as a temporary seal, until a child is co-operative enough to permit the attainment of a dry field for sufficient time.

### Unfilled resins

All the composite filling materials described so far consist of a resin binder incorporating an inert inorganic filler. They are accordingly called **filled resins**. A catalyst makes the resin set, while the filler remains unchanged throughout. This gives the unset material its paste consistency, and the set filling its hardness and durability.

Thus it is only the resin and catalyst which are actually involved in the setting process. Several brands of composite make use of this fact by providing a liquid base containing just the resin without a filler. This is called an **unfilled resin** and sets in the same way as all the others by using the same catalyst. These unfilled resins (e.g. Delton) are available in chemical-cure or light-cure brands.

The advantage of an unfilled resin is its liquid consistency. Both resin and catalyst are liquids and the mixture can be easily flowed over acid etched enamel, into fissures, or mixed with a filled resin paste to give any desired consistency.

Unfilled resins are accordingly used as fissure sealants, and for surface glazing.

### Dentine-bonding agents

Although acid etching can satisfactorily bond older composite materials to enamel, it cannot bond them to dentine. Small undercuts are therefore required for adequate retention of composite fillings.

A new group of dental materials are now available which can bond composites to dentine and enamel. There is such a bewildering range of products available, with such a confusing pattern of instructions for use, that no consensus on the ideal type of product seems to have been achieved. However, the ideal simplest and best product would be one that is a single component, one-stage application to enamel and dentine, without any need to keep the prepared tooth dry. Some light-cured products that approach these ideals are already available, e.g. Optibond Solo Plus, Solobond M.

### Glass ionomer cements

Glass ionomer cement (GIC) consists of a powder and liquid which are mixed together on a paper pad. The powder is a glass-like mixture of **aluminosilicates**. The liquid contains **polyacrylic acid** (or polymaleic acid) and is similar to polycarboxylate cement liquid. Calcium hydroxide lining is unnecessary unless the cavity is very deep.

GIC has many different uses which depend on two outstanding properties:

■ It releases fluoride and thereby prevents recurrence of caries in and around the cavity
■ It bonds directly to enamel, dentine and cementum without acid etching

This chemical bond to tooth substance means that undercuts are not essential and makes it suitable for filling unretentive cavities, deciduous teeth, fissure sealing, a dentine substitute for restoring excessive loss of tooth substance, cavity lining, and as an adhesive cement for inlays, crowns and orthodontic bands.

## Permanent fillings

Older types of GIC are not strong enough for filling cavities which are exposed to the full force of mastication, so they are unsuitable for class I or II fillings in posterior teeth. Although GIC is tooth-coloured, its appearance is not as good as composite fillings as it is slightly darker and less translucent. Composites accordingly remain the material of choice for class III and IV fillings in anterior teeth.

The most useful application of GIC is for the permanent filling of class V (cervical) cavities anywhere in the mouth. Such cavities are naturally saucer-shaped, unretentive and not easy to undercut, and were accordingly very difficult to fill satisfactorily. GIC, e.g. ChemFil, Ketac-Fil, has provided the answer to this problem. Its darker colour is less important in cervical cavities in anterior teeth and does not matter in posterior teeth. Minimal cavity preparation is required and the filling provides its own retention by bonding directly to the cavity.

Cavities in deciduous teeth are also very suitable for filling with GIC as its natural retention allows minimal cavity preparation. Although it cannot withstand prolonged masticatory abrasion, the limited lifespan of deciduous teeth lessens the importance of this weakness.

Wherever and whenever it is used, its ability to release fluoride helps prevent further caries and, in that respect, it is superior to other filling materials.

## Cavity lining

As GIC is not very irritant to the pulp, and bonds naturally to dentine, it is suitable as a cavity lining beneath any permanent filling material. It is the strongest of all cavity linings and, together with calcium hydroxide, is superseding the traditional lining cements described earlier.

## Dentine substitute

The restoration of teeth which have lost much of their natural crown poses a retention problem. One way in which this can be overcome is to replace most of the lost dentine with amalgam to form a core on which a gold veneer crown (Chapter 18) can be fitted. However, amalgam does not bond to tooth substance, so retention in such cases often requires the insertion of pins into the remaining dentine prior to building up an amalgam core.

GIC can avoid the need for a pinned amalgam core as it bonds directly to dentine and can therefore be used as a dentine substitute. The core is accordingly made entirely of GIC without pinning, and when set it is trimmed to shape ready for the crown impression. However, there must be sufficient remaining natural crown structure to support the core. The same proviso applies to GIC crown cores in root-filled teeth.

## Adhesive cement

Inlays, crowns and orthodontic bands can be cemented into place with zinc phosphate or polycarboxylate cement, but a luting GIC (e.g. Aquacem) is better as it forms a stronger bond with tooth substance. Furthermore it is the only luting cement which releases fluoride and thereby has a **cariostatic** (caries preventive) effect.

## Fissure sealing

Fissures can be sealed with composites or GIC. The advantage of composites is their superior strength, and the ability of unfilled resin to be flowed into, and over, acid etched fissures. GIC is too viscous for that and it is consequently necessary to widen the fissure slightly with a pointed diamond bur. It can then be inserted into the fissure.

The advantages of GIC for fissure sealing are its fluoride release which provides a cariostatic effect and that there is no need for acid etching. This is particularly important when treating young children, as etching is ineffective if moisture contamination cannot be prevented. However, in practice, the two materials can be combined. If a part of the occlusal fissure system has already become carious, that part may be filled with GIC. The remaining sound fissures and the GIC are acid etched and the entire occlusal fissure system is then sealed with composite.

## Advantages

- Adhesive to enamel, dentine, and cementum; so minimal cavity preparation is required.
- It is therefore ideal for class V cavities, where cavity preparation is likely to expose the pulp.
- It has excellent marginal seal, which can be further improved by the use of **conditioners** (either polyacrylic acid or tannic acid).
- Releases fluoride over time, so it has a cariostatic effect.
- Modern products with metal powder added are strong enough to use for core build-ups – these are called **cermets**.
- GIC has better aesthetics than amalgam.

■ Modern, light-cure products are now available which overcome the moisture contamination problems of older cements.

## Disadvantages

■ Low strength compared to amalgam and composites.
■ Very exacting handling is required for correct placement, and easily ruined by moisture contamination.
■ Surface requires protection from moisture during full setting by varnish or resin.
■ Technique-sensitive while being mixed; exact proportions of powder and liquid are required to produce the optimal set.

## Technique

Although GIC forms a direct *chemical* bond with tooth substance, it can only do so if the cavity walls are clean and free of cavity preparation debris (the **smear layer**). Cavities are accordingly *conditioned* with polyacrylic acid before inserting the cement. This must not be confused with the use of phosphoric acid for acid etching, which only provides a *mechanical* bond.

Complete saliva control is necessary at all stages and this is best achieved by the use of rubber dam. After preparing the cavity, the polyacrylic acid conditioner is applied for up to thirty seconds depending on the product used, then thoroughly washed off and dried before insertion of the GIC.

### Mixing

GIC may come in the form of powder and liquid which are mixed on a waxed paper pad. The liquid constituent (polyacrylic acid) is usually dehydrated and included in the powder. This **anhydrous** version (e.g. Aqua-Fil), only needs mixing with water. Alternatively it can come in the form of a capsule containing powder and liquid (e.g. ChemFlex), for use in a mechanical mixer such as the amalgamator used for mixing amalgam capsules.

Manufacturers of hand-mixed brands supply measuring spoons to ensure that the correct proportions are used and proper consistency achieved – creamy for cementing and fissure sealing; thicker for fillings and linings. As GIC is so hard, an abrasion-resistant spatula, such as *agate* or stainless steel, is preferable for hand-mixing.

### Insertion

Deep cavities are lined with calcium hydroxide before the conditioning of the cavity walls. Hand-mixed materials are inserted and manipulated with non-stick plastic instruments, whereas mechanically mixed brands are provided with a special injection gun similar to that used for composite compoules. Permanent fillings are contoured to the tooth surface with a clear matrix strip which is held in place with a crocodile clip. Special shaped and contoured adhesive cervical matrices are available for class V cavities.

It is essential to avoid moisture contamination while setting, and to avoid dehydration through water loss after setting. Thus the cement must be covered with a waterproof varnish immediately the matrix is removed. A convenient varnish for this purpose is a light-cured unfilled composite such as Scotchbond.

## Finishing

Any removal of excess material, or polishing, should be deferred for at least one day as the heat produced during such instrumentation may dehydrate and weaken the filling. Ideally, trimming and polishing should be avoided altogether by inserting an exact amount of cement and relying on the matrix strip to give a polished surface. However, this cannot always be achieved and some finishing may be necessary. The cement manufacturers' recommended abrasive discs, strips and white stones should be used and dehydration avoided by lubricating the abrasives with petroleum jelly or the unfilled resin mentioned in the section on insertion.

## Resin-modified GIC

The introduction of light-cured composite fillings, which gives the dentist complete control of the setting process, has revolutionised the use of composite restoratives. This *command setting* has now been extended to some brands of GIC (e.g. Fuji LC) by adding some of the light-cured resin contained in composite filling materials.

The main advantage of such products seems to be the immediate setting that results from light-curing, as this allows polishing of the GIC at the same visit.

## Compomers

As the name implies, compomer is a term used to describe some of the new products which combine the advantages of composites and GIC in one material (e.g. Dyract, Compoglass).

Compomers are supplied in ready-to-use syringes for direct injection into the prepared cavity. They differ from resin modified GIC in so far as the latter are GIC plus some resin to make them light-cured, whereas compomers are composites plus some GIC component to provide fluoride release and chemical bonding.

# 17 Endodontics

Endodontics is the term used for all forms of root canal therapy. Non-surgical endodontics includes root filling, pulpotomy, and pulp capping, while surgical endodontics is correctly called apicectomy.

## Principles of endodontics

As explained in Chapter 11, pulpitis leads to pulp death. This in turn eventually leads to an acute alveolar abscess, which is a very painful condition. To prevent this chain of events, endodontic treatment or extraction is required whenever the pulp is irreversibly inflamed or dead, or when an alveolar abscess is already present.

The aims of root canal therapy are as follows:

- Complete removal of the pulpal contents – **extirpation**
- Shaping of the root canal to allow thorough irrigation
- Irrigation with antibacterial disinfectants such as sodium hypochlorite or chlorhexidine
- Removal of these irrigants and any residual bacteria from the root canal
- Filling of the root canal with a non-irritant, impermeable material – **obturation**
- This seals any further bacteria off from the periapical tissue fluids
- Allow the restoration of the tooth to full function, either by filling or by cementing a crown or inlay

The same procedure provides drainage and complete cure of an existing abscess. The root filled tooth will then function just as well as one with a normal pulp. Success depends on achieving a leak-proof seal at each end of the root canal, and thereby preventing micro-organisms from entering or leaving it.

There are many causes of pulpitis and pulp death but the treatment is similar in each case: either extraction or endodontics.

## Causes of pulpitis

The commonest cause of pulpitis is **exposure** of the pulp. This allows mouth bacteria to enter the pulp chamber and infect the pulp. Exposure of the pulp may be caused by:

- Caries
- Accidental exposure during cavity preparation
- Fracture of the crown

Even when the pulp is not exposed, pulpitis can still occur. The causes are:

- Irritation from an unlined filling
- Excessive heat during cavity preparation, such as the use of an air turbine handpiece without water spray
- Impact injury

Impact injuries are common in children with prominent anterior teeth. The crown may fracture and expose the pulp. Alternatively the crown remains intact but the blow damages the apical blood vessels and pulp death ensues. Treatment of a tooth which is completely knocked out (avulsed) is described in Chapter 20.

## Choice of treatment

In deciding whether to treat by extraction or endodontics, several factors are considered, as follows:

- The feasibility of restoring the tooth to function after endodontic treatment
- The medical history of the patient
- The usefulness of the tooth in occlusion
- The patient's wishes, especially where costs are involved
- The dental health of the patient. If this is poor then advanced dental treatment is likely to fail

Many technical difficulties beset the endodontic treatment of multi-rooted teeth and for this reason they often used to be extracted rather than root treated, although advances in rotary endodontic instruments has made treatment of these teeth easier nowadays. Endodontic treatment on anterior teeth is easier as they are more accessible and have only one root canal to treat. It is consequently simpler and more likely to be successful than on posterior teeth. Furthermore, most patients would prefer to save a front tooth rather than have it extracted. Although premolars and molars are frequently extracted, they can be saved by endodontic treatment when necessary.

## Importance of the medical history

Some medical conditions make the patient more likely to develop infective endocarditis (Chapter 4) following the bacteraemia that will occur during endodontic treatment, and these are:

- Acquired valvular heart disease
- History of rheumatic fever
- Congenital heart defects
- Patients wearing a pacemaker

These patients should be given a prophylactic antibiotic one hour before the endodontic treatment – either a single 3 g dose of **amoxicillin** or a single 600 mg total dose of **clindamycin**, if they are allergic to penicillin-type antibiotics. However, patients with a history of infective carditis, rheumatic fever or valve replacements should not be administered prophylactic antibiotic cover (as recommended by NICE).

Patients with diabetes should also be treated with caution, as their condition tends to make them prone to poor wound healing and infections. Other medical conditions will contraindicate the extraction of a tooth, as follows:

- Epilepsy – these patients should not wear dentures if possible
- Bleeding disorders – especially clotting disorders where haemostasis may be difficult to achieve
- Cleft palate

### Vitality tests

The dentist's decision on whether to treat a decayed tooth by an ordinary filling, endodontics or extraction depends on the state of the pulp. If it is dead, endodontics or extraction is necessary. If it is alive and unexposed, an ordinary filling will suffice.

The state of the pulp is not always apparent and vitality tests are often required to determine whether it is alive or dead. These tests depend on the painful response of the pulp to certain stimuli. If there is a response the pulp is vital, if not, it is probably dead. The following tests are used.

- *Heat.* A stick of **gutta percha** (GP) is heated in a flame and applied to the crown of the tooth. A film of petroleum jelly should be applied to the crown before the placement of GP to prevent it sticking to the tooth and causing excessive pain.
- *Cold.* Cotton wool moistened with **ethyl chloride**, or an ice stick, is applied to the crown.
- *Electricity.* An electronic pulp tester is applied to the crown.

■ *Drilling*. Cavity preparation without LA is painful when the pulp is vital, but this procedure is not considered best practice nowadays.

■ *X-ray*. Alveolar abscess on a dead tooth will show on an X-ray film as a widened periodontal ligament or an actual radiolucent periapical area.

The symptoms of **acute irreversible pulpitis** are as follows:

■ The patient experiences spontaneous intermittent spasms of pain
■ The pain becomes throbbing and continuous with time
■ The tooth is no longer stimulated by temperature changes or sweet foods
■ The tooth becomes hypersensitive to vitality testing, but is not tender to percussion (TTP) when tapped by the dentist

## Root filling or pulpectomy

The object of root filling is to remove the inflamed or dead pulp from a tooth and replace it with a sterile non-irritant, insoluble root canal filling that seals off the entire canal and thereby prevents any recurrence of apical infection. It is often done in two stages: the first to prepare the canal; the second to insert the root filling. If no difficulties arise, both stages can be completed in one visit.

At the first visit:

1   The pulp is extirpated, using a **barbed broach**
2   The root canal is reamed and filed to enlarge and shape it using **reamers and files**, then cleaned and disinfected to prepare a dry, smooth, empty canal which tapers gradually from the pulp chamber towards the apex
3   An **antiseptic dressing** and temporary filling is inserted to seal the entrance to the empty root canal, to kill any residual bacteria and prevent contamination of the canal between visits

At the second visit:

1   The temporary filling and dressing are removed
2   If the root canal is still clean and dry, it is **obturated** with **gutta percha** (GP) to seal off the entire canal to within a millimetre of the apex

### Root filling instruments

Special instruments used for root filling are barbed broaches, root reamers, root canal files, pluggers and rotary paste fillers (Figure 17.1).

**Barbed broaches** are single use disposable hand instruments for removing the pulp. They consist of a fine wire with multiple barbs. When the broach is inserted in a root canal and rotated, its barbs engage the pulp, whereupon the pulp can be withdrawn with the broach.

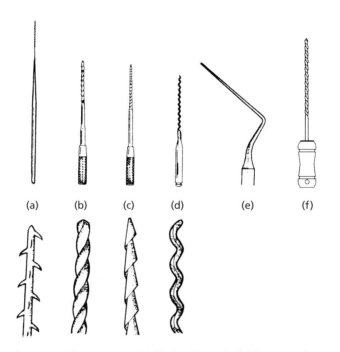

**Figure 17.1** Root canal instruments. (a) Barbed broach. (b) Root canal reamer.
(c) Root canal file. (d) Rotary paste-filler. (e) Root canal finger spreader.
(f) Flexible hand K file.

**Root reamers** resemble wood drills and are used for enlarging root canals in a circular fashion so that a filling can be inserted. They are made in standardised sets – all of the same length, but with an increasing range of widths. Each reamer is numbered or colour-coded to indicate its size. The reamer is inserted in the canal and advanced by hand or by specially adapted handpieces for use with rotary endodontic instruments.

**Root canal files** are hand or handpiece instruments which are similar to reamers but are flexible, and they are made in the same standardised range of sizes (Figure 17.2). Their function is to smooth and clean the walls of enlarged root canals and remove debris, and their flexibility allows them to negotiate curved root canals. They are inserted in the canal and used with an up-and-down filing action against the canal walls. Many practitioners use files exclusively instead of reamers, but in the same sequence of sizes.

Reaming and filing root canals by hand is laborious and time consuming. However, the introduction of flexible nickel-titanium root canal instruments, used with modern variable speed handpieces, allows dentists to undertake these procedures far more easily and precisely. They are particularly useful for the curved canals of multi-rooted teeth.

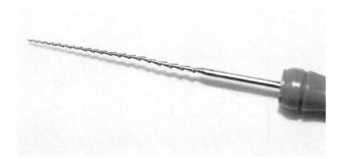

**Figure 17.2** Endodontic hand file.

**Root canal pluggers** or **spreaders** have a long, tapered smooth point used to condense the GP filling against the canal walls and obliterate any gaps.

**Rotary paste fillers** are engine instruments for inserting pastes into a root canal. They consist of a spiral wire which fits in a handpiece and propels the required material to the full length of the root canal.

## Preparation

As the root canal must be disinfected before it is filled, all instruments and dressings must be sterile. A convenient arrangement is to keep a sealed container holding a complete sterilised root filling kit ready for immediate use at any time. Rubber dam (Figure 17.3) is essential to achieve the following:

- To prevent ingress of micro-organisms from the mouth into the root canal
- To prevent accidents such as inhalation or swallowing of small root canal instruments
- To improve access and visibility for the dentist

Non-latex purple or blue rubber dam should be available for use on patients who are, or may be, sensitive to latex, otherwise the regular green latex dam sheets are used. If, for whatever reason, use of rubber dam is impractical, small root canal hand instruments must have a length of dental floss or a **parachute chain** attached. This allows them to be retrieved if they accidentally slip out of the dentist's hand.

Modern infection control practice stipulates that all endodontic instruments inserted into a root canal must be considered as single use, and safely disposed of in the sharps box after use. A new set of instruments must then be used on the next patient, and disposed of in a similar fashion.

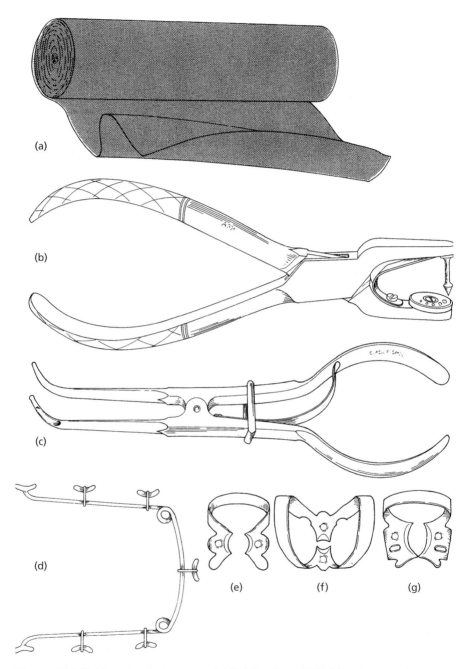

**Figure 17.3** Rubber dam instruments. (a) Rubber dam. (b) Rubber dam punch.
(c) Rubber dam clamp forceps. (d) Rubber dam frame. (e) Premolar clamp.
(f) Incisor (butterfly) clamp. (g) Molar clamp.

Procedure

As mentioned earlier, more than one visit may be necessary. The following description is for a two-visit procedure.

1   Local anaesthetic is used if the pulp is still vital.
2   Rubber dam is applied. The tooth and rubber dam are then swabbed with a disinfectant such as chlorhexidine.
3   Access to the root canal(s) is gained by drilling open the pulp chamber. A Gates-Glidden bur (Figure 17.4) is safe and convenient for this purpose.
4   Any intact pulp tissue can be extirpated with a barbed broach. Patients at risk of infective endocarditis (Chapter 4) require antibiotic cover.
5   The length of the root canal must be measured before any further instrumentation is undertaken – this is called the **working length**. This is done by taking a diagnostic periapical X-ray with a root reamer or file of known length inserted in the canal. It may also be done with an electronic apex locator, but should be confirmed with an X-ray. Once an X-ray shows the required length of canal preparation (1 mm short of the apex), all subsequent reaming and filing is kept to this length by fitting a stopper to each instrument before insertion. This prevents penetration of the apical foramen or too short a preparation of the canal.
6   The walls of the root canal are smoothed and cleaned with files to produce a smooth-bordered canal which tapers from a wide entrance to a narrow apical end. It is achieved by using a wide file at the root canal entrance followed by successively narrower files until the preparation reaches its end point, 1 mm short of the apical foramen. This results in a wide entrance to the root canal, with adequate visibility and access for instrumentation, and a progressively narrower taper towards the apex.
7   Throughout reaming and filing, the canal is irrigated with a disinfectant such as sodium hypochlorite or chlorhexidine to remove debris and disinfect the canal. A special sterile disposable syringe, with a blunt end and a side bevel (Monoject syringe), is used for this purpose. The side bevel prevents the irrigation solution from being injected through the apex into the surrounding tissues – this is especially undesirable when sodium hypochlorite is used.
8   The canal is then dried with absorbent **paper points** and its entrance covered with dry sterile cotton wool, or if infection was present before cleaning, an antiseptic-soaked paper point can be left in the canal.
9   The pulp chamber is sealed off with a temporary filling to prevent contamination of the empty, clean, dry root canal between visits.
10  At the next visit, if the root canal is still clean and dry, or all signs of infection have gone, it is ready for insertion of the permanent filling. A **gutta-percha point** that most closely matches the root canal taper is selected. This is called the master point and has to be sealed to the apical end of the canal with cement.

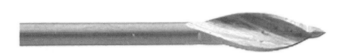

Figure 17.4 Gates-Glidden bur.

11  Various proprietary brands of root canal sealers are available, many being based on a modified zinc oxide eugenol cement, e.g. Tubliseal. The canal walls and the end of the master point are coated with sealer and the point inserted into the root canal.

12  The gap between the canal walls and the master point is filled by **condensing** successive GP points against the canal walls with a **finger plugger or lateral condenser** (Figure 17.1e) until no space is left. Warming the spreader softens GP and assists condensation against the canal walls. The use of self-locking tweezers facilitates handling of paper and GP points. An alternative technique uses pre-heated GP and pluggers to provide easier and effective sealing by vertical condensation (Thermafil, Alphaseal); whichever method is used, it must ensure that each end of the root canal has a leak-proof seal.

13  An X-ray is taken to ensure that the root filling is satisfactory and to check subsequent progress.

14  Having completely filled the root canal with GP, the access cavity and pulp chamber are lined with glass ionomer cement and filled with composite or amalgam.

If, at step 10, the root canal is not dry, it means that apical infection is still present. In that case the canal is irrigated again with disinfectant, dried with paper points and another temporary dressing is inserted in the access cavity. It should then be ready for a permanent root filling at the next visit. If not, a temporary root dressing of non-setting calcium hydroxide paste is inserted until the next visit. The paste can be made by mixing calcium hydroxide powder with sterile water or local anaesthetic solution. The paste is inserted into the canal with a rotary paste filler.

Instruments

- Mirror, probe and tweezers
- Local anaesthetic equipment
- Rubber dam equipment, aspirator and saliva ejector
- Handpiece and burs
- Barbed broaches, root reamers, files, spreaders and pluggers, rotary paste fillers
- Locking tweezers, paper points and cotton wool
- Syringe for irrigation with sodium hypochlorite
- GP points and sealer cement
- Ruler for measuring length of root canal

## Pulpotomy

In adults, the conservative treatment of an exposed vital pulp is by root filling. But in children, growth of the root is not yet complete and an exposed tooth may still have a wide open apex, instead of the minute apical foramen. Root filling is unnecessary for these teeth as pulp death does not always occur. The wide open apex allows blood circulation through the pulp to continue, without being cut off by a build-up of inflammatory pressure. Instead of total removal of the pulp, followed by root filling, it is only necessary to remove the infected part of the pulp in the pulp chamber – a procedure known as **pulpotomy**. The very rich blood supply through an open apex allows healing to occur. The pulp survives and growth continues to its natural completion. In fully grown teeth, such healing is rarely possible and that is why the entire pulp must be removed and a root filling inserted.

The procedure in pulpotomy is similar to root filling only in so far as a sterile technique is necessary. The pulp tissue is removed from the pulp chamber within the crown of the tooth only. The amputated pulp stump at the entrance to the root canal is then covered with a calcium hydroxide dressing. This stimulates the pulp in the root canal to form a layer of secondary dentine over itself. The pulp is thereby completely sealed off again, as it was before the exposure occurred, and normal growth continues until apical formation is complete. It may then be necessary to do a full root filling.

### Procedure

The procedure is the same as root filling for steps 1–3.

4   The pulp in the pulp chamber only is removed by a sterile slow-speed bur.
5   The pulp at the entrance to the root canal is covered with calcium hydroxide paste and sealed with a temporary filling.

### Instruments

1–5: as for root filling.

6   Sterile cotton wool
7   Calcium hydroxide and sterile water, or pre-mixed paste
8   Temporary filling

### Open apex root filling

Pulpotomy is only successful if the exposed pulp is vital and can separate itself from the exposure site by laying down a secondary dentine bridge. A dead tooth with an open apex must be root filled as no secondary dentine will form, but this cannot be done in the same way as one with a closed apex, because the GP points will be too small to seal the open apex and will perforate the apical foramen instead. A method that seals the open apex before filling the rest of the root canal is used.

■ Antibiotic cover and local anaesthesia are used if necessary.
■ Rubber dam is applied and the working length of the canal is determined.
■ The dead pulp is removed with barbed broaches.
■ The root canal is cleaned with hand files and irrigated with saline, taking care not to proceed beyond the open apex.
■ The prepared canal is dried with paper points.
■ A spiral root canal filler is then used to fill the entire canal with a special non-setting calcium hydroxide paste (e.g. Hypocal). This disinfects the canal, shows on X-rays and does no harm if it goes slightly beyond the open apex.
■ After an X-ray to confirm adequate filling of the canal, a reinforced zinc oxide eugenol temporary filling is inserted to seal the root canal entrance.
■ After a *pulpotomy*, the calcium hydroxide in the pulp chamber forms a hard tissue bridge that seals off the root canal entrance. However, in the open apex root-filled tooth it only seals off the apex, closing down the size of the apical foramen. This may take up to six months, after which, the calcium hydroxide filling is removed and replaced with a conventional root filling.

## Pulp capping

When a vital pulp is exposed, either root filling or pulpotomy is necessary to conserve the tooth. This cannot always be done immediately as pulp exposure often occurs unexpectedly, or presents as an emergency.

In such cases pulp capping is a valuable temporary measure. The exposure is covered with calcium hydroxide paste or Ledermix and the cavity is filled with a temporary cement. This prevents pain and protects the pulp from infection until root filling or pulpotomy is performed.

## Apicectomy

Apicectomy is a surgical procedure to remove an infected apex and the surrounding infected tissue. The purpose of apicectomy is to save the tooth in cases where root filling is either unsuccessful or impossible. It is the final alternative to extraction and is done for the following reasons:

■ Root filling unsuccessful
  – Incomplete filling of inaccessible canal
  – Continued pain and infection after pulpectomy
  – Continued presence of a chronic sinus tract
  – An enlarging periapical area on subsequent radiographs

- Root filling impossible
  - Canal blocked by broken instrument
  - Alveolar abscess on tooth with post crown
  - Persistent periapical area following re-root filling
  - Removal of excess root filling material from the periapical area
  - Elimination of curved or fractured root apices

## Procedure

1  Under local anaesthesia, an incision is made through the gum and a flap raised off the bone with a periosteal elevator.
2  Using a straight handpiece and burs, a window is cut in the overlying bone to expose the infected apex.
3  The apex is cut off and infected tissue surrounding it is scraped away with a **Mitchell trimmer or curette** (Figure 17.5), which resembles a large excavator.
4  The cut end of the root is then examined to see if the remaining root filling is deficient. If so, a bit more filling is inserted in the cut end. Reinforced zinc oxide eugenol or GIC is usually chosen and the procedure is known as **retrograde root filling**. A promising new type of sealant cement for this purpose has recently become available, called MTA (Pro-Root MTA), but has not been in use long enough for long-term assessment.
5  Debris is removed by syringing with sterile saline and the gum flap is sutured back into place.
6  Sutures are removed a few days later and an X-ray is taken for record purposes. By comparing this X-ray with future ones, the progress of healing can be observed.

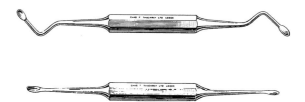

**Figure 17.5** Curettes.

## Instruments

Set out on sterile towel:

- Aspirator tubes or saliva ejector
- Mirror, probe and tweezers
- Local anaesthetic equipment
- Scalpel, periosteal elevator and swabs

- Straight handpiece and surgical burs
- Curettes or Mitchell trimmer
- Retrograde amalgam carrier
- Disposable syringe and sterile saline
- Dissecting forceps, needle-holder, sutures, scissors

## Use of antibiotics in endodontics

The aim of endodontic treatment is to attempt to save the tooth from extraction. When a patient presents with obvious signs of an acute infection, a course of antibiotic therapy may be required before treatment of the tooth can commence. The signs of an acute infection are as follows:

- The presence of pus
- A raised body temperature (**pyrexia**)
- Obvious debilitation of the patient
- Severe pain and loss of function of the affected tooth
- Swelling, either intra-orally or extra-orally

The dentist will attempt to begin treatment and alleviate these symptoms if possible, by either **lancing** the intra-oral abscess or opening the root canal and placing the tooth on **open drainage**. At the same time, antibiotics will be prescribed:

- **Amoxicillin 250 mg four times daily**, or **erythromycin** if allergic to penicillin derivatives
- **Metronidazole 200 mg three times daily**, given at the same time if a severe infection is present

# 18 Inlays, Crowns and Bridges

Plastic fillings such as amalgam and composites are normally completed in one visit, but pre-constructed restorations such as inlays, crowns and bridges require a minimum of two visits with one laboratory stage between them:

- First visit: tooth prepared
- Laboratory: restoration constructed on model of prepared tooth
- Second visit: restoration cemented

As these restorations cannot utilise undercuts for retention, tapered burs (see Figure 16.10) are used as they are less likely to produce undercuts. Any undercuts on the preparation are blocked out with the lining cement.

## Gold inlays

Gold inlays are used as stronger alternatives to amalgam fillings. They are generally confined to teeth which have lost cusps, undergo heavy occlusal forces, or are otherwise too weak to be satisfactorily restored with amalgam. Small uncomplicated cavities do not usually warrant the extra time and expense of gold inlays. The advantages of gold are that it does not tarnish and has great strength which is superior to that of other filling materials. Consequently much less tooth substance need be drilled away.

The disadvantages are the extra time and expense involved and, like amalgam, it is unsuitable for front teeth where it would show. As gold is so expensive, alternative ceramic or composite materials have been tried, but their long-term durability for inlays is less than that of gold.

### First visit

The cavity is made retentive with parallel cavity walls and an impression is taken with an accurate elastic material, such as a silicone or polyether. This is sent to the laboratory, together with a recording of the occlusion. A temporary filling is then inserted and the patient is given an appointment for fitting the inlay. The temporary fillings described in Chapter 16 are not suitable for this purpose as they cannot be removed without drilling. An elastic material which can be removed in one piece is best, e.g. Fermit, Clip.

## Laboratory

A technician uses the impression to make a model of the prepared tooth and then constructs a wax inlay on the model. This is done by softening a stick of blue **inlay wax** over a flame and pressing it into the inlay cavity on the model. The wax is trimmed to the original shape of the tooth with a **Ward carver** (see Figure 16.15) to make a **wax pattern** of the required restoration. The wax pattern is then cast in gold, polished, and returned to the surgery for fitting.

## Second visit

The temporary filling is removed and the inlay fitted. Before cementing the inlay, the occlusion is checked and any high spots are removed with a Carborundum stone. The edges are burnished to give a good marginal fit and the inlay is cemented with glass ionomer cement (GIC), zinc phosphate, polycarboxylate, or one of the dual-cure GIC materials now available (Figure 18.1).

This procedure, whereby the wax pattern is made in the laboratory from an impression, is called the **indirect method** of construction. The **direct method** is a procedure whereby the dentist makes the wax pattern in the surgery and the technician casts it directly in gold. For all but the simplest inlays, the direct method can be far more difficult and time-consuming for a dentist than taking an impression. For this reason it has been virtually superseded by the indirect method. All crowns and bridges are made by an indirect method.

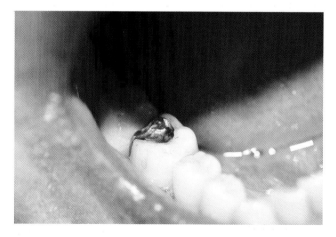

Figure 18.1  Cemented gold inlay.

## Impressions

The elastic impression materials used for inlays, crowns and bridges are called **elastomers**, e.g. Impregum, Aquasil. They consist of two components – base and catalyst – which are mixed together and loaded into a metal impression tray (Chapter 19). In the mouth they set into a solid rubbery consistency. There are many different types of elastomer, such as **addition silicones** and **polyethers**, but they are all used in much the same way.

## Mixing

For hand-mixing the base and catalyst are supplied in tubes of different colours. They are mixed with a spatula on a pad, in the recommended proportions, to give a mix of uniform colour. Most makes are available in two different consistencies: *light-bodied* for syringing over a prepared tooth; and *heavy-bodied* for filling the impression tray.

Some brands use a putty for the heavy-bodied material. This is mixed with its catalyst by kneading in a gloved hand, but some of these materials cannot be used with every brand of glove.

Most elastomers are also supplied in cartridges which are inserted into a special gun and are extruded, ready-mixed, directly into the cavity or impression tray. This is obviously the most convenient, accurate and quickest procedure and is superseding traditional hand-mixing methods.

## Technique

Before the impression is taken, the gum must be eased away from the cavity margin to keep it dry and permit a good impression. This is done by packing the gum margin with **gingival retraction cord** which consists of string or cord impregnated with an astringent, such as adrenaline or alum. It shrinks the gum away from the cavity margins, so that the impression material can reach every part of the preparation.

With such a wide range of these impression materials there is a corresponding range of techniques, but a typical procedure is as follows:

1   Pack gingival retraction cord into the gingival crevice
2   Mix light-bodied material and load into syringe
3   Mix heavy-bodied material and load into metal tray
4   Remove retraction cord
5   Syringe light-bodied material into cavity, ensuring that it covers the entire preparation and its margins
6   Insert impression tray of heavy-bodied material
7   Remove tray when material has set

For putty materials an impression is taken with the kneaded putty. Light-bodied material is then mixed and placed over the putty or syringed over the prepared tooth. The impression is then reinserted to provide the final impression, this is called a **two-stage technique**. Alternatively both these stages may be combined into one by loading the tray with putty and covering it with a wash of light-bodied material before insertion, or by syringing the light-bodied material onto the prepared tooth and inserting the loaded tray over it – this is called a **one-stage technique**. A relatively new impression tray system called a **triple tray** allows an impression of the prepared tooth, the occluding teeth and their occlusion to be recorded at the same time. This system has the following advantages:

- Uses less impression material
- Quicker technique
- Less uncomfortable for the patient than full mouth impressions

The disadvantage is that the dentist must ensure the patient bites accurately together while the impression material sets, otherwise the occlusion will be recorded incorrectly and the restoration may require a remake.

As elastomers do not adhere to conventional impression trays, it is necessary to either use a perforated tray, or apply a tray adhesive before loading, to ensure the safe withdrawal of the impression. It is then washed in running water, immersed in a disinfectant such as 10% sodium hypochlorite, rinsed in water again then blown dry before despatch to the laboratory.

The advantages of elastomers are their combination of elasticity, strength and accuracy. This ensures an **accurate undistorted** impression of undercut areas and allows several cavities to be included in one impression. Their disadvantages are the elaborate technique required, long setting time and the sticky consistency before setting.

## Occlusal records

Having obtained an impression of the prepared tooth, the next step is to record the occlusion between the prepared tooth and those which bite against it, unless a triple tray system has been used. An alginate (Chapter 19) or putty impression of the opposing teeth is taken and this provides the technician with a model of the opposing teeth as well as the prepared tooth. However, an additional record may be needed to show the technician how the two models occlude together. This can be done by softening a sheet of pink or silver wax in a flame and placing it over the prepared tooth. The patient then bites into the wax to give an imprint of the opposing teeth on one side of the wax and the prepared tooth on the other. This wax **squash bite** allows the technician to fit the two models together in their natural occlusion and thereby produce a wax pattern in correct contact with its adjacent tooth and correct occlusion with its opposing teeth.

For a single inlay, a wax squash bite is usually sufficient, but for multiple-inlay preparations, crowns and bridges a more accurate recording than a squash bite is necessary. This is achieved by using an elastomer occlusal impression material instead of wax, e.g. Blu-Mousse, Futar D. However, the most accurate way of showing the correct occlusion is a pair of models that articulate together precisely without having to use a separate occlusal record. As this cannot be ascertained at the time of taking the impressions, an occlusal record is taken in case the technician is unable to articulate the upper and lower models with complete certainty.

## Crowns

A crown is a laboratory constructed, artificial restoration which replaces at least three-quarters of the natural crown of the tooth. There are various types, made of various materials, and they require at least two visits.

At the first visit the tooth is prepared, using diamond discs, wheels and tapered burs (Figure 16.10). An elastomer impression and occlusal records are then taken and, for anterior teeth, the shade is recorded. A temporary crown is then cemented and the patient is dismissed. In practice it is best to prepare the temporary crown before taking the impression, so that it is ready for immediate cementation at the end of the visit.

At the second visit, the temporary crown is removed and the permanent one positioned. It is then checked for appearance and occlusion before cementing with ordinary or dual-cure GIC, zinc phosphate or polycarboxylate. Finally, any excess cement is removed with hand instruments. This also applies to bridges and temporary restorations; this task may be delegated to a hygienist or therapist.

### Temporary crowns

Temporary crowns are used for the following reasons:

- To maintain appearance
- To prevent sensitivity between visits
- To maintain the correct space between adjacent teeth
- To maintain the correct occlusion between opposing teeth

Temporary crowns are made by fitting a **crown form** over the prepared tooth.

For anterior teeth a clear plastic crown form such as an **Odus pella** may be used. It is trimmed with **crown scissors** (Figure 18.2) and filled with a material which matches the teeth, such as composite. Alternatively, tough tooth-coloured **polycarbonate** crown forms are used, such as **Directa**, and these only need trimming with slow burs.

Metal crown forms made of aluminium or stainless steel are used on posterior teeth.

Trimmed temporary crowns are cemented with a material which is adhesive, but easily and cleanly removed for fitting the permanent crown, e.g. Temp Bond NE, Procem, or ProTemp.

Stainless steel crown forms, cemented with GIC, are also used as the best restoration for large cavities in deciduous molars instead of a conventional filling.

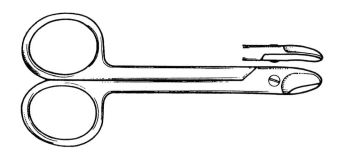

Figure 18.2 Beebee crown scissors.

## Jacket crown

A jacket crown is used for anterior teeth which are too mutilated to be restored by ordinary fillings, and include cases with very extensive caries, fracture of the crown, and severe pitting, discoloration, or deformation of the crown.

The outer coating of the natural crown is removed to leave a stump of dentine with a well-defined cervical shoulder, on which the artificial crown fits like a jacket (Figure 18.3).

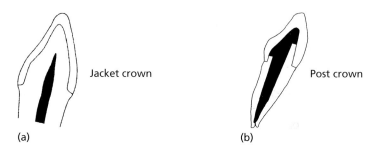

(a)    (b)

Figure 18.3 Crowns. (a) Jacket crown (reproduced with permission from: *A Clinical Guide to Crowns and Other Extra-coronal Restorations*. Wassel, Walls, Steel & Nohl, *British Dental Journal*). (b) Post crown (reproduced with permission from: *Essential Endodontology: Prevention and Treatment of Apical Periodontitis*, 2nd edn, D. Ørstavik & T. Pitt Ford, 2008, Blackwell Publishing, Oxford.

End-cutting burs (see Figure 16.10) are often used for preparing the shoulder for such crowns. Jacket crowns are usually made entirely of **porcelain** (PJC). However, this is liable to fracture under a heavy bite, and such cases require a **porcelain-bonded crown** (PBC) which has a porcelain facing bonded to a gold backing (Figure 18.4). Alternatively, the more modern **all-ceramic crowns** may be used, which are stronger than conventional PJCs. Temporary or semi-permanent jacket crowns are made of acrylic (Chapter 19).

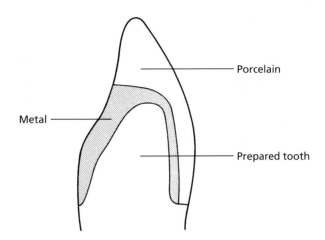

**Figure 18.4** Porcelain bonded crown.
Source: *The Restoration of Teeth*, 2nd edn, T.R. Pitt Ford, Blackwell Science Ltd, Oxford.

## Post crown

When a crown is required on a tooth which has been root-filled, a post crown is generally used. The filled root canal is prepared to accept the appropriate type of post, and as much of the natural crown dentine as possible is retained as the crown core. If there is insufficient core dentine left, it is built up with composite or GIC until the core is large enough to support a crown. The completed preparation is shown in Figure 18.3.

The post may be a gold casting or preformed in stainless steel, or a tooth-coloured fibre-reinforced composite. After cementing the post, a crown core may be built up on the post with composite or GIC. The final stages are an impression and cementation of a temporary crown.

## Veneer crown

A veneer crown is a thin gold (or palladium alloy) shell used in the construction of bridges (Figure 18.5). On posterior teeth it covers the entire crown and is called a **full gold crown** (FGC), (Figure 18.6) while on anterior teeth it covers all but the labial surface and is called a **three-quarter crown**.

**Figure 18.5** Full veneer crown.

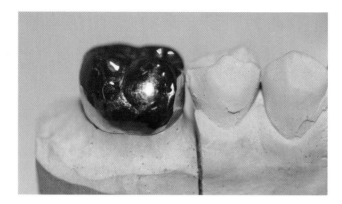

Figure 18.6  Full gold crown on model.

Apart from bridges, full veneer crowns are also used to restore teeth which are unsuitable for amalgam, such as badly broken down teeth and split teeth. In the latter case the crown acts as a splint. On badly broken down teeth the full crown forms a protective shell covering the amalgam or composite core which restores most of the bulk of the natural crown.

Amalgam cores can be retained by metal dentine pins which are screwed into the amalgam. However, this is a potentially risky procedure, as the pins can perforate the root canal, and is considered no longer necessary. The modern bonding agents mentioned in Chapter 16 can bond amalgam to dentine, and are superseding any further need for dentine pins.

Full crowns on premolars may be made with a porcelain-bonded buccal surface to improve their appearance. These PBCs are often used instead of three-quarter crowns for front teeth (Figure 18.7).

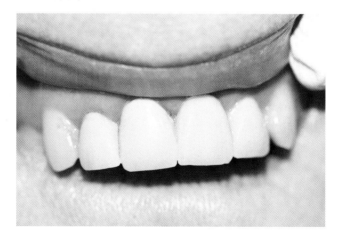

Figure 18.7  Porcelain bonded crowns.

# Bridges

A bridge is a *fixed* replacement for one or a few missing teeth. The artificial tooth filling the gap has a gold backing or a gold base which is soldered to crowns on adjacent teeth. The artificial tooth is called a **pontic** and the supporting teeth are called **abutments**. The crowns on the abutment teeth are called **retainers**. Thus a bridge consists of one or more pontics soldered to gold retainers on the abutments, and is inserted by cementing the retainers on to the abutments (Figure 18.8). An elastomer impression is used when constructing a bridge, as all the teeth involved can be included in one impression. Full occlusal records are then taken and a temporary bridge is fitted between visits.

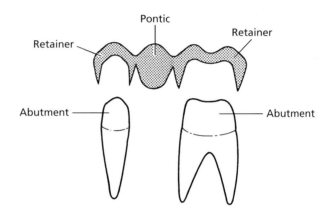

**Figure 18.8** Bridge components.

At the fitting stage, the occlusion must be correct before a bridge is cemented. Any high spots are found by closing the teeth together on a very fine film of articulating foil or mylar (shimstock). These are conveniently and firmly held in place with **Miller forceps** (Figure 18.9) and accurately mark any high spots by leaving coloured marks on the bridge after the patient has bitten into their occlusion.

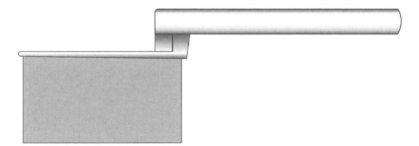

**Figure 18.9** Miller forceps and articulating paper.

A bridge has the following advantages over tooth replacement with a denture:

- Good retention as it is cemented to the teeth
- More hygienic, as minimal soft tissue coverage is involved
- Functions as a normal tooth

However, bridges are far more expensive to construct than dentures, and if the abutment teeth are occlusally overloaded due to a poor bridge design, they may well fracture or become symptomatic and ultimately have to be extracted.

Bridges fixed at each end (Figures 18.8 and 18.10) are described as **fixed-fixed**; those fixed at one end only are called **cantilever** bridges. Bridges can also be made by using **implants** as abutments (Figure 18.11). This saves having to make retainers on natural teeth and is described in Chapter 19.

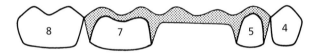

**Figure 18.10** Posterior bridge with sanitary pontic.

**Figure 18.11** Implant replacement of missing lateral incisor.

## Anterior bridges

Bridges replacing anterior teeth usually have pontics consisting of a porcelain jacket crown on a gold stump. This permits easy replacement of the crown without having to remove the bridge. To prevent any gold showing, three-quarter or porcelain-bonded crowns may be used as retainers on abutment teeth.

A cantilever bridge is usually preferred for replacement of a single missing incisor, but this is liable to put an excessive strain on the joint with the abutment tooth. In such cases a **fixed-movable** bridge can be used instead. This is fixed at one end, like a cantilever, while the other end fits loosely on to its abutment tooth, rather like an occlusal rest on a partial denture (see Chapter 19); thus it shares the strain with the fixed end. Alternative restorations for missing front teeth are covered later in this chapter.

## Posterior bridges

Bridges replacing posterior teeth usually have full veneer crowns on the abutment teeth. If the pontic is near enough to show, it has a tooth-coloured facing and its mesial retainer would be a three-quarter or porcelain bonded crown. If it is sufficiently far back, a **sanitary pontic** is preferred. This consists of a gold occlusal surface which spans the space between the abutments just like a real bridge. A large hygienic space is left between the base of the pontic and the gum which minimises food stagnation and facilitates cleaning by the patient (see Figure 18.10).

## Temporary bridges

A temporary bridge is necessary between visits to prevent sensitivity, space closure, tipping or over-eruption of the abutment teeth. It is made as given below.

1   Before the abutment teeth are prepared, the gap of the missing tooth is filled with a piece of cotton wool roll. A putty or heavy-bodied elastomer impression of the bridge area is then taken, the cotton wool discarded, and the impression put aside.
2   The abutments are then prepared and an impression for the permanent bridge is taken.
3   The first impression is now used to make a temporary bridge. A composite-type resin (e.g. Temphase) is placed in the part of the impression containing the abutment teeth and pontic area, and the impression is then reinserted until the resin sets.
4   On withdrawal of the impression, the temporary bridge is removed, trimmed, and cemented back into place with a temporary cement until the permanent bridge is cemented at another visit.

   This direct method of making a temporary bridge is facilitated by new dual-cure materials (Chapter 16) utilising cartridges and a special gun for automatic mixing and application into the impression (e.g. Provipont DC). Similar materials are also available as temporary cements (e.g. Provilink).

## Surgery procedure

As bridges are effectively one or more crowns joined together, the surgery procedure is the same as that involved in the indirect method of inlay and crown construction. However, the following extra steps may be required:

■   Study models and X-ray films are first taken to decide the best design and plan the number and length of appointments needed
■   A try-in visit for the crowns, to check their fit and occlusion, followed by an overall impression with crowns in place to facilitate soldering the pontic to the retainers

# Direct-bonded restorations

Chapter 16 described composite filling materials and bonding agents, and acid etching – which allows composite materials to bond directly to enamel, porcelain and metal surfaces. This technique enables small anterior bridges to be made without having to crown the abutments. It also allows the use of porcelain veneers instead of jacket crowns in appropriate cases.

## Maryland bridges

These bridges replace just one or two front teeth. The pontic has a porcelain bonded facing while the metal backing has wing-like flanges which rest against the palatal surface of the abutments, and are bonded directly to their acid etched enamel. The fitting surface of the flanges is made retentive by acid etching and sand blasting, and a chemical-cure adhesive resin, such as Panavia Ex, which bonds to both metal and enamel, is used as a luting cement.

These Maryland bridges (Figure 18.12) conserve tooth tissue and are accordingly ideal for younger patients. They are far quicker to make and can be replaced much more easily than conventional bridgework, as they do not have to be cut off the abutment teeth. However, they will not withstand heavy occlusal forces without becoming dislodged, so suitable cases have to be chosen carefully.

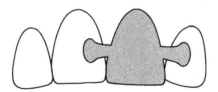

**Figure 18.12**  Direct-bonded bridge – palatal aspect.

## Porcelain veneers

Conventional jacket crown preparation requires the removal of a significant amount of dentine. While this may be harmless in fully developed adult teeth, it could result in pulpal damage in children and adolescents as the pulp chambers are larger in younger patients. In other cases it may be felt that labial enamel defects in incisors, which require a restoration to improve appearance, do not justify a full jacket crown preparation.

In such cases just the outer layer of labial enamel may be removed and replaced by a porcelain veneer to restore normal appearance. After removal of the outer layer, the remaining labial enamel is acid etched and a laboratory made porcelain veneer is bonded to it with a light or dual-cure unfilled composite resin. The porcelain is etched in the laboratory with hydrofluoric acid to provide a retentive surface, but phosphoric acid is used for the enamel.

The surgery stages are as follows:

- First visit:
  1. The porcelain shade is chosen
  2. The outer layer of enamel is removed and an impression of the prepared tooth taken
  3. The prepared surface is covered with a layer of temporary composite or GIC
  4. The impression is sent to the laboratory
  5. The technician constructs a porcelain veneer on the impression of the prepared tooth
- Second visit:
  1. The temporary covering is removed and the veneer checked for correct fit, occlusion and appearance
  2. When the dentist and patient are satisfied, the prepared enamel is etched and the veneer cemented

## Bleaching

Discoloration of front teeth is one of the commonest reasons for making porcelain veneers. There are many possible causes, including:

- Defective tooth structure
- Pulpal bleeding following exposure or impact injury (Chapters 17 and 20)
- Smoking
- Fluorosis (Chapters 11 and 13)
- Tetracycline staining (Chapter 6)
- Surface staining from chlorhexidine mouthwash (although this can usually be removed by scaling and polishing)

The most severe cases may require a porcelain jacket crown, the less severe, a porcelain veneer.

However, both options require removal of a significant amount of enamel. Bleaching the affected tooth structure can treat the least severe forms of discoloration. Using rubber dam, and a protective apron for the patient, a bleaching agent is applied to the tooth surface. Unfortunately, some legal technicalities are currently limiting use of the most effective methods.

# 19 Dentures and Implants

Dentures are *removable* artificial replacements (prostheses) for missing teeth. Fixed replacements include bridges (Chapter 18) and implants. The latter are covered both at the end of this chapter and in Chapter 18. The branch of dentistry concerned with all types of replacements for missing teeth is called **prosthodontics** (formerly called prosthetics).

The reasons for tooth replacement by dentures, bridges or implants are as follows:

- Preventing excessive masticatory force on the remaining teeth, which may cause their eventual fracture
- Preventing over-eruption of the opposing teeth, which may cause occlusal problems
- Preventing tilting of the adjacent teeth into the edentulous spaces, causing stagnation areas
- Preventing soft tissue trauma of the alveolar ridges during mastication
- Allowing adequate mastication and avoid digestive problems and malnutrition, especially in older people
- Providing good aesthetics, especially if anterior teeth are missing

When there are no teeth left in a jaw, it is said to be **edentulous** (edentate) and the artificial replacement is called a **full** or **complete denture**; if some teeth are still present the replacement is called a **partial denture**.

## Denture retention

As dentures are removable prostheses, their retention in the mouth relies not on cements, as it does for bridges, but a combination of the following:

- A **suction film** of saliva between the denture and the patient's soft tissues
- A **post-dam** along the back border of the denture which helps the saliva film to develop
- An **accurate design and fit** of denture, to allow the saliva film to develop adequately without large gaps being present beneath the denture

- **Natural undercuts** in the patient's mouth, such as the alveolar ridge or any natural teeth
- **Stainless steel clasps** incorporated in the denture, to grip around any suitable standing teeth

Sometimes the patient's own teeth can be adjusted to provide better undercuts for denture retention, by any of the following:

- Use of a crown
- Use of a composite build-up
- Changing the shape of an existing restoration

In edentulous patients, the alveolar ridge can be surgically altered to improve retention and comfort, in any of the following procedures:

- **Alveoplasty** – changing the shape of the existing ridge
- **Alveolectomy** – removing sharp ridges and spicules of bone
- **Bone replacement** – using artificial bone substitutes to build up the ridge

## Denture materials

Dentures are usually made of pink or transparent acrylic with acrylic teeth. Chrome cobalt metal is often used for the framework of partial dentures, and for the palate of full dentures if there is a heavy bite.

### Acrylic

Most dentures and orthodontic appliances are made of acrylic. This consists of powder called **polymer** and a liquid called **monomer**. When mixed together they form a plastic mass which has the consistency of dough. This sets into a hard acrylic by a process called **curing**. Curing is effected by heating the dough slowly in a special flask in an oven, or by adding a catalyst which allows it to cure at room temperature. These two methods of curing are known respectively as **heat-curing** and **cold-curing**.

- Heat-cured acrylic is used for dentures and orthodontic appliances.
- Cold-cured acrylic (also called self-cured or auto-polymerised acrylic) is used for temporary crowns, denture repairs and impression trays.

## Patient suitability for dentures

Not all patients are suitable for tooth replacement involving the use of dentures, and the following points will be considered by the dentist for every case before treatment commences:

- Any previous denture experience, and whether it was successful or not
- Any identifiable cause for unsuccessful previous treatment
- Any likely problems with retention that can be remedied by pre-prosthetic surgery or tooth shape adjustment
- Any likely problems with the occlusion, such as a deep overbite directly onto the palate
- Any medical contraindications, such as epilepsy or allergy to the acrylic monomer
- Any dental problems present, such as caries or periodontal disease
- How recently any teeth were lost, as significant bone resorption can occur for up to six months after tooth extraction
- Any likely problems with patient co-operation and perseverance
- Cost of providing the denture

## Stages of full denture construction

Usually, acrylic dentures are made in five stages, with each stage being returned to the laboratory between appointments. The construction is summarised below and described in detail later.

1 **Initial impression** – taken in either a boxed stock tray for dentate patients, or an edentulous stock tray as necessary, using alginate (Figure 19.1).
2 **Laboratory** – models are cast in plaster, and special trays of acrylic or shellac are made for the accurate second (final) impressions.
3 **Final impression** – taken using the special trays and one of the following impression materials: alginate, silicone, impression paste for edentulous patients.
4 **Laboratory** – final models are cast in dental stone so that wax occlusal rims can be constructed.
5 **Bite registration** – occlusal face height of the patient is recorded using a **Willis bite gauge** (Figure 19.2), and the rims are stuck together by warming their wax or by using bite registration paste; the tooth shade and tooth shape are also chosen.
6 **Laboratory** – the joined rims and their model bases are mounted on an **articulator** to mimic the normal jaw movements, and allow the dentures to be constructed so that they function in the patient's normal occlusion; a wax try-in can then be constructed.
7 **Try-in** – wax try-ins with the shaded teeth set to the recorded occlusion, and tried for fit, shade and occlusion; minor adjustments can be carried out at the chairside but major adjustments will require a re-try.
8 **Laboratory** – try-ins and their model bases are sealed into the curing flasks, where the wax is boiled out and replaced by the **heat-cured acrylic** to form the denture bases; any clasps required are now added.
9 **Denture fit** – completed dentures are inserted and checked for comfort, fit and retention; patient care instructions are issued.

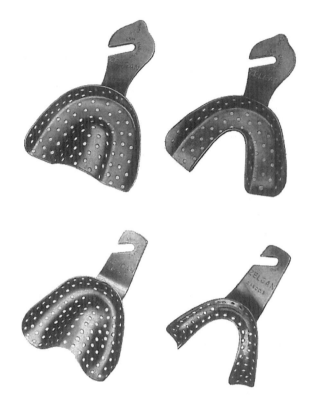

**Figure 19.1** Impression trays. Top row: upper and lower perforated trays for partial denture impressions. Bottom row: edentulous impression trays.

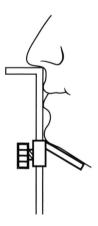

**Figure 19.2** Willis bite gauge. Reproduced with permission from: *The Prosthetic Treatment of the Edentulous Patient*, 4th edn, R.M. Basker & J.C. Davenport, 2002, Blackwell Publishing, Oxford.

Dentures are made in a dental laboratory on models of the jaws. The technician makes these models by pouring **plaster of Paris** into an **impression** of the patient's jaw. The impression is taken by the dentist in an **impression tray** which is filled with impression material and held in the mouth until set.

Having obtained models of each jaw, they must be mounted in the same spatial relationship to each other as they are in the mouth, i.e. the upper and lower models are mounted in such a position that the distance between them, vertically and hor-izontally, is exactly the same as that between the jaws when the mouth is at rest. In order to achieve this, **occlusion rims** are constructed in the laboratory. They consist of a **baseplate** with a wax rim. A baseplate is a temporary plate made of acrylic, shellac or wax, which the technician moulds to the model and trims to the exact outline of the intended denture. The wax rim is attached to the baseplate in the same position as the teeth would be. These occlusion rims are then sent to the surgery, where they are worn by the patient while the dentist records the normal relationship of the jaws at rest. Although this stage is commonly referred to as *taking the bite*, more correct terms are **recording the jaw relationship** or **occlusal registration**.

The models and occlusion rims are then returned to the laboratory where the technician mounts them on an **articulator**. This is essentially a hinged mechanism for keeping models in their correct relationship as obtained at the occlusal regis-tration stage. It can open and close to simulate some of the movements of the jaws. Once the models are mounted on an articulator, the wax rims are removed from the baseplates, and the acrylic teeth fixed on, with wax, in their place. The baseplates with teeth attached are then fitted in the surgery to see that they occlude together correctly and are of satisfactory appearance. This is called the **trial inser-tion** stage or *try-in*. As the teeth are only embedded in wax, any alterations in arrangement or shade can easily be made at this stage.

These *waxed-up* **trial dentures** are now returned to the laboratory to be made into finished dentures, which are then fitted in the surgery.

## Prevention of cross-infection

In order to prevent cross-infection of patients, surgery and laboratory staff, all work for a laboratory must be disinfected (and labelled as such) before despatch. Similarly, all work received from a laboratory must be disinfected before use. Immersion in 10% sodium hypochlorite for 10 minutes is suitable for most mater-ials, but this cannot be used for aluminium impression trays. Chrome-cobalt can only withstand short periods of contact with hypochlorite. Alternatives in such cases are chlorhexidine and several other proprietary disinfectants, such as Perform. However, equipment and materials manufacturers are required to provide instructions for sterilisation or disinfection of their products, and these should always be followed. Gloves should be worn by personnel handling labora-tory work.

# Impressions

## Surgery procedure

The dental nurse sets out:

- The patient's records
- Laboratory prescription pad
- Bowl of water for patient's existing dentures
- Mouth mirror, impression trays and impression material ready for preparing and loading into a tray
- A large kidney dish in case the patient is sick: patients known to be prone to sickness can be helped by giving them a surface anaesthetic mouthwash, spray or lozenge beforehand; ear or point of chin acupuncture can be successful in patients who do not respond to the former remedies

After removal from the mouth, impressions are rinsed in cold running water to remove saliva and any blood, then disinfected by immersion in the appropriate disinfectant, and rinsed again in running water. Eye protection should be worn in case of splashing.

As the impression must reach the laboratory in perfect condition, the dental nurse must take great care to handle it correctly. It should be very carefully packed if it is to be sent away to an outside laboratory. It should be labelled as disinfected, and enclose the name of the dentist and patient, prescription of the work required and date for return.

## Impression trays

Impression trays are of two kinds: edentulous and partial (Figure 19.1). Edentulous trays are used for taking impressions for full dentures and are semicircular in cross-section (Figure 19.3). Partial trays are used for impressions for partial dentures and have a box-shaped cross-section to accommodate the remaining teeth. For upper impressions both types of tray have a palatal section, which is, of course, absent in lower trays. Those obtained from dental suppliers are called **stock trays**. They are made of metal for repeated use, or disposable plastic material for single use. They may be perforated or non-perforated, depending on the type of impression material to be used. Metal trays are sterilised in an autoclave. Disposable trays are discarded after the model is made, and no time is lost in having to clean off the impression material. They should be used whenever possible.

Very often it is not possible to obtain an adequate impression with a stock or a disposable tray. In such cases the model obtained from the first impression is used to make a **special tray**. With this *made to measure* individual tray a perfectly accurate final impression can be taken. Special trays are usually made of shellac baseplate or an acrylic material.

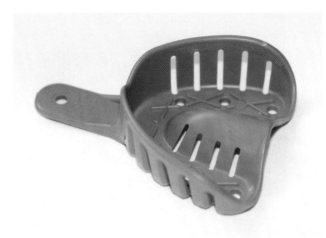

Figure 19.3 Boxed impression tray.

### Laboratory procedure

The technician pours plaster into the impression to make a model of the patient's jaw. If required, this model is then used to construct a special tray. The impression taken in this special tray is used for making the final (working) model, which is an exact reproduction of the required part of the patient's jaw.

### Impression materials

The choice of impression material to be used depends on various factors, such as the condition of the jaws and the presence or absence of teeth. Each type of material has a different method of preparation and use, and the manufacturer's instructions must be carefully followed if a satisfactory impression is to be obtained. Impressions for full dentures are called edentulous impressions while those for partial dentures are known as partial impressions.

The most widely used impression materials for dentures are alginate, impression paste and elastomers.

### Alginate

Alginate impression materials, e.g. CA 37, Blueprint, are elastic and can therefore be used for all impressions, partial or edentulous. They give an accurate impression which can be withdrawn from undercut areas without distortion or fracture (Figure 19.4).

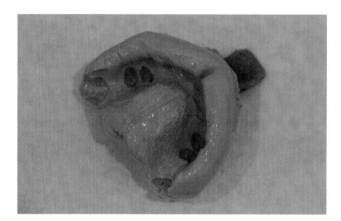

**Figure 19.4** Alginate impression.

Alginate impressions are prepared by mixing the powder and water with a spatula in a flexible plastic bowl. The tin is shaken before opening to loosen the powder but care must be taken to avoid inhaling any. The water should be at **room temperature** to give the correct setting time. Correct measures of powder and water are mixed vigorously to a smooth consistency and loaded into a perforated tray. It sets in a few minutes in the mouth and, on withdrawal, must be wrapped in a wet napkin until the model is made. Some brands change colour during mixing to indicate when it is ready for loading, and then to a different colour when set.

The advantages of alginate are its elasticity and ease of use, which make it the material of choice for most impressions, and allow more than one model to be made from the same impression.

The disadvantages of alginate are:

- If special care is not taken, alginate undergoes dimensional changes which would produce an inaccurate model. It may either absorb water and expand, or lose water and shrink
- To prevent this happening the model should be cast immediately
- If this is not possible, or the impression must be sent to an outside laboratory, dimensional changes can be delayed by wrapping the impression in a wet napkin and sealing it in an airtight plastic bag until the model can be made
- A similar procedure is used for disinfection of alginate impressions:
  - Rinse in cold running water
  - Dip in manufacturer's recommended disinfectant
  - Rinse in water again

Alginate does not adhere to an ordinary tray so a perforated tray is preferable. An ordinary tray will do, however, if a special adhesive is applied. The only other materials requiring a tray adhesive are the elastomers.

Impression paste is a modified form of zinc oxide eugenol. Various other constituents are added to make it suitable as an impression material. It is supplied in
two tubes: one containing the white zinc oxide mixture, and the other containing
the red eugenol mixture. Equal lengths from each tube are mixed together with
a spatula on a paper pad to give a uniform pink mix without any red or white
streaks.

Impression paste is used for final *edentulous* impressions in a number of different
ways.

- First impressions are taken with alginate or putty elastomer and well-fitting
  special trays made. Final impressions are taken in these trays using a wash of
  impression paste.
- For relining loose dentures, the denture is used as an impression tray for the
  paste and is then sent to the laboratory for a new fitting surface to be processed
  in acrylic.
- It is also used as a lining to improve the fit of baseplates in the occlusal registration and trial insertion stages.

*The advantages of impression paste are:*

- The improved fit obtainable by its use in peripherally sealed special trays,
  baseplates or dentures
- Its accuracy can be checked or improved by reinsertion in the mouth and
  adding fresh paste where necessary

Disadvantages are:

- It cannot reproduce undercuts and is therefore unsuitable for partial denture
  impressions
- It tends to stick to the lips and surrounding skin, but this can be avoided by
  smearing them beforehand with petroleum jelly
- Some patients are sensitive to materials containing eugenol; an elastomer is a
  more modern and satisfactory alternative

*Elastomers*

The impression paste techniques just described cannot be used where undercuts
are present as it is not an elastic material. In such cases an acrylic special tray and
a heavy-bodied elastomer (see Chapter 18) are usually preferred. Light-bodied
elastomer is used where the alveolar ridges are too soft and flabby to withstand
distortion by more viscous impression materials. Silicone putty has replaced
composition for first impressions for special trays, as it is just as easy to prepare
and use.

The advantages of elastomers are:

- Elasticity makes them suitable for all types of denture
- Stronger, less liable to tear, and more accurate than alginate
- Less liable to significant dimensional change than alginate

The disadvantages are:

- Their cost
- More complicated technique than other materials

## Composition

Composition sticks are called tracing sticks and they may be green, brown or red according to the brand. The stick is:

- Softened over a flame or hot air jet and quenched in hot water before insertion into the mouth (the dentist checks its temperature with a finger to avoid burning the patient)
- It is used to form the periphery of acrylic special trays or baseplates
- The periphery is built up bit by bit, repeatedly adding more to it and retrying in the mouth, until it forms a perfect peripheral seal with the soft tissue of the buccal sulcus

Thus optimum retention for a full denture is ensured.

## Disinfection procedure

Dentists are legally responsible for ensuring that all work sent from a practice to a dental laboratory has been cleaned and disinfected, and labelled accordingly. Such work includes impressions, repairs, occlusion blocks and trial dentures, etc. Similarly, all work received from a laboratory must undergo the same procedure.

Manufacturers are required to state how their products should be disinfected, including the strength and immersion time for their recommended product.

- Immediately after removal from the mouth, work for the laboratory should be rinsed under cold running water to remove saliva and blood.
- Any residual contamination is removed by immersion in detergent in an ultrasonic cleaner, and it is then rinsed again.
- It is disinfected in accordance with the manufacturer's instructions and rinsed again before dispatch.

# Occlusal registration

## Laboratory procedure

The technician makes occlusion rims on the final models obtained from the impression stage. They consist of wax rims on wax, shellac or acrylic baseplates. The rims represent the alveolar bone and teeth, and their purpose is to allow the dentist to record the patient's jaw relationship or *bite*.

## Surgery procedure

1 The dental nurse sets out: the patient's records, models, occlusion rims; sheets of pink wax, wax knife; shade and mould guides; heat source (gas flame, spirit lamp or hot air jet) for trimming the wax rims; impression material for fixation of occlusal registration; and laboratory prescription pad.

2 The patient is provided with a bib and mouthwash and any existing dentures are placed in a bowl of water.

3 The occlusion rims are removed from their models, rinsed in disinfectant and washed before insertion in the patient's mouth.

4 The sides of the wax rims are trimmed with a **wax knife** (Figure 19.5b) until they represent the correct position of the teeth and give proper support for the lips. A **Le Cron carver** (Figure 19.5c) is used for fine trimming.

5 The wax rims are then reduced or increased in height until the jaws are the correct distance apart when the rims are in contact. A hot flat metal surface, such as an electric iron, is useful for providing a flat even occlusal surface on the wax rims.

6 Some operators use a **Willis bite gauge** (Figure 19.2) to determine the correct height of occlusion rims. This is based on an assumption that rim heights are correct when the distance between nose and chin equals that between eyes and mouth. The bite gauge facilitates comparison and measurement of these distances. Dividers or the more modern **Alma bite gauge** can also be used for this purpose.

7 Once the wax rims are trimmed correctly they must be fixed together to register the correct jaw relationship (Figure 19.6). This can be done by cutting grooves in the rims and placing some registration material, such as a softened wax wafer, impression paste or a quick-setting light-bodied elastomer, between them. When the patient closes together it is squeezed into the grooves and permanently records the correct relationship of the jaws at rest. Marks are also made on the upper rim to indicate the midline of the face and rest position of the upper lip.

8 Best results are obtained if dentures are made on an **anatomical articulator** but it entails extra surgery time at this stage, and extra time in the laboratory. The extra steps required when such an articulator is used are for indicating the movements of the jaws during mastication and consist of the **face bow** and protrusive bite registrations. A face bow is an accessory part of the articulator for recording the position of the upper occlusion rim relative to the mandibular

condyles. The protrusive bite is taken with the mandible postured forward to obtain an occlusal record in the protruded position.

9   Finally the shade, shape and size of artificial teeth to be used in the finished dentures are selected from the manufacturer's shade and mould guide and the laboratory prescription is then written by the dentist. The dental nurse disinfects the occlusion rims in hypochlorite before despatch to the technician.

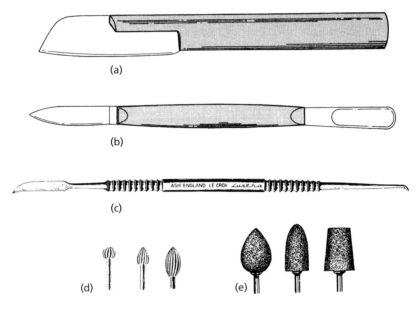

(a)

(b)

(c)

(d)   (e)

Figure 19.5 Prosthetic instruments. (a) Plaster knife. (b) Wax knife. (c) Le Cron carver. (d) Acrylic burs. (e) Acrylic stones.

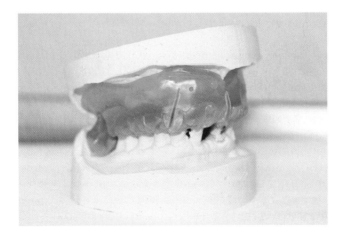

Figure 19.6 Wax rims on working model.

The traditional occlusal registration procedure, just described, is more of an art than a science. However, modern materials offer a more accurate, simpler and far quicker procedure. Using a thin rigid tray and an elastomer impression material (e.g. Blu Mousse) on its upper and lower surfaces, it is now possible to record the occlusion, in one step, without any need for baseplates and occlusion rims.

## Trial insertion

### Laboratory procedure

The technician seals the models and occlusion rims together in exactly the same relationship which the dentist recorded at the occlusal registration stage. Then they are mounted on an articulator to provide the technician with an accurate three-dimensional copy of the required parts of the patient's jaws.

The wax rims can now be removed and are replaced by the actual teeth to be used on the denture. They are mounted in wax on the baseplate in normal occlusion with the opposing teeth. Then the wax is moulded, trimmed and polished to produce a perfect copy of the final denture. This waxed-up denture is called a **trial denture**.

### Surgery procedure

The dental nurse sets out:

- The patient's records
- Articulator with models and trial dentures
- Bowl of disinfectant, bowl of water, bib for the patient
- Pink wax, Le Cron carver and heat source
- Large hand mirror
- Laboratory prescription pad

After the dentist has checked the occlusion of the trial dentures on the articulator:

1 The dental nurse rinses them in disinfectant, washes them in cold water, fits a bib on the patient, and places existing dentures in a bowl of water.
2 The dentist fits the trial dentures in the patient's mouth.
3 The dentures are checked for comfort, stability and occlusion, and the patient is given a mirror to see the shade, shape and arrangement of the teeth. If the patient is dissatisfied with them, they are replaced on the articulator, and any necessary adjustments are made in the surgery.
4 It is emphasised to the patient that such adjustments can only be done at this stage, while the teeth are still embedded in wax. Such alterations cannot be carried out once the dentures are finished.

5   Finally the junction of hard and soft palate is marked on the upper model, together with the extent of the pad of softer tissue in this region. This enables the technician to make a retentive posterior border (**post-dam**) for the final denture.

6   The trial dentures are then disinfected again, remounted on the articulator and the laboratory prescription is written up for the technician.

## Final insertion

### Laboratory procedure

The technician invests the trial dentures in a plaster mould and eliminates all the wax by flushing with boiling water. The space formerly occupied by wax is now filled with acrylic dough and heat-cured in a warm oven. The acrylic dentures are then trimmed and polished ready for fitting.

### Surgery procedure

The dental nurse sets out:

■   The patient's records, and a bib
■   New dentures in a bowl of water
■   Occlusal indicator wax, articulating paper and pressure indicating paste
■   Straight handpiece, acrylic burs and stones
■   Large hand mirror

When the dentist is ready to fit the dentures:

1   The dental nurse fits a bib on the patient, disinfects the dentures and rinses them in water when the dentist is ready to fit them.

2   The dentist fits each denture in turn to check its retention, stability and comfort.

3   Any necessary adjustments to the occlusion are found when the patient bites on articulating paper or **occlusal indicator wax** (Chapter 18). These mark any high spots on the teeth which can then be ground with an acrylic trimming bur or a Carborundum stone in a straight handpiece.

4   High spots on the fitting surface or overextension of the periphery can be localised by painting **pressure-indicating paste** on the fitting surfaces. The offending parts are removed with an acrylic bur or stone (Figure 19.5). The dentist fits each denture in turn to check its retention and stability. Any necessary adjustments to the occlusion are noted by biting on a piece of **articulating paper**, held in **Miller forceps** (see Figure 18.9) **or occlusal indicator wax** (Chapter 18). These mark any high spots on the teeth, which can then be

ground down with a Carborundum stone in a straight handpiece. High spots on the fitting surface, or overextension of the periphery can be localised by painting pressure-indicating paste on the fitting surfaces. The offending parts are then removed with an acrylic trimming bur or stone. The patient is given a mirror to see the appearance of the new dentures and is shown how to insert and remove them.

5   Instructions are given, as follows, on the care of new dentures:
    – They should be cleaned after meals with a toothbrush, toothpaste and cold water, and handled with care as they can break if dropped. When cleaning, partially fill the washbasin with water to act as a cushion and prevent breakage. Very hot water should not be used as it can damage acrylic.
    – At night, or at any other time when dentures are not worn, they must be kept in a glass of water. If allowed to dry out, acrylic is liable to warp and may not fit properly.
    – Wear the dentures daily to allow the soft tissues to acclimatise to them, but leave out at night to allow the soft tissues to recover.
    – Eat soft foods initially until the soft tissues have adjusted to the new dentures.
    – Use hot salt water mouthwashes to ease any soft tissue soreness experienced.

## After care

An appointment is given for a few days later to see how the patient is managing the new dentures. Patients are advised to stop wearing a denture if it is hurting the soft tissues. However, they should wear it again for 24 hours before their appointment so that the dentist can see the sore area and can deal with it.

Articulating paper or occlusal indicator wax is used again to find any high spots on the teeth, and pressure-indicating paste for detecting the causes of soreness or ulceration. A straight handpiece, acrylic trimming burs and stones, polishing paste and brushes are used to trim offending surfaces and leave them smooth and polished. The dentures are then scrubbed with disinfectant, rinsed in water and returned to the patient.

Patients are also told that new dentures do not last for ever, and are advised to have them checked every year. Alveolar bone gradually changes its shape following the loss of teeth and the denture will eventually become too loose. By that time most patients will have learned how to control a loose denture, but the alveolar bone changes can adversely affect appearance as the loose denture may no longer provide adequate support for the lips and cheeks. It is consequently necessary to **reline** the fitting surface of a denture from time to time and perhaps make other adjustments. Relining is usually done with a light-bodied elastomer material, or impression paste.

As already mentioned, patients are advised to clean their new dentures by scrubbing with toothpaste and cold water, and to keep them immersed in water overnight. If such advice is followed the mouth should remain healthy and the use of proprietary denture cleansers should be unnecessary.

If this advice is not followed, the soft tissues covered by a denture may become inflamed. This condition is called **denture stomatitis** and is treated with anti-fungal drugs (Chapter 6) and oral hygiene instruction. Similarly, the dentures may become stained and calculus may form on them. Patients with such dentures are advised to clean them by soaking in hypochlorite (e.g. Milton) for 20 minutes, rinsing thoroughly and immersing in water overnight. Dentures with metallic components should be soaked in non-hypochlorite disinfectants, such as Dentural, instead.

## Partial dentures

There are two types of partial denture. One is made entirely of acrylic; the other consists of a metal framework with the artificial teeth embedded in acrylic and is commonly known as a **skeleton design** denture. Both are made from alginate or elastomer impressions followed by the stages of denture construction already described.

For **acrylic** dentures, alginate impressions usually suffice, and for those replacing only a few teeth, a wax squash bite (Chapter 18) may be adequate to show the technician how the remaining teeth occlude. Otherwise, the full denture occlusal registration procedure is used. The models can then be mounted correctly on an articulator and the trial denture made. This is followed by a trial insertion in the surgery.

Acrylic partial dentures may have stainless steel or chrome-cobalt clasps to improve retention. They spring into the undercut areas of the teeth and prevent vertical dislodgement of the denture. The metal framework of a **skeleton denture** is a chrome-cobalt casting, resulting in a far stronger, less bulky and more hygienic denture that is specially designed to avoid food traps and plaque retention round the gums and teeth.

The remaining teeth are used for support and retention of the skeleton. Clasps are used for retention and **occlusal rests** for support. Occlusal rests are tiny lugs which fit on the occlusal surface of the enamel or in a groove cut into a filling. If there are no suitable fillings or surfaces, seats for occlusal rests may be made by bonding some composite filling material to the enamel.

Skeleton dentures take longer to make and are far more expensive than acrylic ones. Special tray elastomer impressions are necessary to ensure accuracy as it is difficult to make adjustments to metal castings. Extra visits may also be required: before the final impression stage, to prepare seats for occlusal rests, and after the occlusal registration stage, to try in the metal framework before waxing-up the teeth for the trial denture.

The after-care instructions for full dentures also apply to partial dentures but, because of their potential for plaque retention, patients are emphatically advised not to wear them at night, and not to miss their regular check-up appointments.

# Immediate dentures

Dentures are usually made some months after the teeth have been extracted, as this allows time for completion of the initial alveolar bone resorption and gum healing. Many patients, however, are not prepared to wait that long for the replacement of missing front teeth.

In such cases they can be provided with **immediate dentures** which are made *before* their anterior teeth are extracted, and are fitted immediately afterwards. But patients must understand that the rapid remodelling of alveolar bone which follows extractions necessitates relining or replacement of immediate dentures within a year, as they become too loose and ill-fitting.

## Procedure

1   Before any extractions are done, the dentist provides the technician with final impressions, the occlusal registration, and required shade for the new teeth.
2   In the laboratory, the teeth to be extracted are cut off the working model by the technician, and the artificial ones fitted in their place.
3   The denture is then waxed-up and processed in acrylic and disinfected.
4   In the surgery the teeth are extracted and the denture is fitted at the same visit.
5   The patient is given an appointment to attend for check-up the next day, and is instructed not to remove the denture before then. After that it should only be removed for cleaning, and worn full-time until the dentist decides that it can be left out at night.

# Overdentures

An overdenture is one which is fitted on top of standing teeth or retained roots. The advantage of an overdenture is the presence of natural roots remaining in the alveolar bone. These have the effect of greatly reducing the absorption and shrinkage of alveolar ridges which normally occurs after extraction of teeth. When teeth are extracted, the alveolar bone becomes redundant, as it has lost its natural function of providing support for the teeth. It consequently diminishes in size as the bone resorbs and this loss of bone may be so great that it becomes very difficult to make a denture which is not perpetually loose. Lower dentures pose the most awkward problems in this respect.

As long as any roots remain, there is hardly any loss of alveolar bone and these problems of difficult lower dentures are far less common. However, dentures cannot be fitted directly on top of retained roots or teeth. In most cases a certain amount of preparation of the abutment teeth is required to remove undercuts and prevent caries.

Retained roots are root-filled and ground to a dome shape level with the gum. If the root surface is irregular because of previous caries, the dome shape can be restored by fitting an appropriately shaped post crown. Teeth which still have intact crowns are usually treated by reducing the crown to a small tapered stump and fitting a full gold veneer thimble. Having prepared the remaining teeth or roots, the overdenture is then made in the usual way.

Overdentures are usually made as full dentures but they can be used as partial dentures in cases where some of the remaining teeth are unsuitable for the partial denture design. They are also used for patients with cleft palates and for those who have undergone surgical removal of part of their jaw. In such cases the alveolar ridges may be so mis-shapen that properly fitting conventional dentures cannot be made.

Where there are no remaining roots, **implants** can be used to support an over-denture. This is covered later in the chapter.

## Obturators

An **obturator** is an appliance for plugging an abnormal cavity, such as a cleft palate; the space left after surgical removal of part of the jaw following oral cancer treatment or due to a cyst cavity. It usually consists of an ordinary acrylic denture bearing a plug which seals the cavity. This prevents the ingress of food and improves speech. If the cavity is very large, a hollow plug is used to lighten the obturator.

An obturator can be made in the usual way, using an elastic or functional impression material. Alternatively the denture part is made first in acrylic and a temporary plug, made of black gutta percha, or a more permanent soft lining material (e.g. Molloplast), is added. When this has been worn for a while, and moulded itself to the shape of the cavity, it is remade in acrylic.

## Soft linings

The section on impression paste described its use for relining loose dentures: those which have been worn for many years, and immediate dentures which have lost their fit after a few months. Impression paste, as with all other conventional impression materials, sets in a few minutes and reproduces a totally artificial situation where the mouth is wide open and immobile throughout. The real and natural situation in the mouth is one of continual movement and change. Recording this real situation in an impression requires a material which takes hours to set while the denture is being worn and used. Such an impression is called a **functional impression** and it provides a much better fit.

The oldest functional impression material is black gutta percha but this has been superseded by modern materials called **soft linings** which are a type of slowcuring acrylic resin, e.g. Visco-gel, Coe Comfort. They usually consist of a powder and liquid which are mixed together and applied to the fitting surface of the denture for up to six hours. When found to provide a comfortable and satisfactory fit, the denture is sent to the laboratory, to replace the soft lining with heat-cured acrylic. This is necessary as soft linings deteriorate with use, and are only suitable for temporary use. Soft lining material can also be used in the same way by applying it just to the periphery of a full denture, to greatly improve its fit by providing a perfect peripheral seal.

Soft linings can also be used as **tissue conditioners**. These are required when the soft tissues become too sore, swollen or otherwise distorted, to withstand pressure from a denture. A soft lining accommodates any changes in the soft tissues and allows the denture to be worn without discomfort until the tissues have healed or a new denture can be made. Tissue conditioners may also be used when immediate dentures are first fitted, and for relining them during the first few months when the most rapid changes in alveolar shape take place.

## Implants

Overdentures and bridges rely on teeth for retention. If there are no available tooth roots for an overdenture, or suitable teeth for bridge abutments (Chapter 18), artificial tooth roots implanted into the alveolar bone can be used instead. These **implants** are made of titanium and generally consist of threaded cylinders which are screwed into holes drilled in the bone. The cylinders also have an internal thread for a screw which attaches the artificial abutment to the implant (Figure 19.7). Up to six implants may be needed to retain a denture or extensive bridgework.

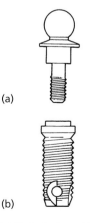

(a)

(b)

Figure 19.7 Implant components. (a) Ball abutment for overdenture. (b) Implant fixture.

## Construction

- A team of oral or periodontal surgeon, prosthetic specialist, and hygienist examine and assess the patient, helped by study models, X-rays or even three-dimensional computer scans. The team can then plan the preparation, construction and maintenance of an implant procedure.
- Local or general anaesthetic is used for the oral surgery procedure of inserting implants into alveolar bone. A gum flap is raised to expose the bone and special low-speed drills are used to prepare holes for the implants. They are screwed into these holes and the gum flap is then sutured back into place to completely bury the implants.
- After a period of up to six months, the implants become firmly embedded in the bone, by a process called **osseointegration**. Under local anaesthesia, a small incision is made in the overlying gum to expose the top of each implant, and the artificial abutments are then screwed on to the implants. Abutments may be in the form of stumps for fitting bridge pontics, or a bar for clipping on a removable overdenture (Figure 19.8).

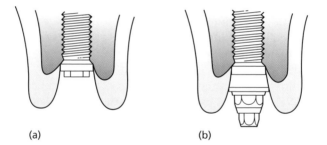

(a)                              (b)

**Figure 19.8** Implant procedure. (a) Stage 1: implant fixture. (b) Stage 2: crown or bridge abutment fitted.

## Procedure

Patients are very carefully selected as implants can only succeed if meticulous oral hygiene and plaque control is maintained before and after the implants are inserted. A thorough medical history, and comprehensive clinical and X-ray examinations, are essential to confirm the feasibility of implants, and to exclude patients who are unsuitable for reasons of general or dental health, motivation or ability to attend for regular check-ups.

Implants and their abutment components are intended to act as natural teeth and it is essential that their supra- and subgingival parts are kept clean and regularly checked in the same way as natural teeth, as described in Chapter 12 on periodontal disease.

## Advantages of implants

They allow full dentures to be worn in cases where there is insufficient alveolar bone to provide adequate retention for a conventional denture. They also permit the construction of bridges without having to crown adjacent abutment teeth.

## Disadvantages

They require a specialist team and a highly motivated patient. They are accordingly very expensive.

# 20 Extractions and Minor Oral Surgery

The removal or extraction of teeth is carried out under local anaesthesia, with or without some form of anxiety control, or under general anaesthesia in dental clinics or hospital departments. The decision on whether to extract or conserve teeth, and the choice of anaesthesia may depend on the patient's medical and dental history. These factors are discussed in Chapters 5, 6, 22 and 23. Teeth are extracted for various reasons but the commonest are as follows:

- Pain which cannot be relieved by conservative measures
- Alveolar abscess – acute or chronic
- Caries – extensive cases that are unsuitable for conservation
- Periodontal disease – cases unsuitable for periodontal therapy
- Prosthetics – teeth detrimental to the fit or appearance of dentures
- Impaction – causing stagnation areas and likely long-term problems
- Orthodontics – misplaced teeth, or to create more space
- Cosmetic – teeth of poor appearance, unsuitable for restoration

## Extraction instruments

Teeth may be extracted as a 'simple' procedure, or as a surgical procedure involving the raising of a gingival flap and alveolar bone removal. Instruments used for simple extractions are forceps and elevators. Surgical extractions are discussed later.

### Forceps

There are two basic types of forceps – roots and molars (Figure 20.1).

**Root forceps** have blades with rounded ends. There are many different patterns and they are named according to the angle which the blade makes with the handle, or the teeth for which they are designed, for example: lowers, straights, Read and bayonets. Every practitioner has particular forceps of choice for individual teeth but, generally speaking, they are used as follows:

- Lower roots – all lower teeth
- Straights – upper incisors and canine

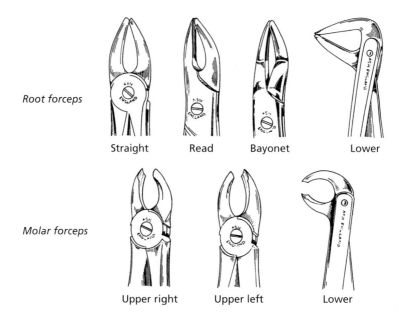

Root forceps

Straight        Read        Bayonet        Lower

Molar forceps

Upper right        Upper left        Lower

Figure 20.1 Extraction forceps.

- Read – upper premolar teeth or molar roots
- Bayonets – upper premolar teeth or molar roots
- Lower molars – all lower molars
- Upper molars – a left molar pattern and a right molar pattern

Some root forceps have narrow blades. These are used for small teeth such as lower incisors and for retained roots.

**Molar forceps** have pointed blades designed to fit the bifurcation (branching) of molar roots. Lower molar forceps have two identical pointed blades which fit the buccal and lingual sides of the bifurcation. Left and right lower molars are extracted with the same pair of forceps. Upper molar forceps have one pointed blade to fit the bifurcation of the buccal roots and a rounded blade which fits the single palatal root (Figure 20.2). Different forceps are needed for each side but dental nurses should have no difficulty identifying them correctly if they understand why the blades are different.

## Elevators

These instruments are designed to elevate a retained root or impacted tooth out of its socket whence it can be easily removed. Many types of elevator are available but perhaps the most well known are Warwick James and Cryer patterns (Figure 20.3). A Coupland chisel is also shown but this is *not* an elevator, although it can be used as one by some dentists.

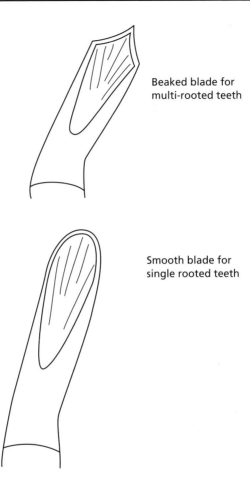

Beaked blade for
multi-rooted teeth

Smooth blade for
single rooted teeth

Figure 20.2 Molar forceps blade patterns.

**Warwick James elevators** are made in a set of three: straight, left and right curved. They are used for retained roots and impacted teeth. **Cryer elevators** are used for retained roots and impacted teeth. They have a triangular sharp end and are made in a set of two: left and right.

A **Coupland chisel** is correctly used for prising between the roots of multi-rooted teeth to separate them, or sometimes for prising between the root and alveolar bone to dilate the socket and facilitate extraction. However, it is sometimes too large for the latter purpose. Much finer instruments that can penetrate deeper into the periodontal ligament are used instead. They are called **luxators** (Figure 20.4) and are much sharper than a Coupland chisel. They also cause far less damage to the alveolar bone and simplify extraction. Many dentists now use them routinely instead of forceps.

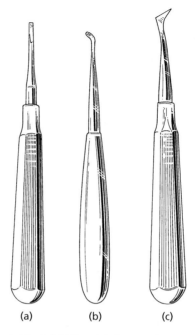

**Figure 20.3** (a) Coupland chisel. (b) Warwick James elevator. (c) Cryer elevator.

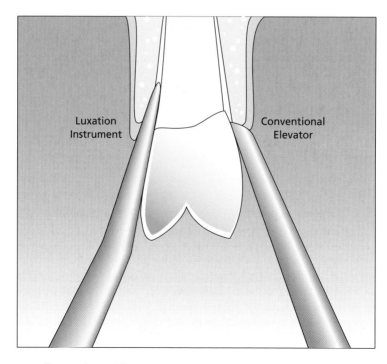

**Figure 20.4** Comparison of Coupland chisel and luxation instrument.

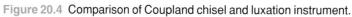

The required instruments are sterilised and placed in a sterile dish ready for use, or they are pre-sterilised and sealed in pouches ready for use. The patient is provided with a sterile disposable waterproof bib to prevent clothing being soiled, a disposable beaker of mouthwash, and a napkin for wiping the mouth after the extraction.

During an extraction the dental nurse may be required to hold the patient's head steady.

After extraction the forceps are carefully cleaned to remove all traces of blood, oiled if necessary, and then sterilised (Chapter 7).

## Care of the patient

Some patients require antibiotic cover to prevent infective endocarditis. This is described in Chapter 6. If an oral sedative (such as **diazepam**) is given to relieve nervousness, it is liable to make the patient quite drowsy. Alternatively, patients may be given inhalation or intravenous sedation for their treatment (Chapter 22). Such patients must be accompanied to the surgery by a responsible adult who stays in the waiting room and returns home with the patient afterwards. Patients are legally forbidden to drive a vehicle or operate machinery for the remainder of that day, and are advised not to take alcohol nor sign legal documents for 24 hours after sedation.

Upon removal of the tooth, the dentist squeezes the socket walls together, places a gauze pad over the socket, and instructs the patient to bite on it for 10 minutes to help to achieve **haemostasis** (stop the bleeding). After treatment the patient is not dismissed until the bleeding has ceased. Post-operative advice is given, as follows, on the steps necessary to prevent bleeding recurring, to avoid infection and relieve soreness.

- For the next 24 hours, *avoid*:
  - Mouthwashing
  - Very hot fluids
  - Alcohol
  - Strenuous exercise.
- Soreness can be relieved by taking some analgesic tablets such as paracetamol, but **not** aspirin as this is an anticoagulant and bleeding will recur.
- After 24 hours, carry out hot saltwater mouthwashes after every meal for several days – a teaspoon of salt in a glass of hot water.
- If prolonged bleeding or severe pain occurs, contact the surgery for advice.

# Complications of extractions

Complications during extraction are: fracture of the tooth; perforation of the maxillary sinus; and loss of a tooth. Complications occurring after extraction are: bleeding and dry socket.

## Fracture

The crown of a tooth may fracture and come away with the forceps, leaving the root behind in its socket. This is most likely to occur when the crown is extensively decayed or heavily filled. Alternatively a root fracture may occur during extraction, leaving the apex behind. This is most likely to occur in teeth with curved or fine roots.

If a crown or root fracture occurs, the dentist may remove the retained part while the anaesthetic is still effective, or defer removal until the extraction wound has healed. If a retained root fragment is small and uninfected it may be decided to leave it alone, in which case the patient is informed and reassured.

The removal of retained roots is minor oral surgery and the technique is described later in this chapter. An X-ray film is necessary before removal is attempted, so that the dentist can determine the position and depth of the root fragment, and plan its successful removal.

## Maxillary sinus

The roots of upper premolars and molars are very close to the floor of the maxillary sinus (Chapter 8). Just how close this relationship is can best be seen by looking at X-ray films of upper teeth, where their roots may be seen forming bulges in the floor of the sinus, or the floor may dip down into the trifurcation of molar roots. In such cases there may only be a thin layer of compact bone separating a root from the sinus (see Figure 14.1).

It is not surprising, therefore, that the floor of the sinus may be perforated during an extraction. In the majority of cases the perforation is small and no harm results as the perforation is protected by the blood clot which fills the socket. Usually, neither the dentist nor the patient is aware of what has happened. However, if the perforation is larger, it may be detected by the presence of air bubbles in the socket, or the patient may notice fluid entering the nose after drinking or rinsing the mouth. A perforation of this kind is called an **oro-antral fistula**, which means an unnatural communication between the oral cavity and the maxillary sinus (antrum). Closure of these perforations is necessary to prevent infection of the sinus and inconvenience to the patient. Small perforations are closed by stitching the socket, but larger ones require coverage by a flap of gum stitched across the perforation.

Attempted removal of a retained root sometimes results in the root being pushed into the sinus, and this again may cause infection of the sinus. X-ray films are necessary to locate a root which has disappeared upwards, as it may be loose inside the sinus or just trapped beneath the mucous membrane lining the floor of the sinus. Appropriate minor oral surgery can then be undertaken to remove the root.

## Loss of a tooth

If an extracted tooth slips out of the forceps it may be swallowed or inhaled. The patient may be aware of swallowing it, or they may cough, which suggests inhalation of the tooth. On the other hand, the patient may not be aware that anything untoward has happened.

When a tooth disappears it must be looked for inside and outside the mouth. If it cannot be found in the mouth, aspirator filter or within the vicinity of the dental chair, the patient must be referred to hospital for a chest X-ray. If it has been swallowed, no action is necessary as it usually passes through the alimentary canal without doing any harm. But if it has been inhaled an urgent operation is necessary to recover it from the airway or lung, before it causes serious complications such as pneumonia or a lung abscess.

Loss of a tooth is more likely to happen under general anaesthesia (GA) as the patient's protective choking reflexes are ineffective and the operative field may be obscured by a copious flow of blood. To help prevent such accidents it is the dental nurse's duty to account for every tooth as it is extracted, and place it in a kidney dish so that another check can be made afterwards.

## Bleeding

This is covered later in the chapter.

## Dry socket

Dry socket (correctly called **localised osteitis**) is a very painful condition which develops a few days after extraction. It is an acute inflammation of the bone (*osteitis*) lining the socket and is caused by microbial invasion of a socket. The natural protective barrier against such invasion is the blood clot which fills the socket immediately after an extraction, so anything which prevents formation of an adequate blood clot can give rise to a dry socket. Such factors are as follows:

- Infection of the blood clot
- Failure of formation of a blood clot
- Disturbance of the blood clot

Infection of the blood clot may occur in neglected mouths where gingival (gum) infection is already present. Hordes of micro-organisms invade the socket, overwhelm the defending white cells, disintegrate the blood clot and set up an acute inflammation of the unprotected bare bone of the socket. Pre-extraction scaling of the teeth reduces gingival infection and may prevent a dry socket. Alternatively, application of chlorhexidine to the gingival crevice (Chapter 8) just before extraction helps to reduce the risk of infection.

Failure of formation of a blood clot may occur in difficult extractions, as pressure on the bone during such an extraction crushes the blood vessels and results in insufficient bleeding to produce a protective blood clot. It is more common in the mandible than maxilla as the former has a thicker layer of compact bone.

Disturbance of the blood clot is caused by too much mouthwashing soon after extraction, or by the patient poking and fiddling at the extraction socket. This breaks away the blood clot and leaves the socket bare.

### Treatment of dry socket

Treatment is aimed at relief of pain and protection of the socket during healing. It is achieved by syringing the socket with sterile water or mouthwash to remove debris, inserting a sedative dressing (e.g. Alvogyl) to relieve pain and prevent ingress of food and by taking an analgesic drug such as paracetamol or ibuprofen.

A previous commonly used sedative dressing was gauze incorporated with a soft paste of zinc oxide and eugenol. However, nowadays there are many different pre-made dressings for treating dry socket and practitioners vary in their method of choice.

Patients are advised that relief of pain and quicker healing can be helped by frequent mouthwashing with hot saline, as discussed in their post-operative instructions. At this stage it is very helpful, as hot saline keeps the mouth clean and increases the blood flow to the area, thus aiding healing. Any evidence of infection of the socket can be treated with metronidazole, which acts on the anaerobic bacteria likely to be involved.

## Accidental extraction

Accidental extraction can happen for a variety of reasons. One example is the removal of an unerupted premolar while extracting its deciduous predecessor. As a premolar crown is surrounded by the deciduous molar roots (Figure 20.5) it can be dislodged or completely extracted together with the deciduous tooth.

Fortunately the accidentally extracted premolar can be saved by immediately replanting it in its socket. The periodontal membrane and pulp should retain their vitality and the tooth subsequently erupts normally. Success is accomplished by immediate replacement, which gives no time for the periodontal membrane to become infected or dried out.

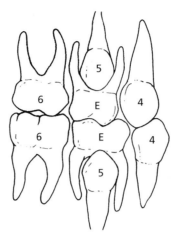

Figure 20.5 Deciduous second molars and unerupted second premolars.
Source: *A Textbook of Orthodontics*, 3rd edn, T.D. Foster, Blackwell Science, Oxford.

The same procedure can be adopted if a child's tooth – usually an incisor – is knocked out by a fall or a blow. Such a tooth is said to be **avulsed**. As long as the periodontal membrane remains vital the tooth can be pushed back into its socket, with complete success in many cases. This type of accident constitutes a dental emergency and it is essential that correct first-aid treatment is applied before the child reaches a dental surgery. The following advice should be given to the person reporting the accident.

- Reassure the child that successful treatment is possible.
- Retrieve the tooth and, holding it by its crown, rinse it gently in warm water. Do not use a disinfectant.
- Put the tooth back into its socket.
- If that is not possible, let the tooth lie loose in the child's own mouth to keep it moist in saliva, although care should be taken with younger patients to avoid choking.
- If that is impracticable, immerse the tooth in a container of milk. Do not wrap it in anything.
- Come to the surgery immediately.

Once the tooth has been replanted in its socket and an X-ray taken, no further treatment may be necessary, but a splint (Chapter 16) is sometimes required to immobilise it for a week or so, followed by root filling. Other injuries to children's teeth are covered in Chapters 16 and 17.

## Minor oral surgery

The term minor oral surgery includes all the procedures listed below.

- **Surgical extractions** – of roots or whole teeth; where a gingival flap has to be raised, or flap raising and bone removal have to be carried out to gain access to the area.
- **Operculectomy** – this is the surgical removal of the gingival flap overlying a partially erupted tooth, especially a lower third molar (Chapter 12).
- **Alveolectomy** – this is the surgical adjustment and removal of bone spicules from the alveolar ridge after tooth extraction, to produce a smooth base for denture seating (Chapter 19).
- **Gingivectomy and gingivoplasty** – this is periodontal soft tissue surgery to adjust the shape of the gingivae and aid oral hygiene measures (Chapter 12).
- **Periodontal flap surgery** – this is the surgical raising and replacing of a surgical flap to enable complete subgingival debridement to be carried out (Chapter 12).
- **Soft tissue biopsies** – the partial (incisional biopsy) or full (excisional biopsy) removal of a soft tissue oral lesion, to be sent away for pathological investigation and diagnosis.

Because of the time involved, these operations are often done under conscious sedation, or in a hospital operating theatre under GA. Those most likely to be carried out in hospital are summarised below.

### Impacted teeth

An impacted tooth is prevented from erupting fully by being jammed beneath another tooth. It usually occurs in jaws which are too small to accommodate all the teeth in their normal position. The commonest example is an impacted lower third molar (Figure 20.6).

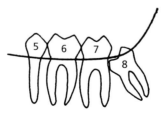

Figure 20.6 Impacted lower third molar.

A unique complication of extraction of impacted lower third molars is damage to the lingual nerve, due to its proximity to the surgical site (see Figure 9.2). It results in numbness or tingling (paraesthesia) of the tongue on the affected side lasting up to six months, or even permanently. The inferior dental nerve may also be damaged but this is less common. Patients must always be warned of the possibility before they give consent to the extraction.

### Cysts

A cyst is a sac of fluid confined within a soft tissue lining. There are many different types found in various parts of the body. In dental practice they are most commonly seen as an abnormal cavity in the bone, at the apex of a dead tooth (**dental** or **apical cyst**), or surrounding and preventing eruption of an unerupted tooth (**dentigerous** or **follicular cyst**). If left untreated a cyst gradually enlarges, causing swelling of the jaw and displacement of other teeth. Whenever possible they are removed, complete with their lining.

### Frenectomy

This means the removal of a frenum. As mentioned in Chapter 8, a frenum is a band of fibrous tissue, covered with mucous membrane, which attaches the tongue and lips to the underlying bone. If the lingual frenum restricts the movement of the tongue so that speech is affected, a lingual frenectomy is performed. If the upper labial frenum is too large it may cause a wide gap to persist between the upper central incisors – this is called a **median diastema**. It can also affect the fit of an upper denture. In such cases an upper labial frenectomy is often undertaken.

### Surgical technique

Although minor oral surgery covers many different procedures, the technique is virtually the same for all of them; so is the order in which each stage of the operation is performed. The following description of the removal of a completely unerupted tooth may be used as a general example of minor oral surgery technique.

1   An incision is made in the gum overlying the unerupted tooth. This is done with a small razor-sharp knife called a **scalpel** (Figure 20.7a). The area of gum outlined by this incision is called the *gingival flap*.
2   The flap is prised away from the surface of the bone with a **periosteal elevator** (Figure 20.7b), which resembles a cement spatula. The flap is then held aside with a **tissue retractor** (Figure 20.7c), or the periosteal elevator itself.
3   This exposes the bare bone covering the unerupted tooth. Some of this bone must now be removed to reveal the underlying tooth. A handpiece

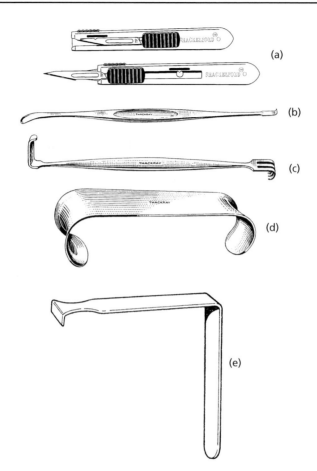

(a)

(b)

(c)

(d)

(e)

**Figure 20.7** Minor oral surgery instruments. (a) Retractable disposable scalpel. (b) Periosteal elevator. (c) Tissue retractor. (d) Kilner cheek retractor. (e) Austin retractor.

and surgical bur, or a **mallet** and **chisel** (Figure 20.8a,b), are used for bone removal.

4  Having removed sufficient bone in this way, the tooth can be loosened and eased out of its socket by gentle leverage with an elevator. It may then be grasped with forceps and removed.

5  Any sharp edges of bone on the socket are removed with **bone forceps** (Figure 20.8d, *rongeurs*) and their margins smoothed with a **bone file** or bur (Figure 20.8e). The socket is then cleared of all debris with a **curette** (Figure 17.5), followed by irrigation with warm sterile saline in a large disposable syringe.

6  Finally, the gum flap is **sutured** (stitched) back into place. The flap is held in position with toothed **dissecting forceps** (Figure 20.9a) and the small curved

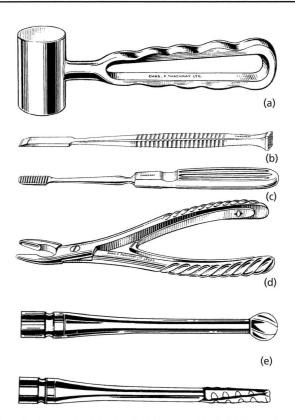

**Figure 20.8** Bone instruments. (a) Mallet. (b) Bone chisel. (c) Bone file. (d) Bone forceps (rongeurs). (e) Surgical (bone) burs.

needle (half circle) is held with special **needle holders** (Figure 20.9b) or alternatively with **Spencer Wells forceps** (Figure 20.9d). Suture needles are supplied in pre-sterilised packs, with the suture material (silk, Vicryl or other synthetic thread) already attached to the needle. The loose ends are then cut off with fine scissors (Figure 20.9e).

A modern alternative to scalpel incisions is the use of a carbon dioxide **laser** beam. This has the advantages of speed of cutting and minimising bleeding. The equipment is very expensive and is accordingly confined to hospitals and specialist practices.

Instruments

- Aspirator tubes; saliva ejector
- Mirror, probe and tweezers
- Local anaesthesia (LA) equipment

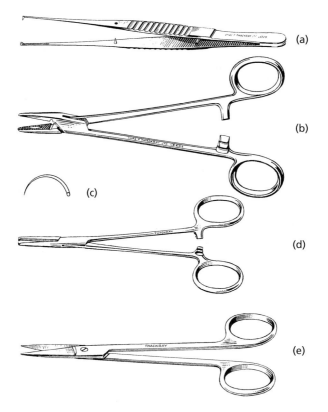

**Figure 20.9** Suture instruments. (a) Dissecting forceps. (b) Needle holders. (c) Suture needle. (d) Spencer Wells forceps. (e) Scissors.

- Scalpel, periosteal elevator and swabs
- Retractors (Figure 20.7d,e)
- Handpiece and surgical burs, mallet and chisels
- Forceps and elevators
- Bone forceps (*rongeurs*), bone files
- Curettes
- Disposable syringe and sterile saline
- Dissecting forceps, needle holder, suture needles, scissors

## Preparation and procedure

A sterile operative field is required. The necessary instruments are autoclaved and transferred on to a sterile towel laid on a trolley or other convenient place, or alternatively they will be pre-sterilised and sealed in pouches. Also placed on the sterile towel are sterile swabs and a dish containing sterile hot saline, together with a sterile disposable waterproof bib for the patient. The patient's X-rays are mounted on a viewing screen and placed where the operator can see them.

A mouthwash is provided and a saliva ejector placed in the patient's mouth. LA is then given and the operation performed.

The dental nurse's duty during the operation is to provide the dental surgeon with a clear operative field. This is done by aspirating the blood and saliva away, and retracting the lip, cheek or tongue as required.

After the operation: all instruments are thoroughly cleaned and sterilised; all traces of blood are removed from work surfaces; and all contaminated zones are disinfected.

### Care of the patient

This is described in the previous section on extractions. Before and during the operation, the dental nurse applies a lubricant, such as petroleum jelly, to the patient's lips to prevent soreness caused by stretching or wide opening, and watches the patient's condition throughout. After operation the patient is given some analgesic tablets, or a prescription for them, and is instructed to return a few days later for the removal of sutures.

## Haemorrhage

Haemorrhage means bleeding, and is classified into three types: primary, reactionary and secondary.

- **Primary haemorrhage** is bleeding occurring at the time of operation, due to blood vessels being cut during the procedure.
- **Reactionary haemorrhage** occurs a few *hours* after operation, due to disturbance of the blood clot.
- **Secondary haemorrhage** occurs a few *days* after operation and is caused by infection at the surgical site.

Reactionary haemorrhage is the most important. Patients suffering from it return to the surgery, up to a day after an extraction, complaining of a bleeding tooth socket. Primary haemorrhage is, of course, seen at the time of operation and the patient is not dismissed until it has ceased, after biting on a bite pack for several minutes. Secondary haemorrhage is not often seen in the dental surgery. It is a complication of dry socket, and is treated as already described for that condition. It is followed by treatment as for reactionary haemorrhage.

### Primary haemorrhage

Primary haemorrhage is obviously caused by the cutting of blood vessels at operation and occurs in all extractions and other surgical procedures. It normally ceases very quickly, as the blood clots, and no treatment is required. But if it is profuse and prolonged, other measures may be necessary.

An additional cause of primary haemorrhage is failure of the blood clotting process. This is an uncommon but very serious matter, occurring in patients taking anti-coagulant drugs and patients with liver disease or some rare blood diseases such as haemophilia. Patients with such conditions should have been identified by the completion of a thorough medical history beforehand, or they may carry a warning card for presentation to any practitioner they attend. In particular, patients with certain heart conditions may be prescribed the anti-coagulant drug **warfarin.** The effectiveness of their blood clotting will be regularly monitored by an **international normalised ratio (INR) score** and this will indicate whether extractions can be safely carried out in dental practice, or whether the patient will require a hospital referral.

## Reactionary haemorrhage

When primary haemorrhage has ceased, the patient leaves the surgery with the tooth socket completely sealed with clotted blood. If anything is done to disturb the blood clot, such as vigorous and frequent mouthwashing with hot fluids on the day of surgery, reactionary haemorrhage may occur later. Similarly an increased blood flow to the part may put an extra strain on the clot and cause it to break away. Strenuous exercise, very hot fluids and alcohol can give rise to reactionary haemorrhage in this way.

Such bleeding is rarely serious, being just a steady ooze in most cases. However, this trivial loss of blood alarms patients because a small quantity of blood, mixed with a large pool of saliva, appears to them as a profuse and dangerous haemorrhage.

## Treatment

The basic principle of treatment of haemorrhage anywhere in the body is application of pressure to the bleeding part. The various measures available for treatment of a bleeding tooth socket depend on this principle. Pressure closes severed vessels and allows blood to clot. Primary and reactionary haemorrhage are both treated in the same way, as detailed below. Each dentist has a preferential method of treatment from the following.

### Pressure pad

A sterile mouthpack or pad of gauze is placed over the bleeding socket and the patient is instructed to bite on it firmly for up to 30 minutes.

### Pressure pad and haemostatic drug

As above but a haemostatic drug is also used, which acts to stop bleeding, e.g. adrenaline (epinephrine); absorbable packs.

Adrenaline is applied to the part of the pad in contact with the socket. Absorbable packs, such as oxidised cellulose (Surgicel), fibrin foam and gelatine sponge (Curaspon) are inserted in the socket before placing the pressure pad.

### Suture

LA is given and a suture inserted. This draws the socket edges together and compresses ruptured blood vessels. An absorbable pack is often inserted in the socket before suturing.

If these measures fail to arrest haemorrhage it may become necessary to send the patient to hospital for treatment and possible investigation.

### Prevention

An updated medical history must be available, with details of drugs taken by the patient and any previous experience of bleeding or bruising following medical or dental treatment. Information suggesting a risk of bleeding may require referral for blood tests or admission to hospital for treatment.

### Primary haemorrhage

If tests show the risk to be slight and that hospital treatment is unnecessary, the precaution of suturing the socket immediately can be taken at the time of extraction. When there is no history of previous haemorrhage, liver disease or anti-coagulant drugs, sutures may still be required if excessive bleeding occurs. This may even be carried out in older patients and those with hypertension, as a precautionary measure. In all cases, however, the patient must not be dismissed from the premises until bleeding has ceased.

### Reactionary haemorrhage

As described earlier, reactionary haemorrhage is caused by increasing the blood flow to the part or disturbing the blood clot. Thus it can be prevented by instructing the patient to avoid mouthwashing, very hot fluids, alcohol and strenuous exercise for the next 24 hours.

## The dental nurse's duty

Sometimes the dentist is away when a patient returns with post-extraction haemorrhage. In such a case it is the dental nurse's duty to reassure the patient that the condition is not serious and can be easily remedied. After obtaining full details about the patient and the extraction, the dental nurse must contact the dentist for instructions.

Meanwhile the patient is made more comfortable by the provision of a mouth-wash to remove the unpleasant taste and clean the mouth. Then, unless instructed to the contrary, the dental nurse may give the patient a pressure pad to bite on until the dentist arrives.

While waiting, the dental nurse should switch on the autoclave and prepare the surgery. Mouth mirror, tweezers, cotton wool, swabs, suction, haemostatic drugs, LA and suture equipment may be required. It should all be ready when the dentist returns.

If the dental nurse is unable to contact the dentist, and a pressure pad is ineffective, help may be sought from an emergency dental service, the patient's doctor or a local hospital.

Extraction is an irreversible procedure. It is therefore essential, when obtaining patients' consent to the extraction or minor oral surgery proposed, to have taken a fully updated medical and dental history (Chapter 15), and to have explained the possible complications, and any alternative treatment, before undertaking the procedure. Furthermore, records of these explanations must be kept. Post-operative instructions given to patients, for prevention of complications, should be given in written as well as verbal form, and should include details of how to obtain emergency treatment outside surgery hours.

# 21 Orthodontics

Orthodontics is the branch of dentistry concerned with the correction of malaligned teeth. When the permanent teeth erupt, parents may notice that the front teeth are crooked or protruding. The condition is known as a **malocclusion** and treatment is sought to improve the child's appearance.

## Aims of treatment

The aims of orthodontic treatment are to reposition the teeth so that appearance is improved and a good functional occlusion obtained. It is important to realise that malocclusion is not a disease, just a deviation from the current cultural perception of good appearance. Children in need of orthodontic treatment are often teased at school and become very anxious about their appearance. Successful treatment is of great psychological benefit in these cases. As far as the dental team are concerned, orthodontic treatment aims to provide the following:

- Correct speech or masticatory function, by aligning the jaws
- Removal of stagnation areas created by crowded teeth
- Reduction in the risk of trauma to proclined ('goofy') teeth
- Psychological well-being of the patient, especially if bullying is a problem

## Normal occlusion

Before learning the types and causes of malocclusion, dental nurses must understand what is meant by normal occlusion, and should refer back to Chapter 8. In *normal* occlusion, all the teeth are well aligned and there is no crowding, no protruding teeth, and no undue prominence of the chin. Upper incisors slightly overlap the lowers vertically and horizontally and special names are given to this overlap: vertical overlap is called **overbite** and horizontal overlap is called **overjet** (Figure 21.1). With the mouth closed and the teeth touching together in occlusion, the position of the first molars and the canines in each jaw determines ideal occlusion and malocclusion. This is called **Angle's classification**. Ideal **class I occlusion**

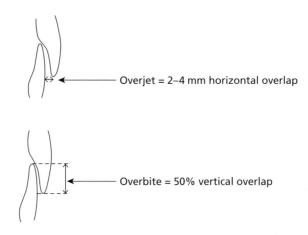

**Figure 21.1** Overjet and overbite.

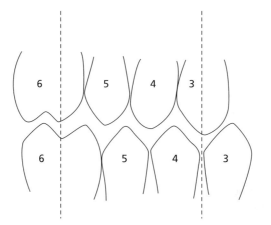

**Figure 21.2** Class I molar and canine relationship.

occurs where the mesiobuccal cusp of the upper first molar lies in the buccal groove of the lower first molar (Figure 21.2). The ideal overjet is 2–4 mm and the ideal overbite is 50%.

For teeth to erupt into normal occlusion, the jaws must be in correct horizontal and vertical relationship to each other, and of sufficient size to accommodate their full complement of teeth. The teeth can then erupt into a normal position of balance between the pressures exerted by the lips and cheeks on their outer side, and the tongue on the inner side.

## Types of malocclusion

The basic types of malocclusion are caused by a combination of any of the following:

- Crowding
- Protruding upper incisors
- Prominent lower jaw

### Crowding

Crowding is caused by insufficient room for all the teeth. It occurs in jaws which are too small to accommodate 32 permanent teeth. The teeth become crooked and overlapping, while those which normally erupt late cannot take up their proper position as there is insufficient room left. Thus the upper canines are usually displaced buccally, lower second premolars lingually and the lower third molars are impacted.

Early extraction of carious deciduous molars also contributes to the crowding in these cases. The gap left by an extraction soon closes, as the remaining posterior tooth drifts forward and takes up some of the space required for the permanent successor.

### Protruding upper incisors

Many children attend for orthodontic treatment because their upper front teeth protrude (**procline**) between their lips. This condition usually arises from a jaw relationship in which the upper teeth are too far forward relative to the lowers. It is commonly associated with an open lip posture and is called a **class II division 1 malocclusion** (Figure 21.3).

When the jaw relationship is not quite so severe, the upper incisors become trapped behind the tightened lower lip and erupt upright, or even pulled back (**retroclined**). This is called a **class II division 2 malocclusion** (Figure 21.4).

### Prominent lower jaw

This condition, in which the chin is unduly prominent, is caused by a jaw relationship in which the lower teeth are too far forward relative to the uppers. It usually results in the incisors biting edge to edge, or with the lowers in front of the uppers, instead of behind them. This is called a **class III malocclusion** (Figure 21.5).

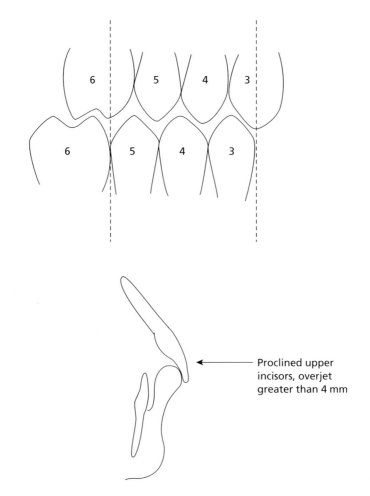

Figure 21.3 Class II division 1 malocclusion.

## Causes of malocclusion

Most kinds of malocclusion are genetic in origin; far fewer are acquired. The most common are inheritance of an abnormal jaw relationship or jaw size. Other genetic factors include supernumerary teeth and missing teeth. The most common acquired causes are early loss of teeth, and thumb sucking habits.

### Jaw relationship

With a normal (ideal) jaw relationship the teeth should occlude in a class I relationship as shown in Figures 21.1 and 21.2. This is the most attractive type of occlusion

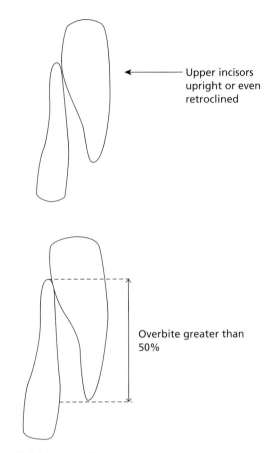

Upper incisors
upright or even
retroclined

Overbite greater than
50%

Figure 21.4  Class II division 2 incisors.

and is accordingly regarded as normal. Other jaw relationships give rise to either a class II or a class III malocclusion.

A jaw relationship in which the upper jaw is too far forward causes two different types of class II malocclusion:

- **Class II division 1** in which the upper incisors protrude, the overjet is increased (Figure 21.3), and the lower lip is trapped inside the overjet
- **Class II division 2** in which the upper central incisors tilt backwards into contact with the lowers, giving a decreased overjet and increased overbite (Figure 21.4), maintained by a strap-like action of the lower lip across the labial surface of the upper incisors

A relationship in which the lower jaw is too far forward causes a **class III** malocclusion. The chin appears prominent and the overjet is reversed, with lower

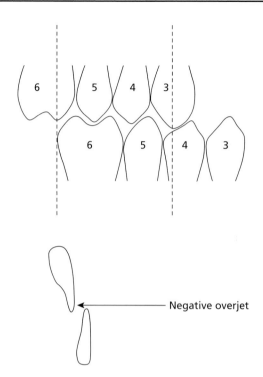

Figure 21.5 Class III malocclusion.

incisors occluding in front of the uppers (Figure 21.5), or in milder cases, edge to edge occlusion.

**Angle's classification** as described above, is based on the relationship of the first molars but this is no longer suitable as early loss of teeth may cause changes in the position of first molars. The incisor relationship is now more convenient.

## Jaw size

Among the commonest abnormalities of all are jaws which are too small to accommodate all the teeth. This is a genetic cause of crowding which is usually localised to the front teeth. The effect of premature loss, described previously, is an acquired cause usually localised to the premolar region. Unfortunately, all causes of crowding often occur together, thus producing an even worse malocclusion.

Jaws which are too large cause spacing of the teeth but this type of malocclusion is not so common.

## Supernumerary teeth

A supernumerary tooth is an extra tooth, in addition to the normal complement of 32 teeth. It occurs most commonly in the upper incisor region as a **mesiodens** and may either prevent a central incisor erupting or cause it to erupt in an abnormal position.

## Congenitally missing teeth

This is the opposite condition to supernumerary teeth where a patient is born with an absence of one or more of their permanent teeth. Upper lateral incisors are often missing and orthodontic treatment may be necessary to close the resultant gaps. Sometimes, instead of being absent, upper lateral incisors are tiny conical teeth, called **peg laterals**. Again the appearance is unsightly and restorative treatment may be required to build up these abnormally small lateral incisors to a more normal size. The other teeth which are most commonly missing are third molars and second premolars. If several teeth are missing, the condition is called **hypodontia**, but this is a rare occurrence.

## Sucking habits

Habits such as finger or thumb sucking can cause displacement of anterior teeth resulting in a decreased overbite and increased overjet. In addition, the sucking action tends to exert excess pressure on the cheeks, so that the upper buccal teeth are forced to develop inside the arch of the lowers. This is called a **cross-bite**. These displacements may correct themselves if the sucking habit is stopped early enough, otherwise orthodontic treatment will be necessary.

## Risks of orthodontic treatment

All orthodontic treatment involves the patient wearing an appliance in their mouth for months or even years, usually 24 hours daily. Their oral hygiene must therefore be meticulous throughout the whole course of treatment, and their diet must be well controlled in relation to non-milk extrinsic sugars and acidic drinks. Otherwise the teeth will be prone to demineralisation and caries.

In addition, root resorption can occur after orthodontic treatment, especially in incisors and other teeth that have undergone trauma or endodontic treatment, or have developed with abnormal root shapes.

In adult patients, unstable periodontal disease may worsen during orthodontic treatment, heavily filled teeth can fracture while fixed appliances are being removed, and temporo-mandibular joint dysfunction may also worsen during or after treatment.

All these points require highlighting and discussing with the patient before treatment begins. Indeed some patients may be advised not to undergo orthodontic treatment because the risks are considered too great.

# Treatment of malocclusion

Orthodontic treatment may involve extractions and the use of any of the following appliances:

- Removable appliance – to carry out simple tooth movements, such as reducing a large overjet
- Fixed appliance – to carry out more complicated tooth movements, especially such as correcting rotations or severe crowding
- Functional appliance – a special type of removable appliance worn in both arches together, to correct the position of the mandible in class II cases while the patient's jaw is still growing

## Extractions

When the jaw is too small to accommodate all the teeth properly, or premature loss of deciduous molars occurs, the permanent teeth become crowded and irregular. This often results in overlapping of the incisors, labially displaced canines, lingually/palatally displaced second premolars, and/or impacted lower third molars. Such malocclusions are treated by extractions. The commonest teeth to be extracted for this purpose are first premolars and the resultant space provides room for straightening the anterior teeth.

If there is an abnormal jaw relationship, such as class II division 1, there may be no apparent crowding, but extractions are still necessary to provide space for moving protruded incisors backwards and thereby improve appearance. Crowded teeth often straighten themselves after extractions, but appliances are usually required to reposition them in good alignment.

## Appliances

Orthodontic appliances may be fixed or removable. They all require a great deal of co-operation from the patient and parents as treatment may last up to two years.

It necessitates wearing an appliance all the time, and maintenance of a high standard of oral hygiene throughout.

Appliances work by applying pressure to the teeth. This results in a remodelling of the alveolar bone surrounding the teeth concerned, allowing them to be guided by the appliance into the desired position. However, appliances cannot be discarded as soon as the teeth have been aligned, as they would simply move back to their original positions. A period of **retention** with an appliance is then required to hold them in their new position until the alveolar bone changes become stabilised, although it is routine nowadays for patients to wear retaining appliances for many years after the completion of their active treatment. Relapse towards the original condition is highly likely if the patient fails to co-operate in this final stage.

## Care of appliances

Many orthodontic appliances utilise delicate wire springs, designed to fit precisely against the teeth to be moved. Patients and parents are accordingly advised to take the greatest care of their appliances and not to miss their regular adjustment appointment. Failure to keep appointments prolongs the overall treatment time, and may even result in the discontinuation of treatment if appointments are cancelled or not attended too frequently.

Removable appliances must only be removed and inserted as directed by the dentist. Careless handling may distort the springs and produce discomfort or undesirable tooth movements. They should be removed and cleaned with a toothbrush, toothpaste and cold water after meals. Patients are warned that failure to do this can result in rapid caries and a sore palate (denture stomatitis).

Fixed appliances are less robust than removable ones and even greater care must be taken over oral hygiene, as discussed later.

Whichever type of appliance is used, patients are instructed to contact the surgery at once if any difficulties arise, without waiting until their next appointment. If attending a different dentist for orthodontic treatment, they must still visit their own general practitioner for routine dental inspection and treatment.

## Removable appliances

A removable appliance resembles an acrylic partial denture but instead of teeth it contains springs made of stainless steel wire. The springs press against the teeth to be moved and guide them in the required direction. The appliance is held in place by stainless steel clasps called **Adams cribs**, which are placed on the first molars and the first premolars usually (Figure 21.6). One of various forms of anterior retention may be used, depending on the tooth movement required. The appliance is made in the same way as a denture, on a model of the jaw obtained from an alginate impression, but special trays, occlusal registration and trial insertion stages are unnecessary.

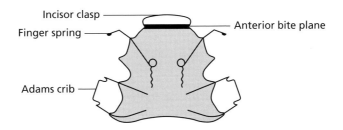

**Figure 21.6** Removable upper orthodontic appliance.

Teeth may be moved into position by finger springs, screws or elastics. When the teeth are satisfactorily aligned, a new appliance may be required to retain them in their new corrected position for at least a year, often for much longer. This appliance is called a **retainer**.

Removable appliances with active springs are now used for simple tooth movement only, such as for correction of upper incisors that have erupted into a negative overjet position behind their lower counterparts. The most important uses of removable appliances are as:

■ Passive space retainers following extractions
■ Retainers
■ An *anterior bite plane* to reduce the overbite

Instruments required to adjust removable appliances are shown in Figure 21.7 and are:

■ **Adams universal** pliers
■ Adams spring forming pliers
■ **Maun wire cutters**

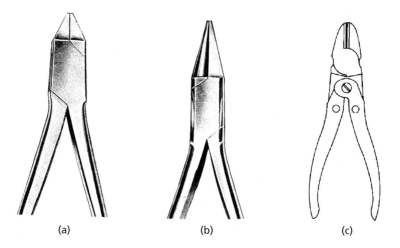

(a)                          (b)                          (c)

Figure 21.7  Orthodontic pliers. (a) Adams universal pliers. (b) Adams spring forming pliers. (c) Maun wire cutters.

The advantages of removable appliances are:

■ Ease of cleaning by the patient, as they can be removed from the mouth
■ Simplicity of construction and repair by the laboratory
■ Short amount of surgery time needed for fitting and adjustment

Their disadvantages are:

- Limited range of tooth movement
- They only achieve tilting of teeth and overbite reduction
- Unsuitable for more severe types of malocclusion where bodily tooth movement or rotation is required
- Unsuitable as lower appliances because their bulk makes them too uncomfortable to wear

## Fixed appliances

Fixed appliances (Figure 21.8) consist of an **archwire** made of springy stainless steel or a flexible nickel-titanium alloy which is bent or preformed into the desired

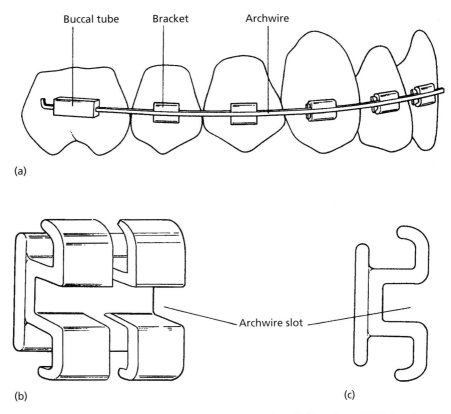

Figure 21.8 Fixed appliance. (a) Archwire in direct-bonded brackets. (b) Edgewise orthodontic bracket. (c) Side view.

ideal shape of the dental arch. When all the teeth are bound to the archwire it forms them into its own ideal shape. It rests in **edgewise orthodontic brackets** which are attached to the labial or buccal surfaces of incisors, canines and premolars. These brackets are made of stainless steel or tooth-coloured materials (Figure 21.8) and are fixed to the teeth by acid etching and direct bonding with a composite or glass ionomer cement (GIC) material.

The distal ends of the archwire fit into **buccal tubes** welded to stainless steel **orthodontic bands,** which are cemented onto the first molars with GIC, polycarboxylate or zinc phosphate. Alternatively, the buccal tubes can be directly bonded to the buccal surface of the first molars with composite.

The archwire is attached to the brackets with fine **ligature wire** or nowadays with tiny elastic rings called **Alastiks**. These are supplied in many different colours which can be changed at each visit, and therefore help to maintain the interest and co-operation of the patient throughout the course of treatment.

## Stages of fixed appliance treatment

- In the first stage, highly flexible nickel-titanium alloy round wires (e.g. Nitinol) are used to align the most displaced teeth without using excessive force.
- The next stage may involve moving the teeth along or around the archwire by means of springs or elastic chains.
- For the final stages of treatment, rectangular-section (edgewise) archwires are used as they fit snugly into the edgewise brackets (Figure 21.8) to exert the greater forces required for bodily movement and/or rotation of teeth.
- A passive fixed or removable retainer is fitted when the teeth are satisfactorily aligned.

## Instruments

Instruments used for fixed appliances are shown in Figure 21.9 and include:

- **Band drivers** and **pushers** for fitting molar bands
- **Molar band removers**
- **Bracket tweezers** for direct bonding of brackets
- **Needle holders** for placing and tightening ligature wires
- **Ligature cutters** or serrated scissors for cutting off excess wire
- **Ligature tuckers** for curling the ends away from soft tissues
- **Fine-ended mosquito forceps** for placing Alastiks and chains
- Smaller versions of removable appliance pliers for adjusting archwires
- A white marking pencil used to indicate adjustment or measuring points on archwires
- Mitchell trimmer for removing excess cement

The advantages of fixed appliances are their precise control over the full range of tooth movement, rapid action and excellent end results. For these reasons they

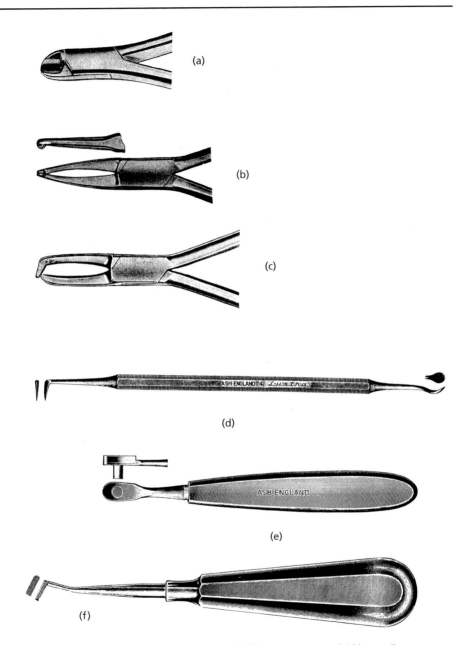

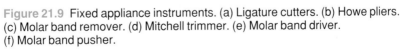

**Figure 21.9** Fixed appliance instruments. (a) Ligature cutters. (b) Howe pliers. (c) Molar band remover. (d) Mitchell trimmer. (e) Molar band driver. (f) Molar band pusher.

have superseded removable appliances for all but the simplest types of orthodontic treatment.

The disadvantages are their susceptibility to damage and the loss of brackets or bands, difficulty in cleaning, and longer surgery visits for fitting and adjustment. The oral hygiene measures required by the patient at least twice daily involve all of the following:

- Routine toothbrushing of the gingival margins and tooth edges of all teeth, using a manual toothbrush or a high quality electric brush such as a Sonicare or an Oral B orthodontic
- Use of an interdental brush to clean each surface beneath the archwire, on each tooth
- Use of Superfloss to clean interproximal areas if necessary
- Use of fluoride mouthwash to counteract any enamel demineralisation

## Functional appliances

These are a removable type of appliance but differ in their mode of action from the type already described. Instead of having springs which engage and actively move the teeth, functional appliances utilise the forces exerted by the muscles around the oral cavity. The most commonly used type of appliance is the **twin block** (Figure 21.10). These are most effective when used during rapid growth, so they are generally limited to the duration of the natural puberty growth spurt. As with the removable appliances already described, they should be worn full time except for during meals.

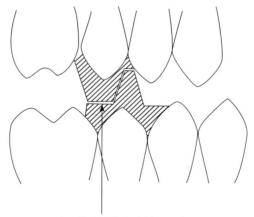

Acrylic blocks hold lower jaw
in class I occlusion when
worn correctly

Figure 21.10 Functional appliance.

The twin block appliance is an effective method of treating those class II occlusions where the arches are uncrowded and the teeth well aligned. As its name implies, it consists of separate upper and lower acrylic bite blocks, which only occlude together comfortably when the lower jaw is postured forward. They have Adams cribs for retention, with an upper labial bow and occlusal coverage to promote the desired tooth movement. As the lower jaw is forced into a forward posture by this appliance, the muscles of mastication are stretched. They react to this by exerting backward pressure on the bite blocks. By careful selective trimming of the occlusal coverage, the upper labial bow retracts the upper incisors while the lower incisors are stabilised. Forward drift of lower back teeth is permitted, together with backward drift of the uppers.

## Surgery procedure

Before orthodontic treatment is provided, a thorough assessment is undertaken to check the occlusion and the desire of the child and parents for treatment. Unless a child is keen to wear an appliance, the prolonged period of co-operation and strict oral hygiene required are unlikely to be forthcoming. Parents must participate, too, by ensuring that appointments are kept, oral hygiene is maintained and instructions for wearing and activating the appliance are followed. These instructions are given orally and in writing. Parents must also realise that time off school for attending appointments may be inevitable.

### Orthodontic examination

Apart from a detailed inspection of the teeth, careful observation of the patient is necessary to assess the effects of lip, tongue and swallowing actions, and to detect any deviations or premature tooth contacts during opening and closure of the mouth. A **calliper gauge** or steel measuring ruler is used to measure overjet, overbite, tooth width and spaces. Photographs are taken at this stage, in addition to X-rays and impressions for study models.

### X-rays

Children usually attend for orthodontic examination before all their permanent teeth have erupted. X-ray films are necessary at this stage to confirm the presence and position of unerupted permanent teeth, and to detect any supernumerary teeth or other abnormalities. Cephalometric, orthopantomographic (OPG), lateral oblique and occlusal films may be taken. These are described in Chapter 14.

### Study models

Models of upper and lower teeth in occlusion are required before, during and after orthodontic treatment. They are often referred to as study or record models. The first models are studied to decide the treatment plan, subsequent models to record progress, and the final models to monitor stability of the end result.

Impressions for record models and appliances are taken in alginate. A wax squash bite may also be necessary to allow the technician to prepare the models in correct occlusion. Disinfection of impressions, appliances and other laboratory work is covered in Chapter 19.

## Removable appliances

Patients usually attend monthly on average to check progress. The dental nurse sets out:

- The patient's records and study models
- Mouth mirror, calliper gauge
- Adams pliers and wire cutters for adjusting springs and clasps
- Straight handpiece and acrylic burs (see Figure 19.5) for trimming the appliance

When a new appliance is fitted:

1 The patient and parent are shown how it works and, with aid of a hand mirror, how to insert, remove and carefully clean it.
2 They are given instructions that it should be worn 24 hours a day, and possibly during meals depending on the type of appliance.
3 It is emphasised that appliances should *only* be removed for cleaning and then reinserted immediately.
4 Instruction is also given, where appropriate, on the use of a key to activate any screws, or the fitting of elastics.
5 The importance of keeping all appointments is stressed and information given on how to contact the surgery if any problems arise between appointments.
6 Reassurance is given that any difficulties with eating or speaking will resolve in a few days, once the tongue has accommodated to the appliance.
7 The next appointment is then arranged.
8 If attending a specialist practice for orthodontic treatment, patients are reminded that they must still continue their normal check-ups and treatment from their own dentist.

## Fixed appliances

Patients usually attend monthly to check progress and make any adjustments. The dental nurse sets out:

- The patient's records, study models, mouth mirror and large hand mirror
- Calliper gauge, and marking pencil
- Pliers, ligature cutters and tuckers, needle holders and serrated scissors

- Mosquito forceps, ligatures or Alastiks and chain
- GIC, polycarboxylate or zinc phosphate cement
- Band driver and pusher, and a **Mitchell trimmer** (Figure 21.9) for removing excess cement

If brackets are to be bonded, bracket tweezers, acid etching and composite or GIC, and bonding materials are needed. In either case, full moisture control is essential, so aspirator tubes, saliva ejectors, cotton wool rolls, absorbent sulcus pads and napkins will be required, together with a bib and mouthwash for the patient.

Procedure when fitting the appliance is as follows:

1   The patient is given a large hand mirror and the orthodontist explains to patient and parent how it works, and how and when to fit and change elastics.
2   They are warned that rapid caries can ensue unless the appliance and teeth are thoroughly cleaned after meals.
3   Instruction is given on how to achieve this by careful brushing.
4   Advice is given to eat a healthy diet and to avoid all sweets, hard foods, and carbonated drinks.
5   They are told that some mild discomfort may occur at first but should wear off in a day or so.
6   The importance of keeping appointments is emphasised; so is the need to contact the surgery immediately if any breakages, loosening of brackets or bands, or any other problems arise.
7   The patient may be given a supply of elastics and some soft wax to mould over any parts of the appliance which cause soreness.
8   Finally the dental nurse arranges the next appointment.

## Referral for treatment

Any dentist without an orthodontic component to their National Health Service (NHS) contract now has to refer their patients to specialists for all but the very simplest of orthodontic treatment; this has resulted in long waiting lists. In order to give priority to the most deserving cases, referring dentists are expected to provide the orthodontic specialist with details of the prospective patient's occlusion and general dental condition before acceptance for treatment is granted. The index of orthodontic treatment need (IOTN) was devised, among other things, as a means of overcoming treatment acceptance problems, by categorising each patient into the degree of severity of their orthodontic treatment need. Only the most severe cases are now eligible for NHS treatment. Special IOTN based referral request forms are available for this purpose (see Figure 21.11).

| TYPE OF APPOINTMENT REQUIRED | NEW PATIENT: ☐ | REVIEW: ☐ |
| --- | --- | --- |

REASON FOR REFERRAL (please tick one or more boxes)

| | |
| --- | --- |
| Overjet ≥ 7 mm ☐ | Contact point displacement > 4 mm ☐ |
| Reverse overjet > 1 mm + functional problems ☐ | Hypodontia ☐ |
| Reverse overjet > 3.5 mm ☐ | Supernumerary teeth ☐ |
| Crossbite with > 2 mm displacement on closure ☐ | Partially erupted impacted teeth ☐ |
| Scissors bite with no functional occlusal contact ☐ | Impacted teeth (excluding 8's) ☐ |
| Open bite > 4 mm ☐ | Cleft lip and palate ☐ |
| Increased overbite with soft tissue trauma ☐ | |

| | |
| --- | --- |
| Oral Hygiene good ☐<br>Caries free ☐ | If these two boxes cannot be ticked, patient will not receive orthodontic appliances. |

Urgent ☐      Reason:

PLEASE TICK IF RADIOGRAPHS ENCLOSED ☐

OTHER INFORMATION (Optional)

Figure 21.11 Orthodontic referral form.

# 22 Pain and Anxiety Control

Since the last edition of this book was written, provision of general anaesthesia in a general dental practice has been legally forbidden, and may now be provided in a hospital setting only. However, dental treatment in a hospital usually requires the assistance of a dental nurse, and patients referred for a general anaesthetic will be handled by a dental nurse, so the relevant areas of the subject are covered here briefly. Similarly, an outline of conscious sedation techniques is provided here, and those dental nurses wishing to pursue the relevant post-certificate qualification run by the National Examining Board for Dental Nurses (NEBDN), are directed to the excellent book *Advanced Dental Nursing* edited by Robert Ireland and published by Blackwell Munksgaard.

**General anaesthesia** (GA) is a state of unconsciousness with complete loss of feeling and protective reflexes (Chapter 4). In the dental chair it was formerly used mainly for short procedures such as extractions and the incision and drainage of abscesses.

**Conscious sedation** is a state of conscious relaxation which enables prolonged treatment to be carried out under local anaesthesia (LA). It is used for patients who are otherwise too nervous to tolerate dental treatment. The patient remains conscious and completely relaxed throughout and retains all protective reflexes against blockage of the airway. It is used mainly for long procedures such as restorative treatments.

Mentally or physically disabled patients, and others who are too unco-operative to accept GA or sedation techniques, can be treated in suitably equipped hospital premises, with critical care facilities, under **endotracheal anaesthesia**. This is the general anaesthetic method normally used in hospitals.

## General anaesthesia

Endotracheal anaesthesia involves delivery of the anaesthetic mixture directly into the lungs through a **nasotracheal tube**. The anaesthetist passes the tube through a nostril, along the floor of the nose, into the nasopharynx. From here, using a special instrument called a **laryngoscope**, the tube is guided by direct vision through the larynx and into the trachea. The oro-pharynx can then be packed with gauze to prevent any foreign bodies, blood, saliva or debris entering the airway.

The advantages of endotracheal anaesthesia are that it gives the anaesthetist complete control over the airway, with no danger of obstruction, and allows use of any resuscitative measures which may be needed, whereas for the operator, it provides perfect anaesthesia with a clean, dry field of work for as long as required.

## Referral for general anaesthesia

Special arrangements must be made for patients who are unable to accept necessary treatment under LA and conscious sedation. Their last resort is usually GA at a hospital day stay dental unit. Such arrangements vary depending on local facilities, and there are strict guidelines for referral.

- The referral letter must justify the use of GA and give the relevant dental and medical history.
- The hospital dentist treating the patient must be satisfied that GA is necessary and appropriate for the patient, and that a thorough and clear explanation of the risks and alternative options is given.
- When the decision to provide such treatment has been agreed by the patient, treating dentist and anaesthetist, the patient's written consent must be obtained.
- Clear and comprehensive written pre- and post-operative instructions must be provided, and detailed records kept of all the procedures undertaken.
- The treating dentist must be satisfied that the facilities for such treatment, and the experience and training of the dental nurse, comply with the appropriate professional requirements.
- Adequate monitoring, emergency and critical care facilities and trained staff must be available. These arrangements must be agreed and documented by all concerned.
- Adequate facilities and trained staff must be provided for patients recovering from GA. They must be monitored continuously until pronounced fit for discharge by the anaesthetist, and provided with written post-operative instructions, before leaving with a responsible adult escort.
- All the team involved in providing dental treatment under GA must train together for dealing with emergencies, and practise such procedures frequently.

The usual reasons for GA referral from a dental practice are as follows:

- Young patients who require one or several extractions of deciduous or permanent carious teeth, and who will not co-operate under LA or conscious sedation techniques
- Older patients who require multiple third molar extractions, especially if a surgical technique is likely due to impaction
- Older patients with severe dental infection, in whom LA cannot be used safely
- Patient request – although this is for extraction only, not restorative treatment

## Conscious sedation

Conscious sedation has replaced GA as a method of pain and anxiety control in general dental practice. Conscious sedation may be defined, in simple terms, as a technique that uses drugs to induce a state of relaxation that is:

- Sufficient to allow injection of local anaesthesia and subsequent dental treatment
- During which verbal contact with the patient is maintained throughout the procedure
- The patient remains conscious, and is able to understand and respond to commands
- The patient retains their protective airway reflexes

Normally in the dental surgery, long procedures such as fillings are done under LA. However, some patients are too nervous or otherwise unco-operative to tolerate LA. In such cases sedation techniques may be used to permit prolonged painless operating time on a relaxed patient. Three methods of conscious sedation can be used in dental practice.

- **Oral sedation** – a sedative tablet is given the night before the dental appointment, and a second one just one hour before treatment begins.
- **Inhalation sedation** – formerly known as 'relative analgesia'; the patient breathes a controlled mixture of nitrous oxide and oxygen through a nasal tube, for the duration of the dental appointment.
- **Intravenous sedation** – a drug is injected into the patient's vein in a controlled manner, so that their anxiety is removed and dental treatment can be carried out.

The advantages of sedation techniques are:

- Patients remain conscious and co-operative throughout
- They retain their protective reflexes against blockage of the airway
- There is no need for a long period of starvation beforehand, as with a GA
- A separate anaesthetist is not required, as the suitably trained dentist can act as both sedationist and operator

However, the General Dental Council (GDC) has issued strict guidelines concerning the experience and training of all surgery staff involved.

- A full medical and dental history (Chapter 15) must be taken before using or referring for conscious sedation. The type of sedation proposed must be explained and appropriate alternatives given.
- Written pre- and post-operative instructions must be provided and written consent obtained, before the procedure (Figure 22.1).

---

**INSTRUCTIONS FOR PATIENTS BEFORE UNDERGOING SEDATION BY INJECTION IN THE ARM**

The technique of sedation by injection in the arm will relax you during your treatment. You will not go to sleep .You will be drowsy, but able to talk and reply to questions. You may not be able to remember much about the treatment afterwards.

The following advice will help you benefit most from this technique:

Make sure you advise your dentist of any changes in your medical history; any medicines you are taking; any recent visits to your doctor.

**ON THE DAY OF TREATMENT**

1.  Please bring with you a responsible adult, who is able to wait and escort you home
2.  At least 2 hours before have only light food prior to intravenous sedation
3.  Take any routine medicines at the usual times
4.  Do not drink any alcohol
5.  Do not wear make up or nail varnish

**DURING THE 12 HOURS FOLLOWING TREATMENT**

1.  Travel home with your escort, by car if possible
2.  Stay resting quietly at home, supervised by your escort
3.  Do not use any complex machinery, e.g. cooker, power tools
4.  Do not drive a motor vehicle
5.  Do not sign any legal or business documents, or make important decisions
6.  Do not drink any alcohol

*If you have any queries or questions regarding sedation, please do not hesitate to contact us at the surgery*

**I HAVE READ AND UNDERSTOOD THE ABOVE INSTRUCTIONS AND UNDERTAKE TO COMPLY BY THEM**

Signed............................................................ Date................................................................

Figure 22.1  Example of an intravenous (IV) sedation consent form.

- Adequate records must be kept, at the time of the procedure, of the technique and drugs used (Figure 22.2).
- As in all other types of dental treatment, dentists must only work within the limits of their own knowledge, training, skill and experience.
- A dentist who undertakes the dual responsibility of sedation and providing the treatment must have completed relevant postgraduate education, training and continuing professional development (CPD). They also must ensure that the most appropriate type of sedation is used, and that the minimum amount of drug is administered to achieve the object of treatment.

NAME              STATUS              AGE              DATE
                                                       IV STARTED AT:


MEDICAL HISTORY          CURRENT MEDICATION          IV SITE: _____

CVS: _____                                      NEEDLE TYPE: _____

LIVER: _____          ALLERGIES: _____      SOL & VOL: _____

RESP: _____                                      DRUGS
                                                       ADMINISTERED: _____
KIDNEYS: _____

OTHER: _____

REASON FOR SEDATION: _____

| TIME | | | | | | | | | | | |
|---|---|---|---|---|---|---|---|---|---|---|---|
| RESP (SA 02) | | | | | | | | | | | |
| HEART RATE (PULSE) | | | | | | | | | | | |
| BLOOD PRESSURE ASA | | | | | | | | | | | |


DENTAL TREATMENT

START _____          COMMENTS: _____

FINISH _____         DENTIST: _____

                             NURSE: _____

INFORMED CONSENT?   YES / NO  MONITOR: _____

Figure 22.2  Example of intravenous (IV) sedation monitoring record sheet.

- A second appropriately trained person must be present throughout the procedure to assist the dentist and be capable of monitoring the condition of the patient, assisting in any complication that may arise and acting as chaperone (Chapter 2). Such a person would ideally be a dental nurse who possesses the NEBDN Certificate in Dental Sedation Nursing, although a qualified dental nurse without this additional post-certificate qualification is currently acceptable.
- Where a second medical or dental practitioner is administering the sedation, the treating dentist must ensure that the sedationist complies with the GDC guidelines already stated.

Conscious sedation guidelines and clinical governance (Chapter 1) also require the following.

- It must only be used when suitable equipment, facilities and drugs are immediately available at the chairside for treating complications.
- All clinical staff are trained, practised and regularly updated to act as a team when using sedation techniques, monitoring patients and managing related complications.
- Supervision and monitoring of patients must be continued in the recovery room until the dentist decides they are fit for discharge, into the care of a responsible adult escort who has been provided with the written post-operative instructions.

## Oral sedation

Some people are so frightened of dental treatment that they are unable to sleep beforehand or co-operate adequately in the dental chair. Such patients can be relieved of their anxiety by the use of anxiolytic drugs such as diazepam, taken orally as a tablet. This is called **pre-medication** and may be used before any form of dental treatment, with or without LA or conscious sedation. The technique is very useful in reducing the 'gag' reflex when impressions are required.

Oral sedation is suitable for adults but not for children, and the drugs involved are addictive if over-used. The patient is far less sedated than with other techniques, as the tablets are absorbed less by the body. However, a suitable escort must still be available for the patient, and a **pulse oximeter machine** should be used to monitor the patient if a prolonged appointment is required (Figure 22.3).

This machine is connected to the patient by a finger probe, and records their pulse rate and oxygen concentration levels in the blood. If either is outside the normal parameters an alarm will sound, and dental treatment must cease while the patient is attended to.

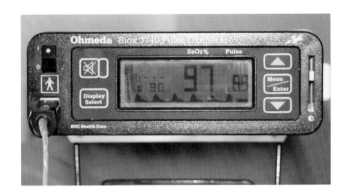

Figure 22.3  Pulse oximeter display.

## Inhalation sedation

This is the safest and best sedation method for children under 16. It uses a mixture of **nitrous oxide** ($N_2O$) and **oxygen** ($O_2$). Nitrous oxide is a powerful analgesic gas that is supplied in light blue cylinders. Oxygen is supplied in black cylinders with a white top. These gases are administered through an autoclavable or disposable nose mask, called a **nasal hood** (Figure 22.4), from a special anaesthetic-type machine that prevents over-dosage of nitrous oxide by limiting its maximum concentration to 50%, and the minimum oxygen level to 30%. The technique was formerly known as **relative analgesia** (RA).

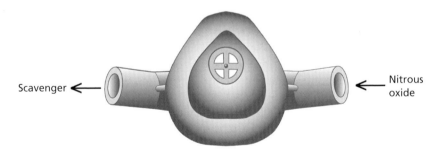

Scavenger ←                         ← Nitrous oxide

Figure 22.4  Nasal hood.

Sedation and analgesia are obtained by continuous inhalation of nitrous oxide and *at least* 30% oxygen. Apart from a small minority of cases, the degree of analgesia is insufficient to prevent pain, but the patient is sufficiently sedated to accept LA.

Before a patient enters the surgery, the following checks are made:

- All equipment is working satisfactorily, with full gas cylinders, spares, resuscitation kit and the scavenging system ready for use

- The patient's records have been read again
- An adult escort has accompanied the patient
- All the pre-operative instructions have been obeyed
- The patient has not got a cold

The patient may then be shown into the surgery and seated in the supine position. The treatment procedure is explained and any questions answered. The patient is shown how to fit the nasal hood and is praised and encouraged throughout the whole of the following procedure.

1   100% oxygen is given at first, followed by 10% nitrous oxide.
2   The patient is told to expect pleasantly relaxing feelings as another increment of nitrous oxide is added.
3   Further increments of 5% nitrous oxide are added until the patient is relaxed enough to accept a local anaesthetic injection and the required dental treatment.
5   When the patient is ready for sedation to be discontinued, the nitrous oxide is switched off and replaced by 100% oxygen for two minutes.
6   During this stage the patient remains receptive to more praise and positive suggestion concerning future treatment.
7   Finally the patient is asked to remove the nasal hood and may then be gently restored to an upright position.
8   After 10–15 minutes the patient should be ready to leave the surgery, but must stay in the company of the escort for another 15 minutes before being discharged with the following instructions for the next 24 hours:
    – Do not drive
    – Do not operate machinery
    – Do not drink alcohol
    – Do not sign legal documents

The advantages of inhalation sedation are:

- Patients may have a light snack up to two hours beforehand
- Recovery is rapid (about 15 minutes) because the sedative drug is exhaled out of the lungs and does not become absorbed into the body
- Electronic monitoring equipment is not required but pulse and respiration must still be checked
- It is the safest and simplest form of sedation, and is the best method for children

The disadvantages of inhalation sedation are:

- It requires a special inhalation sedation machine (e.g. Quantiflex MDM), which prevents less than 30% oxygen, and more than 50% nitrous oxide, from being given

■ It necessitates a scavenging system for exhaled nitrous oxide, so that this does not accumulate in the surgery where it will be inhaled by the dental team

■ In common with most other types of drug treatment, neither inhalation sedation nor intravenous sedation should be given in the first three months (trimester) of pregnancy, although inhalation sedation is suitable for most patients with heart disease and high blood pressure as it reduces their stress levels

■ The nitrous oxide is addictive, so over-use or drug abuse by members of the dental team may be a problem

## Intravenous sedation

A single sedative drug such as midazolam (Hypnovel) is injected intravenously. Although it does not produce anaesthesia or analgesia, it relaxes the patient sufficiently to accept LA. Intravenous (IV) sedation produces **amnesia** (loss of memory of the procedure) and is suitable for patients over 16. A light meal is allowed, not less than two hours beforehand.

The injection is usually given into a vein on the top (*dorsum*) of the hand; or the hollow of the elbow (*antecubital fossa*), and the needle (*cannula*) remains in the vein throughout the procedure, in case any emergency drugs have to be given. To give the injection, the arm is immobilised by strapping it to an arm board attached to the dental chair. A special needle called a butterfly cannula (Figure 22.5) is commonly used. It has flanges to facilitate insertion of the needle (**venepuncture**) and

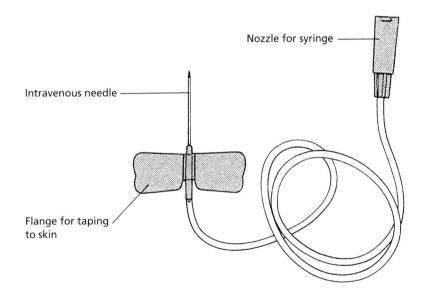

Nozzle for syringe

Intravenous needle

Flange for taping to skin

Figure 22.5 Butterfly intravenous needle (butterfly cannula).

allow it to be taped to the skin, and a flexible tube into which the syringe nozzle fits. This enables additional injections to be given immediately at any time if more sedation or resuscitation drugs are required. A Y-Can is a popular alternative (Figure 22.6).

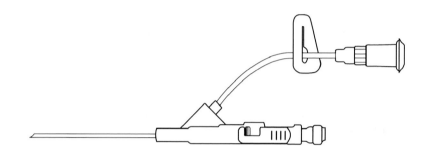

Figure 22.6  Y-Can.

The onset of sedation is recognised by slurring of the speech and difficulty in touching the end of the nose. Monitoring the vital signs is essential throughout and appropriate equipment should be available, together with a resuscitation kit. Two specific requirements in such a kit for IV sedation are the drug flumazenil (Anexate) which is an emergency antidote to an over-dose of the IV sedation agents, and a pulse oximeter machine.

Recovery takes up to an hour and, as for inhalation sedation, the patient must not be left unattended in the recovery room. When the dentist has confirmed that the patient is fit to leave, verbal and written instructions are given for the patient not to drive, operate machinery, take alcohol or sign legal documents for 24 hours.

The advantages of IV sedation are:

■ Better access for the dentist as there is no mask in the way
■ Rapid onset of sedation
■ Supportive patter not required
■ Very effective degree of amnesia
■ No nitrous oxide pollution

The disadvantages are:

■ There is no analgesia so LA is essential
■ Unsuitable for children under 16 and adults over 60
■ Overdose of sedation drug may cause respiratory depression
■ Once injected, the drug cannot be 'switched off', full recovery takes many hours and the patient will need to be supervised for the rest of the day

■ Possibility of complications if drug is accidentally injected into an artery instead of a vein
■ Special monitoring equipment is required

## The dental nurse's duty

Dentists are only allowed to use sedation techniques and act as operator if a suitably trained and experienced dental nurse is present throughout. Such dental nurses must be able to assist the dentist in the preparation and use of sedation agents and equipment. They are required to monitor a patient's condition throughout the procedure and warn the dentist of any impending problems. They are also required to assist efficiently and speedily in any emergencies such as respiratory failure, cardiac arrest or other types of collapse. They must know the uses of all the contents of an emergency kit so that no time is lost in successfully instituting whatever resuscitation measures are needed.

These duties may be listed as given below.

### For inhalation and IV sedation

1 Check that instructions given previously have been obeyed and that the patient is still fit for sedation.
2 Have monitoring and resuscitation equipment ready and check for correct functioning.
3 Use a soothing patter to reassure and calm the patient.
4 Throughout the procedure, check the patient's pulse and observe the respiration rate and colour.
5 Inform the dentist immediately of any changes in the patient's condition.
6 Be prepared, under the dentist's direction, to render immediate assistance in resuscitation procedures.
7 On completion of treatment, assist the patient to a couch in the recovery room, and stay there to monitor and safeguard recovery until the dentist allows the patient to return home with an escort. Before leaving, the dentist or sedation qualified dental nurse will remove any indwelling cannula, apply a dressing, and give verbal and written instructions: not to drive, operate machinery, take alcohol or sign legal documents for 24 hours, or the remainder of the day for inhalation sedation (IH) patients.
8 At the end of a sedation procedure, ensure that all clinical waste disposal complies with legal requirements (Chapters 7 and 23).

### For inhalation sedation

■ Check the machine for correct functioning and cylinder labelling. Have spare oxygen and nitrous oxide cylinders and emergency kit available.

*For intravenous sedation*

- Apply a surface anaesthetic to the intended injection site.
- Lay out an arm board, syringes, drug ampoules, venepuncture needles, cannulae, wipes, dressings and surface anaesthetic. Ensure that syringes filled from ampoules are correctly labelled.
- Lay out mouth props (Figures 22.7 and 22.8), LA equipment and all the dental instruments and materials required.
- Immobilise and prepare the patient's arm for venepuncture.
- Lay out the pulse oximeter and sphygmomanometer.

   Although no special qualifications are currently necessary for adequately trained dental nurses to assist in conscious sedation, they can prove their competence by attending a course and passing the examination for the NEBDN Conscious Sedation Certificate.

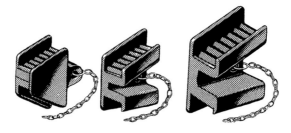

Figure 22.7  Mouth props.

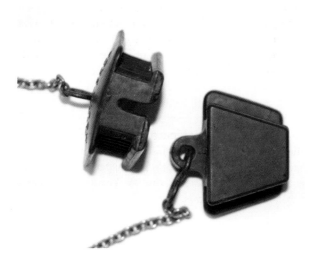

Figure 22.8  McKesson mouth props.

## Care of the patient

Excessive fear of dental treatment is the most common reason for using sedation. Dental nurses should be constantly aware of such patients' anxiety and do everything possible to show them that they understand how they feel. A sympathetic and soothing manner will in itself make the whole procedure less stressful for the patient. Technical expertise alone is not sufficient for treating nervous patients. They require the extra support of the dental nurse who realises that what is a routine day's work for them is a terrifying ordeal for a frightened patient. The dental nurse must be caring, compassionate, calm and approachable, and at all times regard the patient as the most important person in the practice.

It is obvious from this account that dental nurses have an extremely busy time during conscious sedation sessions. Three appropriately trained dental nurses may be required:

- One assisting the sedationist and monitoring the patient
- One assisting the dentist
- One in the recovery room

Arrangements must also be made to ensure that messages, enquiries and telephone calls are dealt with by reception staff to prevent any interruptions or delays to proceedings in the surgery. Dental nurses have an indispensable role in ensuring that the entire session runs smoothly, efficiently and with the maximum consideration for the patient's comfort.

## Monitoring patients

Throughout any conscious sedation procedures it is essential to ensure and check that the circulation is adequately oxygenated. This is done by observing and recording the patient's vital signs: colour, breathing, pulse and blood pressure. This is called *monitoring*, and is made easier by the use of the pulse oximeter. Full monitoring notes must be kept at the time of the treatment, and stored in the patient's record card (Figure 22.2).

## Colour

A patient's colour can be observed by watching the face, fingers, lips or ears. It indicates the state of oxygenation of the blood. A pink colour is normal, whereas a purple tinge (**cyanosis**) denotes deficient oxygenation, and pallor and sweating denote a more severe deficiency. Any such changes require immediate identification and treatment of the cause.

## Breathing

Regular chest movements show that a patient is breathing, and can be seen by watching the reservoir bag on the inhalation machine or by feeling the upper abdomen. The pulse oximeter will also record the blood oxygen saturation levels, when in use.

## Pulse

Feeling the wrist, neck or temporal pulse will indicate the rate, regularity and strength of the heart beats (Chapter 4). The neck (carotid) pulse is found beside the top outer edge of the larynx. The temporal pulse is felt on the zygomatic arch immediately in front of the ear.

## Blood pressure

The pulse gives some indication of blood pressure but it is accurately measured with a **sphygmomanometer** and stethoscope. The sphygmomanometer comes with an inflatable cuff, which is fitted on the upper arm. When inflated it stops the flow of blood through the artery on the inner side of the arm opposite the elbow. This area (the *antecubital fossa*) is the central depression seen between the upper arm and forearm, and it is here that the stethoscope is placed. When the cuff is slowly deflated, blood starts flowing again and this can be heard through the stethoscope. The reading on the instrument scale at which the first sound is heard is noted. This is called **systolic** pressure and denotes ventricular contraction. As deflation of the cuff is slowly continued, the sound increases to a maximum and then disappears. Another reading taken and noted at this point is called **diastolic** pressure, denoting ventricular relaxation between heart beats. The cuff is then deflated and removed until another blood pressure check is required. Sphygmomanometer readings are still measured in units of millimetres of mercury (mm Hg) even though mercury is not often used in modern equipment. Average readings for a healthy young adult are 120/80 mm Hg for systolic/diastolic pressures.

## Continuous monitoring equipment

Traditional methods of monitoring patients' vital signs by observation, feeling the pulse and checking blood pressure can be supplemented, but not replaced, by modern electronic devices, which are standard equipment in hospitals. They give a continuous readout and recording of vital signs. Dentists cannot be expected to have access to all such devices, but a sphygmomanometer and a **pulse oximeter** are required for IV sedation.

A pulse oximeter is a small portable device with a special illuminated clamp (resembling a clothes peg) on the end of a long lead. The clamp is clipped on to the patient's finger or ear lobe and detects the colour of the blood. This enables the instrument to display readings of the pulse rate and oxygenation of the blood. The normal oxygenation reading should be 100%. Immediate investigation, and correction of the cause, is required if it drops below 90%. Similarly, fluctuations of the pulse rate may occur during treatment, and the cause must be found and corrected. The best way to understand the use and readings of a pulse oximeter is to try it on yourself. As the instrument depends on transmission of light through the nailbed or skin, readings may be affected by racial pigmentation or use of nail varnish.

Whichever method or instrument is used for measuring pulse and blood pressure, the readings are noted before and during the procedure. This allows any significant changes to be drawn to the attention of the dentist or sedationist.

The GDC requires dental nurses to be adequately trained and experienced for assisting with conscious sedation treatment. This means that they must know how to monitor a patient's condition with the available equipment, and understand the significance of their findings.

## GA and sedation emergencies

If breathing stops (respiratory failure), air cannot enter the lungs and death will occur in a few minutes. The heart continues beating during these critical few minutes as there is still some residual air in the lungs. It only lasts a few minutes though, after which the heart itself stops beating (cardiac arrest) and death is imminent.

Respiratory failure can occur during GA or sedation and may be caused by blockage of the airway or an over-dose of anaesthetic or sedation agent.

## Blockage of the airway

Blockage of the airway is caused by obstruction of the entrance to the larynx by the tongue or a foreign body. It is recognised by the following:

- Patient's face becomes very blue and congested
- Clammy skin
- Rise in pulse rate and blood pressure
- May also be snoring or wheezing sounds

If the tongue is displaced backwards during GA it blocks the laryngeal entrance. Fortunately this can be easily remedied by pulling the jaw forward, as the base of the tongue is attached to the mandible and moves with it. However, this type of obstruction is normally prevented by the anaesthetist's finger held behind the angle of the mandible, thus making it difficult for the jaw to be accidentally pushed backwards by the operator.

Blockage by a foreign body is an extremely serious matter as it must be located and removed before respiration is possible again. Fortunately it is rare under conscious sedation, as the normal reflexes that prevent such emergencies remain active. However, it may still occur, even with unsedated patients. Before searching for a foreign body, the patient is laid flat with the head lower than the feet; this is called the head-down position. Then 100% oxygen is given.

The foreign body may be a mouth pack, mouth prop, extracted tooth, small instrument, clotted blood or vomited food. The purpose of a mouth pack is to prevent foreign bodies getting past it but these accidents do sometimes occur. Packs and props have a long piece of tape or chain attached which is left dangling out of the mouth, and allows them to be removed easily if they slip backwards and obstruct the airway. Any other foreign bodies are found by feeling behind the tongue with a finger or use of the anaesthetist's laryngoscope and removed immediately, using forceps or suction as necessary.

Whatever method is used to clear the airway, the essential factor is speed. Respiration cannot occur while the airway is blocked, so delay in removing an obstruction may be fatal.

## Overdose of anaesthetic

An overdose of a powerful anaesthetic or IV sedation agent can cause respiratory failure by paralysing the respiratory muscles. The patient is then unable to breathe in enough oxygen from the air or anaesthetic machine. This lack of oxygen is called **hypoxia** and its early stages are indicated by cyanosis (blue complexion). At this stage, IV injection of a remedial drug must be given. In the case of IV sedation with midazolam, the antidote is **flumazenil** (Anexate). It reverses the action of midazolam, and is an essential item for the emergency drugs kit in practices using IV sedation.

If these remedial measures are not taken, breathing will continue to weaken until it stops altogether. The face becomes ashen-grey and the pupils dilate. This will be followed by cardiac arrest unless oxygen can be introduced into the blood, by positive ventilation using emergency respiratory equipment and oxygen. These items are a legal necessity to have on the premises of any dental practice, whether conscious sedation techniques are carried out or not.

## Resuscitation

If collapse (unconsciousness) occurs during conscious sedation in a dental surgery, the essentials of resuscitation are oxygenation of the blood and maintenance of the circulation. This is called **basic life support** (BLS) and is covered fully in Chapter 5.

### Emergency procedure

A state of preparedness is necessary for meeting dental emergencies associated with respiratory failure and cardiac arrest. A sterile, ready-for-use, emergency kit must be immediately available every time conscious sedation or any other treatment is undertaken. Essential items are:

- An efficient suction apparatus for clearing a blocked airway
- Oro-pharyngeal (Guedel) airways (Figure 22.9)
- Manual pulmonary resuscitator, e.g. Laerdal (Figure 22.10)
- Resuscitation drugs, including flumazenil if IV sedation is used
- Syringes and needles for injection of drugs
- An extra non-electric suction apparatus, manual pulmonary resuscitator and cylinder of oxygen must also be part of the emergency equipment

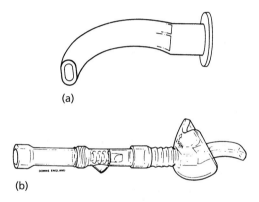

(a)

(b)

Figure 22.9 Airway tubes. (a) Oro-pharyngeal (Guedel) airway. (b) Brook airway.

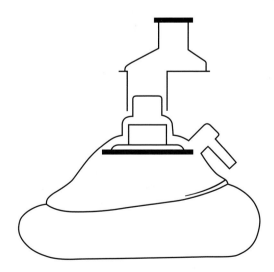

Figure 22.10 Laerdal pocket mask.

## Other forms of anxiety control

Two other forms of anxiety control, which do not rely on the administration of drugs, have begun to have more of a role in dental treatment over the past few years. They are **hypnosis** and **acupuncture.** Although qualifications in either area are not currently a legal requirement for dentists wishing to use these techniques in practice, suitable qualifications are available in both techniques. A brief outline of each discipline is given.

### Hypnosis

This is a technique of anxiety control that relies purely on the skill of the hypnotist to produce an altered state of mind in the patient, so that they are neither fully awake nor asleep. It is achieved by verbally achieving hypnotic suggestion, to produce the altered state. No clear definition of hypnosis is available, but it can be described as 'an altered state of awareness in the patient, so that they are more amenable to suggestion'. When it is successfully suggested to them by the hypnotist that dental procedures are painless, or pleasant or even happy experiences, it is a powerful tool in overcoming a dental phobia.

Full dental hypnosis is not practised by many dentists as yet, but with patients who are already consciously sedated using one of the conventional techniques involving drug administration, it is relatively easy for the depth of their sedation to be accentuated by using hypnotic suggestion as well. The easiest method used is for the dentist to merely alter the tone and depth of their voice while talking to the sedated patient, so that a low and slow, monotone style of speech is used. The desired suggestions are then repeated to the patient in a calm, deep voice, often with key words dragged out in length, so for example the word 'slow' becomes 'sloooow'.

The technique requires lots of practice to be used successfully, and every dentist will develop their own favourite phrases and patter with time. Some examples are as follows:

- '............ and any pain you feel will be just a tiny insect bite ............'
- '....... and all the pain has been sucked away, and everything feels good now ......'
- '. . . . and as you breathe in you can feel yourself becoming more and more relaxed. . . .'
- '. . . and you're lying on a nice sunny beach, and you can hear the waves gently lapping onto the shore . . .'

### Acupuncture

This is a branch of Chinese medicine in which special needles are inserted into the patient's skin for the following reasons:

- As therapy for various disorders
- To produce anaesthesia
- To reduce anxiety

Again, no qualifications are currently required, but the GDC would expect any dentist using acupuncture in the delivery of dental care to have at least attended a validated training course before using the technique on patients. The manner in which acupuncture works is not fully understood, but it is believed to be a combination of the following:

- The needle prick causes the patient's body to release its own painkillers (called **endorphins**) which act as local analgesics
- The technique helps to induce a form of hypnosis in the patient
- The needle prick acts as a distraction from the original source of pain

However it works, acupuncture has been successfully used to carry out dental treatment painlessly, as well as to remove the 'gag' reflex in susceptible patients so that impressions can be taken. It is also used as a technique for long-term management of chronic dental pain in TMJ disorders. Although acupuncture can be used to reduce the anxiety associated with dental treatment, it is currently the least used technique to do so.

## Pain control

There are few invasive techniques involved in dental treatment that do not involve some degree of pain, unless a tooth is non-vital. Consequently, the majority of patients' fears with regard to dental treatment are that they will experience pain during their treatment. The routine use of local anaesthesia (LA) for dentistry has revolutionised the patient experience, and is fully covered in Chapter 9.

# 23 Health and Safety at Work

All dental premises, their staff and patients are covered by the provisions of the **Health and Safety at Work Act**. This legislation seeks to protect staff and patients by making the staff aware of hazards at work, and encouraging them to find the best ways of making their particular premises safer for all concerned.

Dentists are required under this law to ensure, so far as is reasonably practicable, the health, safety and welfare at work of all their employees. Every dental practice is required to:

- Provide a working environment for employees that is safe, without risks to health, and adequate as regards facilities and arrangements for their welfare at work
- Maintain the place of work, including the means of access and egress, in a safe condition
- Provide and maintain safe equipment, appliances and systems of work, including proper seating and eye protection for staff using computer keyboards and monitors
- Ensure safe handling and storage of any dangerous or potentially harmful articles or substances
- Provide such instruction, training and supervision as is necessary to ensure health and safety
- Display the official Health and Safety poster

To comply with these statutory obligations dentists must keep their staff informed of all the safety measures adopted. Practices with five or more employees must produce a comprehensive health and safety policy and provide all staff with a copy. It will classify the practice health and safety procedures and name the persons responsible. It should also list the telephone numbers of all dental, office and essential domestic equipment maintenance contractors, and the local Health and Safety office and emergency services.

## Role of the dental nurse

All dental nurses have a legal obligation to co-operate with their employers in carrying out the practice requirements in respect of these safety measures. They are designed to protect not only the staff and patients, but anybody else using or visiting the premises. In a large practice or clinic, a dental nurse may be appointed as *safety representative* under the Act for the purpose of improving liaison within the practice about health and safety matters.

However, many dental nurses begin their careers as young trainees in the dental environment, so the following two sets of regulations are also important in protecting their welfare:

- **Health and Safety (Young Persons) Regulations 1997**
- **Management of Health and Safety at Work Regulations 1992**

These sets of regulations dictate that a **risk assessment** of the dental environment has to be carried out, with particular regard to the protection of younger staff members, by taking into account the following points:

- The inexperience and immaturity of young persons
- Their lack of awareness of any risks to their health and safety
- The fitting and layout of the practice and surgery, with regard to the safety of young personnel
- The nature, degree and duration of any exposure to biological, chemical or physical agents within the work environment
- The form, range, use and handling of dental equipment
- The way in which processes and activities are organised
- Any health and safety training given, or intended to be given

Full compliance with the Health and Safety Act for all dental practices, clinics and hospital departments involves all of the following:

- **Fire Precaution (Workplace) Regulations**
- **Health and Safety (First Aid) Regulations**
- **COSHH – Control of Substances Hazardous to Health**
- **RIDDOR – Reporting of Injuries, Diseases and Dangerous Occurrences**
- **Environmental Protection Act**, in relation to **Special Waste and Hazardous Waste Regulations** (Chapter 7)
- **Ionising Radiation legislation** (Chapter 14)
- General safety measures
- General security measures

## Fire precautions

The relevant regulations require the employer to risk assess the fire precautions that are needed for their own particular work premises, as these will vary from one practice to another. For instance, a ground floor practice will be considered less dangerous to staff and patients in the event of a fire than one that is in a multi-storey building.

In particular, the areas of fire safety discussed below must be complied with.

## Emergency routes and exits

- These must be kept free from all obstructions to allow immediate evacuation from the premises if necessary – in particular, they must be kept **unlocked** during normal working hours.
- Fire exits must lead directly to a place of safety.
- They must be clearly marked by green 'Fire Exit' signs, with an accompanying pictogram of a running man.
- Emergency lighting should be provided if necessary – this applies to hospitals rather than individual practices.
- Emergency doors should open manually in the direction of escape, and should *not* be operated electrically.
- Sliding or revolving doors should *not* be used as fire exits.

All practices now have to submit to a **Fire Safety Inspection**, so that the premises can be formally recorded as having carried out the necessary risk assessment. Although several companies provide the means for this to be carried out by post, a visit by a suitably qualified inspector from the Fire Service will hold more weight if a fire does occur, and the practice is held to account for its compliance.

The inspection will give advice with regard to the following:

- The number and positioning of **smoke detectors**
- The number and positioning of **fire extinguishers**
- Written records of staff training in the use of fire extinguishers
- The types of fire extinguishers to be provided, with at least two types present in all practices

All extinguishers are coloured red nowadays, but have accompanying labels to advise on the type of fire that each is safe to be used on:

- **Water extinguisher (red)** – for use on all *but* electrical fires
- **Carbon dioxide extinguisher (black)** – for use on all fires
- **Dry powder extinguisher (blue)** – for use on all fires

The extinguishers must all be inspected and certificated yearly, and replaced as necessary. Other forms of fire fighting equipment are fire blankets, fire hoses (in larger premises), and fire buckets containing sand or water. In addition, the practice must have a written **Fire Safety Policy** with which all staff are familiar and practised in, to ensure that a set procedure for evacuation is known and followed by all. In general, the policy should be a variation of the instructions given below.

## On discovery of an outbreak of fire

1   Raise the alarm on the premises.
2   If safe to do so, use the fire equipment provided to tackle the fire.
3   If the fire cannot be contained immediately with the equipment available, call the Fire Service as an emergency.
4   Evacuate the premises, checking all rooms for persons if possible.
5   Do not use lifts or electric doors for evacuation exits.
6   Switch off gas and electric supplies if possible.
7   Close all doors as the premises are evacuated, to contain the fire.
8   Assemble all evacuated persons at the fire assembly point, and check for any missing persons against the day list.
9   Inform emergency personnel of any additional dangers, such as the location of oxygen cylinders and gas canisters.
10   No risks should be taken to salvage personal possessions.

## First aid

In addition to the identification of the signs and symptoms of the medical emergencies that may occur in dental practice (Chapter 5), and their correct management, the whole dental team is required to be able to deal with basic first aid procedures too. These are summarised below, but in line with clinical governance guidelines (Chapter 1), every practice must also be compliant with the following:

- All staff must be trained and certificated in basic life support (Chapter 5)
- All practices must have a **first aid kit** available, besides the full range of emergency drugs and emergency oxygen cylinders required under clinical governance guidelines
- All practices must have an **accident book,** which is used to record all except any major accidental events that occur on the premises to staff, patients or visitors
- In the event of a medical emergency, the dental team must be able to reassure and help the casualty until the professionals arrive, and this may include Basic Life Support (BLS) to maintain life if necessary

The general first aid emergencies that the dental nurse may be required to deal with are all of the following:

- Severe bleeding
- Burns and scalds
- Poisoning

- Electrocution
- Bone fractures

These are summarised below.

### Severe bleeding

- The first aid principle is to **restrict the blood flow to the wound and encourage clotting to reduce blood loss**.
- Arterial bleeding will spurt rhythmically and be cherry red in colour.
- Venous bleeding will gush quickly and be dark red or purple in colour.
- Capillary bleeding will ooze slowly and be dark red in colour.
- The required treatment is to raise the injured part above the level of the heart if possible, and apply direct pressure to the wound for up to 15 minutes using a clean dressing.
- Any foreign objects present should *not* be removed from the wound.
- As a last resort, severed arteries can be compressed against the underlying bone for up to 15 minutes, using a tourniquet.

### Burns and scalds

- A **burn** is an injury caused by **dry heat**, **chemicals** or **irradiation**.
- A **scald** is a wet burn caused by **steam or hot liquids**.
- The first aid principles are to **prevent infection** of the underlying tissues and to **prevent clinical shock developing** due to the loss of blood serum.
- The required treatment is to remove the casualty from the source of danger if possible, and to reassure them if they are still conscious.
- The injured part should be placed under cold water for a minimum of 10 minutes to reduce blistering.
- Any restrictive jewellery should be removed before any swelling occurs, but clothing should be left in place as its removal may cause tearing of the tissues.
- Seek medical help for all but minor burns or scalds, and be prepared to carry out BLS if clinical shock develops in severe cases.

### Poisoning

- The first aid principle is to **limit the exposure of the casualty to the poison**, and maintain life if necessary.
- Consult any available COSHH documentation for the required first aid advice.
- The required treatment is to remove the casualty from the source of the poison, without endangering other lives.
- Vomiting should not be induced, as caustic poisons will burn the digestive tract each time they pass through.
- Maintain the airway and carry out BLS if necessary.
- Seek urgent medical help.

## Electrocution

- Electrocution is caused by an electrical current passing through the body, causing burns and possibly affecting the electrical conduction of the heart itself.
- The first aid principle is to **remove the casualty from the electrical source and maintain life until help arrives**.
- The required treatment is to isolate the electrical supply if it is safe to do so, treat any surface burns and minimise the effects of clinical shock.
- Carry out BLS if necessary.
- Seek urgent medical help.

## Fractures

- These are usually caused by external trauma or a fall.
- The first aid principle is to **prevent further tissue damage by restricting the movement of the casualty**.
- The required treatment is to not move any injured part of the body, to cover any open skin wounds with clean dressings and control bleeding as necessary.
- Seek urgent medical help.

## COSHH

Under the COSHH regulations, all dental practices are legally required to carry out a risk assessment of all the chemicals and potentially hazardous substances used in the workplace, to identify those that could harm or injure staff members. COSHH stands for the **Control of Substances Hazardous to Health**. Harm may be caused if an accident occurs to expose personnel to an unusually large amount of a chemical, or if a chemical accidentally gains entry to the body (for example, by being inhaled), or merely just by the dangerous nature of even small amounts of a chemical (for example, mercury). Once risk assessed, a report can be written for each chemical showing all of the following:

- The hazardous ingredient it contains
- The nature of the risk, ideally by indicating the risk category using recognised symbols (Figure 23.1)
- The health effects of the hazardous ingredient
- The precautions required for the safe handling of the product
- Any additional hazard control methods required
- All necessary first aid measures required in the event of an accident

The reports are then kept in a COSHH file for quick reference as necessary, and updated regularly. They should be available to the whole dental team for reference, and each staff member should sign to say they have read and understood the information. An example of a COSHH assessment sheet is shown in Figure 23.2.

Know your hazardous chemical products. Below are the four health categories:

**TOXIC**
**– can cause damage to health at low levels**
*for example, mercury is toxic by inhalation*

**HARMFUL**
**– can cause damage to health**
*for example, some disinfectants /tray adhesives are harmful by inhalation*

**CORROSIVE**
**– may destroy living tissue on contact**
*for example, phosphoric acid (etchant) causes burns in contact with skin*

**IRRITANT**
**– may cause inflammation to skin and/or eyes, nose and throat**
*for example, some disinfectants and x-ray developer can irritate the eyes and skin*

**Note:**
For packaged hazardous chemical products, the label (depending on the size) should contain a symbol (as above) and simple information about the hazard and the precautions required. The Safety Data Sheet will provide more detailed information and the supplier is obliged to provide this if the substance is hazardous to health and is used at work.

Figure 23.1  Risk categories for COSHH assessment.

The risk assessment is carried out using a procedure similar to that detailed below, for each substance used in the dental practice – ranging from specific dental materials through to general cleaning agents.

- **Identify those substances which are hazardous** – by reading the manufacturers' leaflets and instruction sheets enclosed with the product, or shown on the label.
- **Identify who may be harmed** – this is likely to be anyone who uses the substance, although public access must be taken into consideration too.
- **Identify how they may be harmed** – is the product hazardous on skin contact, or by inhaling fumes, or an eye irritant, etc.?
- **Evaluate the risk** – is the substance only harmful if misused, or is it harmful with every use?

| Name of Substance | | | | |
|---|---|---|---|---|
| **Hazardous Ingredients** | | | | |
| Used for | | | | |
| By whom | | | | |
| Frequency | | | | |
| Amount | | | | |
| | | | | |
| **Nature of Risks** | Chemical | Flammable | Poisonous | Biological |
| **Exposure Limits** | OES (MEL if applicable) | | ppm | mg m$^{-3}$ |
| | Long term (8 hr TWA) | | – | |
| | | | – | |
| Other | | | | |
| | | | | |
| **Health Effects** | | | | |
| Eye contact | | | | |
| Skin contact | | | | |
| Inhalation | | | | |
| Ingestion | | | | |
| | | | | |
| **Precautions for Safe Handling and Use** | | | | |
| Spillage | | | | |
| Waste disposal | | | | |
| Storage | | | | |
| | | | | |
| **Control Measures** | | | | |
| Ventilation | | | | |
| Eye protection | | | | |
| Respiratory protection | | | | |
| Gloves | | | | |
| Health monitoring | | | | |
| Staff training | | | | |
| Other | | | | |
| | | | | |
| **First Aid Measures** | | | | |
| Eye contact | | | | |
| Skin contact | | | | |
| Inhalation | | | | |
| Ingestion | | | | |

**Dentists and staff members to sign to confirm these Control Measures are carried out:**

1 ................................  4 ................................  7 ................................
2 ................................  5 ................................  8 ................................
3 ................................  6 ................................  9 ................................

Figure 23.2 Example of COSHH assessment sheet.

- **Determine whether health monitoring is required** – for example, exposure to mercury, or nitrous oxide gas.
- **Control the risk** – by ensuring the substance is not misused, or reduce the risk as far as possible if it is harmful with every use – this may involve changing the product.
- **Inform all staff of the risks** – by staff meetings, and introduction of the COSHH sheets to be read and signed for by all.
- **Record the risk assessment** – keep documented evidence that the assessment has been carried out, with review and update dates recorded as necessary.

While the dental nurse is an integral part of the risk assessment procedure as a member of staff, more senior dental nurses may take over the role of maintaining the COSHH files and updating them as necessary, once suitable and documented training has been given.

Some general safety points with regard to hazardous substances are given below.

## Storage

All chemicals should be stored in cupboards with separate storage for inflammable substances and poisons. Mercury must be stored in a cool cupboard in properly sealed containers.

Oxygen and nitrous oxide cylinders should, ideally, be stored outdoors, but if this is not possible a well-ventilated fire-resistant store should be used. An appropriate trolley should be available for moving heavy cylinders.

## Ventilation

Adequate ventilation is essential to minimise any risk of dangerous or irritant vapours from mercury, disinfectants, nitrous oxide and laboratory chemicals.

## Disinfectants

Some disinfectants used in dental practice can irritate skin, airway and eyes. Personal protective equipment (PPE) consisting of gloves, mask and glasses should be worn when handling them, and working areas must be well ventilated to avoid irritation of the airway. Manufacturers' instructions must be followed.

## RIDDOR

Accidents that occur in the workplace fall into one of two categories:

- **Minor accidents** – these result in no serious injury to persons or the premises, and are dealt with 'in-house' by analysing the incident to determine how it occurred and preventing recurrence, and by recording the event in the **accident**

**book** – examples include a trip or fall, a needlestick injury, and a minor mercury spillage

■ **Major accidents** – these result in a serious injury to a person, or severe damage to the premises, and are **notifiable incidents** that must be reported to the Health and Safety Executive under RIDDOR (www.hse.gov.uk/riddor)

Notifiable incidents do not include those occurring to a patient while undergoing dental treatment, but do cover all persons on the premises otherwise. Once notified, the Health and Safety Executive will carry out an investigation into how the incident occurred, to determine whether it was purely an accident or whether the practice or a staff member were at fault. Advice will then be given on how to avoid similar incidents in future, but in serious cases prosecution may follow. Dental nurses should remember that under General Dental Council (GDC) registration, they are personally responsible for their own errors and acts of omission – so it may be that they are the ones who are prosecuted. The injuries that must be reported under RIDDOR are as follows:

■ Fracture of the skull, spine or pelvis
■ Fracture of the long bone of an arm or leg
■ Amputation of a hand or foot
■ Loss of sight in one eye
■ Hypoxia severe enough to produce unconsciousness
■ Any other injury requiring 24-hour hospital admission for treatment

The dangerous occurrences that must be reported are as follows:

■ Explosion, collapse, or burst of a pressure vessel (an autoclave or compressor)
■ Electrical short circuit or overload that causes more than a 24-hour stoppage of business
■ Explosion or fire due to gases or inflammable products that causes more than a 24-hour stoppage of business
■ Uncontrolled release or escape of mercury vapour due to a major mercury spillage (Chapter 16)
■ Any accident involving the inhalation, ingestion or absorption of a hazardous substance which results in hypoxia that is severe enough to require medical treatment
■ Any case of acute ill health due to cross-infection from pathogens or infectious materials

It is obvious then that RIDDOR should only be relevant when a genuine and unforeseen accident occurs on the dental premises, as all other incidents should be avoided by the correct instigation of policies and protocols covering the following:

■ Waste disposal (Chapter 7)
■ Recognition of surgery hazards

- Infection control (Chapter 7)
- Safe handling and storage of mercury (Chapter 16)
- Ionising radiation (Chapter 14)
- Safe use of conscious sedation techniques (Chapter 22)

Although all the above are covered elsewhere as indicated, key areas are repeated here for the sake of completeness.

## Waste disposal

Surgery waste is classed as hazardous waste and must not be included or collected with normal domestic waste. It must be segregated into hazardous waste (including sharps waste) and special waste.

- Hazardous waste implies contamination with blood, saliva and other body fluids. It includes **empty** local anaesthetic cartridges.
- Special waste consists of:
  - Prescribed medicines
  - Irritant, harmful, corrosive and toxic substances
  - Cartridges that still contain some local anaesthetic
  - X-ray developer and fixer
- Liquid special waste must not be emptied into sinks or drains.
- Both types of waste must be put into separate specially labelled rigid containers and records kept of their contents and collection.
- Sharp waste, such as syringe needles and scalpel blades, must also be put into special rigid puncture-proof containers. Only authorised waste disposal contractors may be used for collection and incineration of such waste.

Non-hazardous (office and domestic) waste is stored in black plastic sacks to distinguish it from hazardous waste, and the normal domestic waste-collection service should be used for its disposal.

Amalgam and mercury waste, including extracted teeth with amalgam fillings, cannot be incinerated as this would release toxic mercury vapour. Special arrangements are necessary; these are covered in Chapter 16. Records must be kept by the practice of all hazardous waste disposal procedures.

## Staff protection

Staff should be provided with waterproof aprons, gloves, masks and glasses for handling irritant chemicals, disinfectants and X-ray processing solutions. Biological hazards such as exposure to blood-borne infection are covered by the practice cross-infection procedure.

## Surgery hazards

The most important hazards facing dental staff arise from cross-infection, use of mercury and taking X-ray films. Sedation techniques are potentially hazardous procedures for patients and they, too, must be protected under the Health and Safety at Work Act. All these are covered in the previous chapters.

Other risks in dental practice include:

- Use of toxic or corrosive materials
- Inhalation of waste nitrous oxide
- Injury from faulty or improper use of autoclaves and air compressors

These particular risks are also covered in other chapters, but in general they may be guarded against as follows:

- Correct storage, handling and use of drugs – these must be kept in a separate locked cabinet
- Good ventilation and a scavenging system for nitrous oxide during inhalation sedation
- Meticulously following manufacturers' instructions on use and maintenance of all equipment and material
- Wearing personal protective equipment

All the required health and safety procedures throughout the premises are included in the practice quality assurance system.

### Personal protective equipment

Gowns, masks and gloves minimise the transmission of infection from patient or instruments to staff. Surgical gloves prevent absorption of mercury when handling amalgam, and will also prevent irritation of sensitive skin by X-ray processing solutions. Heavy-duty gloves protect against injury when scrubbing instruments prior to sterilisation.

Protective glasses with full lenses and side-shields, or face visors, can prevent eye damage from infected material or amalgam particles when a water spray is used. Glasses should also be worn by patients undergoing treatment in a supine position, where they are at risk of injury from dropped instruments, acid-etching liquids and other materials. Dark glasses or shields may be necessary when using curing lights.

Jewellery, wrist watches and open-toed shoes should not be worn in the surgery as they pose a cross-infection and/or mercury hazard.

## Infection control

Dental staff are at constant risk of cross-infection from patients and used instruments. The sources of infection are:

- Direct contact with a patient's blood or saliva
- Droplet infection from a patient's exhaled breath
- The aerosol cloud produced by a water spray when using a high-speed handpiece or ultrasonic scaler
- Instruments awaiting sterilisation
- Inoculation injury such as needlestick; this is covered in detail in Chapter 7

Pathways by which infection is transmitted to staff are skin cuts or abrasions, the airway and eyes. Ways of avoiding these risks would be outlined in the practice infection control policy (Chapter 7), issued to all members of staff to clarify their duties and should indicate who is responsible for dealing with them. The following precautions are taken to prevent cross-infection of staff and patients.

- Wear protective clothing at all times in the surgery:
  - Uniform coat or gown
  - New mask and gloves for each patient
  - Protective glasses for staff and patients
- If any blood splashes on to an exposed part of the body, wash it off with water immediately.
- Use an efficient aspirator whenever water spraying equipment is used.
- Use rubber dam whenever possible to minimise the infected aerosol effect of water spray and compressed air.
- Keep the surgery well ventilated.
- Use disposable material whenever possible.
- Wear heavy-duty waterproof gloves when cleaning instruments prior to sterilisation.
- Sterilise instruments for the correct time at the correct temperature.
- Work surfaces should be cleaned and disinfected between patients or covered with a new waterproof disposable sheet.
- Great care must be taken to ensure that sterile instruments are not contaminated before use on a patient.
- Hands must be washed and new gloves worn before laying up for the next patient or handling clean instruments.
- Laboratory work should be disinfected with sodium hypochlorite.
- All hazardous and amalgam waste disposal must comply with legal requirements as covered in Chapters 7 and 16. The waste must be packed in heavy-duty yellow plastic sacks and approved sharps containers ready for incineration.
- Re-sheathing devices must always be used for local anaesthesia syringes.
- Autoclave instruments must be at the correct settings.
- Laboratory work must be disinfected and labelled accordingly.

Special care must be taken if child patients have been in contact with virus infections such as mumps and rubella (German measles). The virus is present in saliva before any signs of illness are apparent, and surgery staff may become infected in this way from an apparently fit child.

- Rubella in the first three months of pregnancy can cause serious physical defects in the unborn child, and there are strong medical grounds for advising the termination of pregnancy in such cases.
- Mumps can cause sterility in mature males.

If there is any evidence of contact with these diseases, treatment of the children concerned should be postponed. This will protect staff, and adult patients in the waiting room, from any risk of infection.

Staff must be immunised against hepatitis B, mumps, measles, rubella (MMR), poliomyelitis, and bacterial infections such as pertussis (whooping cough), diphtheria, tetanus and tuberculosis, as a minimum.

## Hepatitis B and C and acquired immune deficiency syndrome (AIDS)

Hepatitis B and C and AIDS can be fatal and are transmitted by contact with the blood of a sufferer or carrier. Special care must accordingly be taken when known sufferers or carriers are being treated. The basic safety principle involved is the avoidance of any contact with the patient's blood or blood-stained saliva. The hepatitis B and C viruses (HBV and HVC) and the AIDS virus (human immunodeficiency virus (HIV)) can infect via the skin, mucous membrane, eyes or airway.

The precautions already given for prevention of cross-infection must be followed for *every* patient seen in a dental practice because the majority of carriers are either unaware of their condition or unwilling to disclose it. However, for known carriers or sufferers some extra precautions have been recommended.

- Reserve the last appointment of the day for their treatment. This allows ample time after completion of treatment for sterilisation of instruments and disinfection of the surgery.
- Move all unnecessary equipment and furniture away from the working area.
- Regard all steel burs used as disposable.
- Items which cannot be sterilised by heat, or disinfected with hypochlorite, should be immersed in an appropriate alternative disinfectant (e.g. Mikrozid).
- If any blood splashes on to an exposed part of the body, wash it off with water immediately.
- All staff must be vaccinated against HBV, MMR, and other serious diseases (Chapter 6).
- Patients with the active disease, or carriers requiring procedures involving much loss of blood, should be referred to a specialist unit.

Dental equipment must be prevented from contaminating the public water supply. It should accordingly be modified if necessary to comply with local requirements.

There is a high use of mercury in dentistry, as it is a key constituent of amalgam filling material. It is highly toxic and the dangers around its usage cannot be over-emphasised, as it is odourless and invisible and can enter the body in the following ways:

- **Inhaled** as a vapour or as an aerosol during amalgam removal from a tooth
- **Absorbed** through the skin by direct contact
- **Ingested** if eaten or swallowed

Vapour is released at ordinary room temperature, but the amount released increases significantly as the temperature rises. Except in the case of a mercury spillage, the main exposure to the dental team occurs during the use of amalgam in restorative dental procedures. Simple precautions taken at the time will reduce the staff exposure to a negligible level:

- Wear full PPE during restorative procedures involving amalgam
- Good surgery ventilation to prevent vapour accumulation
- Good high speed aspiration during amalgam placement or removal procedures
- Use of capsular amalgam to avoid the need for liquid mercury
- Careful handling to avoid spillages
- Use of the mercury spillage kit for small spillages to be dealt with effectively
- Correct waste amalgam and capsule storage in mercury absorption containers, before collection
- Use of a registered and certificated special waste handler
- Adherence to the Health and Safety policy by all staff, to prevent accidents

The actions to follow in the event of a mercury spillage are covered in detail in Chapter 16. Major spillages require evacuation of the premises, reporting of the incident to the Health and Safety Executive, and full co-operation with them and the Environment Agency while the spillage is cleared away.

## General safety measures

These relate to any work premises where staff are employed to provide a service to the public, and therefore apply to all dental practices, clinics and hospital departments. They are all common-sense precautions aimed at preventing injury to anyone using or visiting the premises, and include all of the following:

- A safe means of entry which is adequately lit and unobstructed, including for disabled people
- Non-slip floor coverings which are secure, to prevent tripping
- No dust traps in the décor of surgical areas, such as those present with embossed wallpaper coverings
- No sharp edges on furniture and fittings
- Guards around fires and heaters to avoid burns
- No trailing electrical cables that could cause tripping
- All portable electrical appliances must be inspected annually for wear and tear problems – this is called PAT testing, and may be carried out by any approved person as long as written records are kept
- Gas and electric supplies should be disconnected overnight as a matter of routine, although this may not be possible if items such as a fridge are on the premises
- A fully stocked first aid kit should be available for minor injuries

## General security measures

Although it is unusual for dental practices to have just one or two staff on the premises during normal working hours, because of the need for the dentist to be chaperoned during treatment (Chapter 2), it may happen during holiday periods. In the interests of staff safety, the premises should remain locked during these times if only one member of staff is present, so that they are not vulnerable to attack.

In addition, the following points should be applicable to improve the safety of all staff, and the security of the workplace.

- All staff are trained to be caring and sympathetic to patients, so that confrontations do not occur.
- All visitors should also be treated with respect and spoken to courteously at all times.
- Have a policy in place with regard to assault and violence towards staff in the workplace.
- Advertise the existence of this policy, so that patients and visitors are aware of the 'zero tolerance' attitude encouraged by the National Health Service (NHS).
- Have adequate alarm and security systems in place – these are likely to be a requirement by insurers anyway.
- Keep the number of key holders to a minimum.
- Ask unexpected visitors to the premises for some form of identification, such as the ID cards usually carried by utility personnel.
- Have accurate patient day lists, so that unexpected visitors are easily identified as such.

- Ensure that the burglar alarm is set correctly at the end of each day, so that break-ins are detected immediately.
- Bank all monies daily, so that the incentive for opportunist burglars is removed.
- Lock away all drugs, prescription pads and supplies of needles and syringes to reduce burglary.

## Safety signs

Safety signs in the practice should include:

- Fire safety exits, fire alarms and location of fire fighting equipment
- Location of first aid facilities
- Doors of controlled areas and darkrooms
- Stocks of hazardous substances

All signs must contain a pictorial symbol of their purpose as well as safety information. Doors to controlled areas and darkrooms should also have warning lights to indicate that X-ray exposure or film processing is in progress.

The correct application of all these health and safety issues is regulated by clinical governance guidelines, which are in place to ensure that all dental practices operate to a level of 'best practice' at all times, for the safety of the patients and in their best interests. This issue is discussed in Chapter 1.

# 24 Patient Management

Successful patient management is the responsibility of the whole dental team, not just the dentist, and it involves all of the following areas:

- Reception of the patient into the practice
- Appointments
- Communication skills
- Equality of dental care
- Patients with special needs
- Dental emergencies

The dental nurse has a key role in ensuring that the dental experience of each patient is a pleasant one, whether working at the chairside or in a reception and administrative position.

## Reception of patients into the practice

Most dental practices have one or more dental nurses who 'double up' as receptionists for at least part of their working week, although it is possible to have staff with purely administrative duties. The obvious problem with this latter situation occurs when patients are asking for dental advice or for further information about specific dental treatments, as the administrative staff will have limited dental knowledge. For this reason, most practices prefer a dental nurse to carry out reception duties.

The word 'reception' illustrates the main role of these personnel – to 'receive' the patient into the practice as the first point of contact in the dental environment. It is vital that the dental nurse in this role has all of the following attributes:

- Pleasant disposition
- Friendly and welcoming attitude
- Knowledgeable about dentistry, but only to the limit of their training
- Efficient and accurate at reception duties
- Work well under pressure, without becoming flustered
- Pleasant telephone manner

- Caring and considerate attitude
- Well presented, and neither too loud nor too softly spoken

As very few dental practices, and no hospital clinics, have no computerisation of at least some part of their working system, IT skills are also an imperative requirement for the modern dental nurse. However, the increasingly extensive use of computers in dentistry and dental practice management does not replace the need for the dental nurse to also have legible, neat and accurate handwriting skills. This is especially important when giving written information such as appointment details to patients.

A friendly disposition is invaluable when greeting nervous and anxious patients onto the premises, and is often all that is required to allay the fears of most patients. While this tends to come naturally when dealing with younger patients, it should be remembered that many older patients are just as anxious – whether they try to hide their feelings or not. Being friendly and welcoming to all patients should come as second nature to all of the dental team, so that the patient's dental experience is of a consistently high standard for the whole visit.

## Appointments

Booking appointments for patients takes up a large part of the working day, and during busy periods it can be the one area that causes many problems. When several patients are hovering in a reception area, and one or more telephones are ringing with enquiries from other patients, it is quite easy for members of the dental team to be overwhelmed by the demands of their role and for mistakes to happen. In larger practices and hospital clinics, it is usual for more than one staff member to be responsible for appointment bookings, and without a written protocol in place for the task to be carried out in a consistent manner by all, mistakes can easily be made.

A successful appointments booking system can easily be established by any dental practice or clinic if the following points are considered and adapted for use as necessary.

- Ensure that all staff working at the reception area have been fully trained in all of their necessary duties.
- Have written protocols to be followed by all staff.
- Ensure the booking system is sensible, easy to follow and is explained clearly during training sessions.
- If manual appointment books are used, rather than a computerised system, ensure alterations and cancellations are deleted in a tidy manner, so that the day list is still readable by all staff.
- If possible, delegate the simpler reception duties to other staff so that one senior person remains in control of appointment bookings, as this will lead to fewer mistakes.

- Ensure all staff are aware of how each dentist and dental care professional (DCP) prefers their appointments to be booked, especially the length of time required for various procedures.
- Be considerate but firm with patients when booking appointments; sometimes it may not be possible for them to have the time slot they request.
- If a problem does occur, attempt to rectify it to everyone's satisfaction as soon as possible, but try to uncover the cause of the problem so that it will not be repeated in the future – this shows maturity and common sense.

## Communication skills

Good communication between the dental team and patients is crucial if the patients are to take an active role in managing their own oral health. Not only is it a necessity if any consent given for treatment is to be valid, but it will also lead to greater understanding between all parties, especially if the patient is unsure about treatment options or even refuses to have treatment as advised by the dentist.

An open relationship must exist at all times, so that the patient feels they can ask for advice, query options given, or explain why they do not wish to have certain treatments. All of this depends on the dental team showing good communication skills, and this is especially important for the dental nurse as patients often prefer to discuss matters with them than with the dentist.

Communicating means 'to give or exchange information', and this can be done both verbally and non-verbally, as follows:

- **Talking** – either directly or by telephone
- **Written explanations** – which reiterate any verbal information given
- **Information leaflets or posters** – which can be read and then discussed verbally as necessary
- **Body language** – which can be open and friendly, or defensive and 'stand offish'
- **Eye contact** – maintaining eye contact shows attentiveness, while breaking eye contact indicates the patient is being dismissed
- **Facial expressions** – again, these can be friendly or not
- **Body position** – sitting to listen to the patient is more attentive than standing, especially if the body position of the listener is turned away from the speaker too
- **Touching** – this is sometimes used to reinforce points, although it is not acceptable in some situations and with some patients

A friendly staff member will obviously appear more approachable to patients than one who seems unfriendly, but often an unfriendly demeanour occurs without the staff member realising it. When unexpected situations arise, such as an equipment failure, or a very busy appointments session, staff can seem abrupt, harried or even dismissive towards patients as they try to deal with the unexpected situation. Continuing to carry out tasks while being spoken to, especially if eye contact is not made, can appear extremely rude and dismissive to patients. On the other hand, standing too close to a patient ('invading their personal space') or making inappropriate physical contact, may be construed as threatening or offensive by the patient. Some individuals have naturally good communication skills, but for other dental staff a training course or 'in house' experiential learning, by following the lead of good communicators, is vital in the development of their own skills.

Communicating with patients whose first language is not English will present severe problems for the dental team in some circumstances, and wherever possible a family member or friend should be encouraged to attend and act as an interpreter. Valid consent cannot be given for treatment if the patient does not understand the language being spoken, and the relevant points have not been translated for them. The National Health Service (NHS) issues patient information leaflets in various languages nowadays, and they can be ordered and delivered to dental practices for free quite easily.

## Equality of dental care

As discussed in Chapters 2 and 15, the dental nurse has a legal responsibility to behave equally towards all patients without showing any form of discrimination. This can occur in all of the following areas:

- **Sex discrimination** – between male and female patients
- **Age discrimination** – especially between elderly patients and others
- **Ethnic discrimination** – between ethnic minorities and white British patients, especially where there is a language barrier too
- **Socio-economic discrimination** – between the perceived social class and economic status of various patient groups

In particular regard to sex discrimination, the development of inappropriate relationships between members of the dental team and patients is particularly frowned upon by the profession, and more importantly by the General Dental Council (GDC). No favouritism should be shown towards any patient by a staff member because they are attracted to them – problems are likely to occur, which may result in dismissal or even a charge of serious professional misconduct. Staff only have to read the annual misconduct reports issued by the GDC to determine the seriousness of these charges.

The dental team need to be aware of any likely cultural differences between ethnic groups, some of which are of dental relevance, as shown below. The team must accept these differences in an appropriate manner, while offering oral health advice as necessary. Religious beliefs may prevent a patient from undergoing oral examination at certain times, such as the Muslim period of Ramadan, and again the dental team must accommodate the belief to allow the smooth running of the practice. Other relevant religious beliefs are as follows.

- **Hindus** – they have no beef in their diet and are often vegan or vegetarian. Their diet tends to be high in saturated fats, and they observe many days of fasting throughout the year.
- **Sikhs** – they eat meats other than beef and pork, but are often vegetarian with a relatively high intake of dairy products.
- **Muslims** – they have strict food laws, including no pork or alcohol but lots of fish, and long periods of fasting (Ramadan continues for a full month).

In addition, in all Asian groups, women tend to breast-feed their babies for up to two years, and sugar is routinely added to feeds. For this reason, oral health advice to this group is very important in an attempt to avoid a high caries incidence in young Asian children.

## Patients with special needs

There are many patients who can be considered to be disabled in relation to dentistry and dental treatment, because of a **physical**, **mental**, **social** or **dental problem**. Some of these special needs patients who are likely to be treated in a general dental practice setting, rather than in a specialist dental clinic, are as follows:

- **Older patients**
- **Patients with learning disabilities**
- **Patients with physical disabilities**
- **Patients with certain medical problems**
- **Patients from low socio-economic backgrounds**

### Older patients

The number of people living longer is steadily increasing as medical treatment improves and healthier lifestyles predominate. These older patients also tend to retain at least some of their natural teeth for life, as dental treatments and materials are expanded and advanced. Some of the reasons for these patients experiencing difficulties in accessing dental care are as follows:

- Immobility, or poor mobility, making regular attendance at a dental practice difficult or impossible
- Poor mobility may restrict access to ground floor surgeries only
- Complicated medical problems, which may limit the dental treatments available to them

- Complicated drug regimens, some of which may interact with dental anaesthesia and medicaments
- Various degrees of senile dementia, which may make it difficult for them to understand explanations of dental treatment
- Various degrees of visual impairment or hearing loss, which can again make explanations difficult

The Disability Discrimination Act 2004 has gone some way to assisting with some of these problems, such as by requiring the use of a telephone 'loop' system where necessary to assist those with hearing difficulties. Even simple points such as using certain colours to highlight doorways for the visually impaired, or the instalment of double handrails on staircases to assist those with poor mobility, makes some considerable difference to many patients. However, dental practices are expected to take only reasonable measures to comply with the Act, and there is still a great need for access to basic dental care via **domiciliary visits** (home visits with limited portable dental equipment) or **special needs clinics**.

The provision of dental care to older patients has developed into a specialty called **gerodontics**.

In addition to any infirmities that elderly patients may experience, their age also causes potential treatment problems for the dental team, as follows:

- Deteriorating denture retention, as the alveolar ridges resorb with time
- Age-related dry mouth (xerostomia), which is associated with increased risks of both caries and periodontal disease
- Shrinkage and sclerosis of the pulp chambers within the teeth, making endodontic treatment difficult or even impossible
- Associated difficulties with extraction, as the teeth become more brittle and more likely to fracture
- Age-related darkening of the teeth, making shade matching of anterior restoratives difficult
- More pronounced gingival recession, increasing the risk of root caries developing
- Development of age-related conditions such as osteoporosis, which make jaw fracture during extraction more likely
- Conditions affecting manual dexterity, such as arthritis, which make good oral hygiene difficult to achieve for many older patients

## Patients with learning disabilities

These are patients who have significant problems associated with learning and socialising with others, due to inherited mental disorders such as Down's syndrome and Asperger's syndrome, or acquired but permanent disorders following severe head injury. Those with mild impairment are likely to access dental treatment via general practice, while the more severe cases are likely to be referred for specialist dental care in special needs clinics.

Often (but not always), patients with learning disabilities exhibit a reduced level of general intelligence which presents the following problems to the dental team:

- They have a short attention span, so explaining treatment plans and gaining valid consent is often difficult
- Poor memory retention requires information and advice to be repeated many times
- Reduced level of understanding may cause problems in gaining the trust of the patient before dental treatment can be provided
- Careful explanations of treatment must be given, which are in basic and non-threatening terms
- The link between diet, oral hygiene and dental disease is often impossible to explain satisfactorily, making co-operation in the management of their oral health very difficult
- Some dental staff may slip into a type of 'baby talk' with these patients, which is particularly offensive to those with acquired learning disabilities

## Patients with physical disabilities

This is a wide-ranging group of patients, including those who are paralysed and wheelchair bound, through those with visual or auditory impairments, to those who have acquired medical conditions which affect the level of dental care they are able to receive. Again, the more severely disabled patients tend to be treated in specialist units rather than general dental practice, the latter being able to accommodate the milder cases to varying levels of efficiency. Some of the more common problems that these patients present to the dental team are as follows:

- Hearing impaired patients often rely on hearing aids or lip reading to understand when being spoken to by the team, so the lowering of masks and face to face contact is very important in communicating to them
- Visually impaired patients like to touch and feel, or listen to the sound of, dental equipment before it is used on them, and the dental team should accede to these requests at all times
- Some physical disabilities will require the patient to be treated in downstairs surgeries only, with wheelchair access available too
- Any disabilities causing variations in muscle tone may restrict the ability of the patient to sit comfortably in the dental chair, and may also require the use of muscle relaxants to achieve adequate access to the oral cavity
- Stroke victims may have difficulty communicating if their speech ability has been affected, and may rely on family or carers to make themselves understood
- Arthritic patients, and those with upper limb deformies (such as thalidomide victims or those with dwarfism), may find adequate oral hygiene impossible to achieve without special adaptations to toothbrushes, etc.

Dental nurses interested in these areas of patient management can study for the post-certificate qualification in Special Care Dental Nursing, once they have achieved their National Certificate, or NVQ Level III, qualification.

## Patients with certain medical problems

As well as the conditions already mentioned, such as arthritis and Down's syndrome, there are some less apparent medical conditions that predispose the sufferer to a greater risk of dental problems.

- **Epilepsy** – the required medication (Epanutin) causes gingival hyperplasia, and prevents a good standard of oral hygiene from being regularly maintained.
- **Diabetes** – this condition is associated with poor wound healing, making patients more likely to suffer from oral infections such as dry socket and abscesses.
- **Digestive reflux disorders** – this includes conditions such as hiatus hernia and bulimia, which are both associated with tooth erosion (Chapter 11) and require advice from the dental team to avoid excessive sensitivity or even tooth loss.
- **Dental phobias** – these sufferers often require some form of anxiety control (Chapter 22) before they are able to undergo all but the simplest of dental treatments.
- **Xerostomia** – this condition of a persistent dry mouth may be due to various medications, or be age related, but the effects on the oral tissues can be catastrophic.
- **Rheumatic fever** – a history of this condition can leave patients at risk from infective endocarditis (Chapter 4) unless they are given prophylactic antibiotics before all invasive dental treatments are carried out.
- **Pregnancy** – while not a medical problem, the hormone changes that occur during pregnancy do have a hyperplastic effect on the gingivae (**pregnancy gingivitis**), which can lead to oral health problems in many patients.

Obviously, all of these problems and conditions should be routinely identified while taking and updating the patient's medical history.

## Patients from low socio-economic backgrounds

There has been a lot of research that tends to suggest that patients from low socio-economic backgrounds may be categorised as having special needs for the following reasons.

- They are the least likely group of patients to attend for routine and regular dental examinations, so there is little preventive input from the dental team.
- Their associated poor diet, usually high in carbohydrates, predisposes them to general poor health.

- The high rate of smoking and alcohol use in this group of patients tends to predispose them to periodontal disease and oral cancer (Chapter 12).
- Dental ignorance, often compounded by low self-esteem, prevents their own oral health from being a high priority.
- Their high carbohydrate input tends to be related to the expected high caries incidence and early tooth loss.
- Some of these patients feel intimidated by professionals, and are least likely to seek dental advice, especially in relation to information regarding lifestyle changes.
- Some people may also have difficulty understanding oral health advice.

## Dental emergencies

Even with the very best dental care, emergencies do arise from time to time. Since April 2006 it has been the responsibility of the Primary Care Trusts (PCTs) to provide out-of-hours emergency dental care to all patients, whether they are NHS, private, regular or irregular attenders. It is operated through a telephone **triage** system, by organisations such as *NHS Direct*, where calls are received from patients and categorised into a range of severity. Each PCT will determine the most severe incidents that require emergency treatment, but the following are likely to be included by all:

- **Severe dental pain** – which is not controlled by analgesics
- **Severe swelling** – of the oral soft tissues, which is at risk of compromising the patient's airway
- **Uncontrolled bleeding** – after an extraction or minor oral surgery procedure

Less severe emergencies, such as swelling with no airway implications, are passed to the 'on-call' dentist for an opinion on whether the patient should be seen within 12 or 24 hours, by either their own dentist or by the emergency dentist. As the system is intended to operate during evenings, weekends and public holidays, it may be that treatment will be required before the patient's own dentist is available. In these cases, they will be directed to a local *dental access centre* for emergency treatment such as lancing an abscess, placing a tooth on open drainage, or placing a dressing. The patient can then seek full treatment from their own dentist at a later date, or find a dentist willing to undertake their treatment if they receive no regular dental care.

Private patients may be members of various private dental plans, such as Practice Plan or Denplan, and member dentists will often provide emergency care for less serious incidents, such as re-cementing a crown or bridge. Each practice will have their own emergency protocol to follow for all eventualities, and the dental nurse has a key communication role to play when dealing with patients in these situations.

When emergency calls are received during normal working hours, it is the responsibility of the practice to provide care as it deems necessary, although since the new NHS dental contract system began in April 2006, the situation has become less clear. This is because the new system indicates that NHS patients are no longer registered with a practice or a dentist, and can attend any practice they choose if the dentist is willing and able to provide treatment for them. It could be interpreted then that between courses of dental treatment, the practice has no responsibility towards any patient for the provision of emergency dental care. The vast majority of dentists tend to show goodwill to all regular attenders, however, and are more than happy to provide emergency care for them as necessary. Various different management systems of allowing for dental emergencies during working hours may be operated. Some examples are:

- **Double booking appointment slots** – this saves unbooked time slots, but is disruptive to the running of the appointment system and often results in the dentist 'running late'
- **Set aside emergency time slots** – this is less disruptive, but can result in unbooked surgery time
- **In-house triage system** – the practice determines what constitutes an emergency, and the dentist decides which patients require treatment that day; the patient is then slotted into any unbooked appointment time, or is seen after normal hours
- **Ad hoc system** – all emergency treatment requests are received and slotted into any available appointment slots; again this saves unbooked time but can cause disruptions if a high number of calls are received

Most practices and clinics will run a combination of the above management systems, but the most effective methods of reducing the number of emergencies is for the dental team to work as follows:

- Provide consistently good quality dental care to all patients, to reduce the incidence of predictable emergencies – for instance, if a new crown does not fit well, it should be remade as fitting a poor fitting crown is likely to fail
- Have a written emergency dental call protocol for all to follow, and stick to it without exception
- Have an accepted triage system in place, that is used by the whole dental team
- Ensure that patients are made aware that they will only receive emergency treatment initially, and will have to re-attend for further treatment in a routine appointment slot
- Be aware of the regular patients and their dental histories – an emergency call from a regular attender is more likely to be a **genuine** emergency than one from a patient who routinely fails appointments and ignores oral health advice

The dental nurse has a vital role in running a successful emergency management system, as it is this team member who is the first point of call for what is often a distressed and anxious patient, and one who is quite likely to be in pain. A sympathetic and caring attitude must always be adopted, but a firm hand may also be required for the successful management of those relatively few patients who will not accept advice alone, and insist upon an immediate appointment with the dentist. If all else fails, the handling of these patients may have to be transferred to a senior staff member, or to the dentist. No matter what, the dental nurse should not be intimidated by any patient into breaking the emergency call protocol of the practice.

# Appendix:
# National Examining Board for
# Dental Nurses
# National Certificate Syllabus

(Reproduced with kind permission of the National Examining Board for Dental Nurses (NEBDN))

The syllabus is arranged in the following sections:

1   Health and Safety and Infection Control in the Workplace
2   Emergencies in the Clinical Environment
3   Legal and Ethical Issues in the Provision of Dental Care
4   Anatomical Structures and Systems Relative to Dental Care
5   Oral Diseases and Pathology
6   Patient Care and Management
7   Assessing Patients' Oral Health Needs and Treatment Planning
8   Oral Health Promotion and Preventive Dentistry
9   Restorative Dentistry
10  Oral Surgery
11  Orthodontic Procedures
12  Dental Drugs, Materials, Instruments and Equipment
13  Pain and Anxiety Control in Dentistry
14  Radiography
15  Communication

## HEALTH AND SAFETY AND INFECTION CONTROL IN THE WORKPLACE

1.1   Describe the following aspects of current health and safety legislation and regulation in the workplace in relation to own and other team members' responsibilities:

1.1.1   risk assessments and the Health and Safety at Work Act 1974
1.1.2   Fire Precaution (Workplace) Regulations
1.1.3   Health and Safety (First Aid) Regulations
1.1.4   Control of Substances Hazardous to Health Regulations in the workplace (COSHH)
1.1.5   Reporting of Injuries, Diseases and Dangerous Occurrences Regulations (RIDDOR)

1.1.6 Environmental Protection Act

1.1.7 Special Waste and Hazardous Waste Regulations

1.2 Describe own and other team members' responsibilities in relation to:

1.2.1 avoiding hazards and taking precautions in the dental environment

1.2.2 the safe disposal of clinical waste, sharps and hazardous chemicals

1.2.3 working with hazardous and non-hazardous waste

1.3 Describe infectious diseases, their agents and routes of transmission and methods for preventing cross infection

1.4 Explain:

1.4.1 the principles and methods of sterilisation and disinfection and aseptic techniques

1.4.2 types of micro-organisms, the meaning and significance of the terms pathogens and non pathogens

1.4.3 explain the principles of Universal Precautions

1.5 Explain how personal protection measures are used to control infection

1.6 Explain how the clinical environment should be prepared and maintained prior to, during and after treatment sessions

1.7 Describe and demonstrate the safe disposal of dental instruments, sharps and equipment, and out-of-date drugs and materials

## EMERGENCIES IN THE DENTAL SURGERY

2.1 Describe the signs, symptoms and causes of common medical emergencies and explain the actions to be taken should the following particular events occur:

2.1.1 faint

2.1.2 cardiac arrest

2.1.3 respiratory arrest

2.1.4 asthmatic attack

2.1.5 epileptic seizure

2.1.6 diabetic coma

2.1.7 angina/myocardial infarction

2.1.8 dental haemorrhage

2.2 Identify the hazards associated with the use of drugs and their interaction with other medicaments in dentistry

2.3 Describe the records which have to be kept in the event of a health emergency and explain the reasons for this

2.4 Demonstrate knowledge of first aid

**LEGAL AND ETHICAL ISSUES IN THE PROVISION OF DENTAL CARE**

3.1 Describe the following aspects of current legal and ethical legislation and regulation in the workplace in relation to own and other team members' responsibilities:

    3.1.1 General Dental Council – Standards Guidance
    3.1.2 Dentists Act 1984 (Amendment) Order 2005
    3.1.3 Access to Health Records
    3.1.4 Freedom of Information Act
    3.1.5 Department of Health guidance
    3.1.6 Data Protection Act
    3.1.7 Caldicott Regulations

3.2 Explain what is meant by the term 'valid consent' and discuss related issues for different patients

3.3 Explain the reasons for, and methods of, maintaining confidentiality in relation to:

    3.3.1 duty of care for patients in relation to records and treatment
    3.3.2 colleagues
    3.3.3 the employing organisation

3.4 Describe the importance of Data Protection and access to patient records in relation to own and other team members' responsibilities

3.5 Describe the importance of keeping up-to-date patient records, the medico-legal implications and handling of complaints

3.6 Describe how the practice of dentistry is regulated and how these regulations affect own role and that of other members of the oral health care team in:

    3.6.1 responsibility
    3.6.2 registration
    3.6.3 reporting
    3.6.4 delegation
    3.6.5 professional relationships

3.7 Demonstrate understanding of dental nurses' responsibilities in relation to continuing professional development and lifelong learning

## ANATOMICAL STRUCTURES AND SYSTEMS RELATIVE TO DENTAL CARE

4.1 Have knowledge of the function and structure of general anatomy as relevant to dental nursing:

4.1.1 the circulatory system
4.1.2 the respiratory system
4.1.3 the digestive system

4.2 Describe:

4.2.1 the basic structure of the oral cavity including the:

- nerve and blood supply of the teeth and supporting structures
- mandible and maxilla
- muscles of mastication
- salivary glands

4.2.2 the structure and morphology of deciduous teeth and their eruption dates
4.2.3 the structure and morphology of permanent teeth and their eruption dates
4.2.4 the structure of supporting tissues in the oral cavity
4.2.5 the functions of teeth

## ORAL DISEASE AND PATHOLOGY

5.1 Describe the inflammatory process and the effects of the disease process in all patients including elderly people and children on:

5.1.1 hard dental tissues
5.1.2 supporting dental tissues
5.1.3 other areas of the oral cavity

5.2 Describe the aetiology and progression of:

5.2.1 dental caries
5.2.2 periodontal disease
5.2.3 other oral diseases including tooth surface loss, such as erosion, attrition and abrasion

5.3   Describe micro-organisms and their role in the disease process, especially those associated with:

    5.3.1   dental caries
    5.3.2   periodontal disease
    5.3.3   other oral diseases

5.4   Know the aetiology in the progression of oral cancer

## PATIENT CARE AND MANAGEMENT

6.1   Describe and demonstrate effective ways of providing chairside support in all clinical procedures to:

    6.1.1   patients
    6.1.2   other members of the oral health team

6.2   Describe the special care needs which different patients may have and how these needs can be met effectively:

    6.2.1   young patients
    6.2.2   elderly patients
    6.2.3   patients with medical problems
    6.2.4   patients with disabilities

6.3   Understand the social, cultural, environmental and psychological factors that can affect patient management

6.4   Explain effective ways of dealing with anxious and vulnerable patients

6.5   Describe and demonstrate effective ways of providing emergency dental care

6.6   Be familiar with the problems of drug abuse and its effects in dentistry

## ASSESSING PATIENTS' ORAL HEALTH NEEDS AND TREATMENT

7.1   Describe the reasons for recording personal details of patients and effective methods of doing this

7.2   Demonstrate effective methods of recording medical, dental, and relevant social details of patients:

    7.2.1   UK – National Health Service Chart
    7.2.2   International Dental Federation (FDI)

7.2.3   information technology
7.2.4   other international charts

7.3   Demonstrate effective methods of recording soft tissue conditions using periodontal charts

7.4   Describe the importance of discussing, explaining and recording different treatment options with the patient, including the cost implications and the patient's NHS or other welfare entitlement

7.5   Describe the maintenance of study models and diagnostic reports

7.6   Be familiar with how referral procedures work locally

## ORAL HEALTH PROMOTION AND PREVENTIVE DENTISTRY

8.1   Describe how diet may affect oral health, including non carious tooth surface loss

8.2   Describe how the dental team can help a patient to improve their oral condition

8.3   Describe and demonstrate methods/aids that can be used in maintaining oral hygiene

8.4   The prevention and control of periodontal diseases and dental caries covers:

- observing/monitoring the hard and soft tissues
- applying fissure sealants
- the use of antimicrobial agents
- scaling (hand and ultrasonic)
- polishing
- topical and systemic fluorides

For each of the above:

8.4.1   identify the instruments and equipment used in the procedure, and describe their use and order of use during the procedure
8.4.2   describe the different stages undertaken during the procedure
8.4.3   identify the materials used during the procedure and demonstrate their use
8.4.4   explain the pre- and post-operative care of patients

**RESTORATIVE DENTISTRY**

9.1 Cavity preparation
Explain why cavities are restored and the different ways this may be done:

- provisional restorations
- amalgam restorations
- composite, glass ionomer restorations and compomers
- inlays – gold/porcelain
- veneers

For each of the above:

9.1.1 identify the instruments and equipment used in the procedure, and describe their use and the order of use during the procedure
9.1.2 describe the preparation of a cavity prior to restoration
9.1.3 identify the materials used during the procedure and demonstrate their use
9.1.4 explain the pre- and post-operative care of patients

9.2 Endodontics
Explain the reasons for endodontic treatment and the different procedures that may be used:

- conventional root canal treatment
- apicectomy and retrograde root filling
- pulpotomy/pulpectomy/pulp capping

For each of the above:

9.2.1 identify the instruments and equipment used in the procedure, and describe their use and the order of their use during the procedure
9.2.2 describe the different stages during the procedure and the reasons these are undertaken
9.2.3 identify the materials used during the procedure and demonstrate their use
9.2.4 explain the pre- and post-operative care of patients

9.3 Fixed prostheses
Explain the reasons for providing fixed prostheses and the different procedures that may be used:

- crowns and bridges, both permanent and temporary
- dental implants

For crowns and bridges:

9.3.1   describe their types and uses
9.3.2   identify the instruments and equipment used in the procedure, and describe their use and the order of use during the procedure
9.3.3   describe the preparation of a tooth prior to construction of a fixed prosthesis
9.3.4   describe the laboratory stages required to construct a fixed prosthesis
9.3.5   identify the materials used during the procedure and demonstrate their use
9.3.6   explain the pre- and post-operative care of patients

9.4   Removable prostheses
Explain the reasons for providing removable prostheses and the different types that may be used:

- full dentures
- partial dentures (metal base and acrylic base)
- immediate dentures
- repairs, relines and additions

For each of the above:

9.4.1   describe their types and uses
9.4.2   identify the instruments and equipment used in the procedure, and describe their use and the order of their use during the procedure
9.4.3   describe the surgery procedures required to construct a removable prosthesis
9.4.4   describe the laboratory stages required to construct a removable prosthesis and the need for effective communication with the dental laboratory
9.4.5   identify the materials used during the procedure and demonstrate their use
9.4.6   explain the pre- and post-operative care of patients

9.5   Periodontal surgery
Explain why periodontal surgery may be necessary and give details in simple terms of the different types of procedures:

- gingivectomy
- flap operations

For each of the above:

9.5.1   describe the procedure in simple terms
9.5.2   identify the instruments and equipment used in the procedure

9.5.3   identify the materials used during the procedure
9.5.4   explain the pre- and post-operative care of patients

## ORAL SURGERY

Explain why teeth need to be extracted and the complications that may arise during each procedure:

10.1   Extraction of deciduous and permanent teeth

10.1.1   identify the instruments and equipment used in the procedure, and describe their use and the order of their use during the procedure
10.1.2   describe the post-operative problems which may occur and explain how they are treated
10.1.3   explain the pre- and post-operative care of patients

10.2   Minor oral surgical procedures

- extraction of erupted and partially erupted teeth
- extraction of buried and impacted teeth and roots
- removal of roots
- investigation of hard tissue lesions
- investigation of soft tissue lesions
- intraoral suturing

For each of these areas:

10.2.1   describe the different minor oral surgery procedures and the different stages within them
10.2.2   identify the instruments and equipment used in the procedure, and describe their use and order of use during the procedure
10.2.3   explain the pre- and post-operative care of patients

## ORTHODONTIC PROCEDURES

11.1   Describe the major orthodontic classifications of teeth and jaws

11.2   For removable, fixed and functional orthodontic appliances:

11.2.1   be aware of each of their different uses
11.2.2   accurately record and provide chairside support during assessments
11.2.3   provide chairside support during fitting of appliances, including instrument selection
11.2.4   pre-treatment care and post-operative instructions

## DENTAL DRUGS, MATERIALS, INSTRUMENTS AND EQUIPMENT

12.1   Describe the drugs and materials commonly used in dentistry and explain their use

12.2   Demonstrate the correct manipulation of materials commonly used in dentistry

12.3   Describe the hazards associated with materials commonly used in dentistry and explain how to minimise the risks associated with these materials

12.4   Describe the actions to be taken in the case of mercury spillage

12.5   Demonstrate methods of recording, labelling and storing drugs and materials

12.6   Describe the legislation applicable to drugs and materials in dentistry (including their safe disposal) in relation to their own and other team members' responsibilities

12.7   Describe and demonstrate the care and maintenance of instruments and equipment used in dentistry

## PAIN AND ANXIETY CONTROL IN DENTISTRY

13.1   Be familiar with the management of different forms of facial pain and anxiety control

13.2   Describe:

13.2.1   the different types of local anaesthetic agent and the contents of a local anaesthetic cartridge
13.2.2   the methods of administering local anaesthetic agents
13.2.3   the hazards associated with local anaesthesia
13.2.4   how to treat emergencies associated with local anaesthesia

13.3   Be familiar with:

13.3.1   the differences between conscious sedation and general anaesthesia
13.3.2   the regulations which govern the administration of conscious sedation and general anaesthesia
13.3.3   other techniques of anxiety control in dentistry, such as hypnosis

## RADIOGRAPHY

14.1  Describe the following aspects of current radiography legislation and regulation in relation to own and the clinical team's responsibilities

14.2  Describe:

14.2.1  the use of radiography in assessing oral health needs
14.2.2  the hazards associated with radiation in the dental surgery
14.2.3  the precautions taken to limit radiation hazards
14.2.4  principles and techniques of taking dental radiographs (including digital) and demonstrate the processing, recording and maintenance of dental radiographs
14.2.5  faults that can occur in processing radiographs
14.2.6  how dental radiographic films and chemicals can be stored safely, and demonstrate the care of dental radiographic equipment
14.2.7  the regulations which govern the taking of dental radiographs

## COMMUNICATION

15.1  Describe and discuss methods of communicating clearly and effectively with patients and colleagues

15.2  Discuss the reception of patients into the dental environment and the role of the dental nurse in this procedure

15.3  Explain how dental appointments can be organised effectively

15.4  Discuss working in a team environment and the role of the dental nurse

15.5  Provide evidence of using information technology

# Index

The most important references are printed in **bold** type.